Adolescent Health
SOURCEBOOK

Health Reference Series

First Edition

Adolescent Health
SOURCEBOOK

*Basic Consumer Health Information about Common
Medical, Mental, and Emotional Concerns in
Adolescents, Including Facts about Acne, Body
Piercing, Mononucleosis, Nutrition, Eating Disorders,
Stress, Depression, Behavior Problems, Peer Pressure,
Violence, Gangs, Drug Use, Puberty, Sexuality,
Pregnancy, Learning Disabilities, and More*

*Along with a Glossary of Terms and Other Resources
for Further Help and Information*

Edited by
Chad T. Kimball

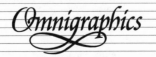

Omnigraphics

615 Griswold Street • Detroit, MI 48226

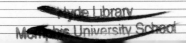

Bibliographic Note
Because this page cannot legibly accommodate all the copyright notices, the Bibliographic Note portion of the Preface constitutes an extension of the copyright notice.

Edited by Chad T. Kimball

Health Reference Series

Karen Bellenir, *Managing Editor*
David A. Cooke, MD, *Medical Consultant*
Elizabeth Barbour, *Permissions Associate*
Dawn Matthews, *Verification Assistant*
Carol Munson, *Permissions Assistant*
Laura Pleva, *Index Editor*
EdIndex, Services for Publishers, *Indexers*

* * *

Omnigraphics, Inc.

Matthew P. Barbour, *Senior Vice President*
Kay Gill, *Vice President — Directories*
Kevin Hayes, *Operations Manager*
David P. Bianco, *Marketing Consultant*

* * *

Peter E. Ruffner, *President and Publisher*
Frederick G. Ruffner, Jr., *Chairman*
Copyright © 2002 Omnigraphics, Inc.
ISBN 0-7808-0248-9

Library of Congress Cataloging-in-Publication Data

Adolescent health sourcebook : basic consumer health information about common medical, mental, and emotional concerns in adolescents, including facts about acne, body piercing, mononucleosis, nutrition, eating disorders, stress, depression, behavior problems, peer pressure, violence, gangs, drug use, puberty, sexuality, pregnancy, learning disabilities, and more; along with a glossary of terms and other resources for further help and information / edited by Chad T. Kimball.-- 1st ed.
   p. cm. -- (Health reference series)
  Includes bibliographical references and index.
  ISBN 0-7808-0248-9
   1. Teenagers--Health and hygiene. 2. Teenagers--Psychology. 3. Consumer education. 4. Adolescence. I. Kimball, Chad T. II. Health reference series (unnumbered)

RJ140 .A335 2002
613'.0433--dc21

            2002025249

Table of Contents

Part II: Physical Health Issues Affecting Adolescents

Part III: Adolescent Sexual Health

Part IV: Drug Abuse in Adolescents

Part V: Social Issues and Other Parenting Concerns Affecting Adolescent Health and Safety

Preface

About This Book

Adolescence is a turbulent time associated with many challenges for teenagers, parents, and caregivers. For example, research indicates that teenagers participate in high risk behaviors more often than other age groups. In the last three years, approximately 24 percent of 12th graders used marijuana and 32 percent of 12th graders and 24 percent of 10th graders reported heavy drinking. High risk behaviors, however, are not the only influences on adolescent health and well being. Significant emotional, hormonal, and physical changes also affect nearly every aspect of development.

This *Sourcebook* provides parents and caregivers with a basic understanding of many of the issues that affect adolescent health and well being, including peer pressure, depression, eating disorders, behavior problems, violence, and other mental health concerns. It also includes information about puberty, teen pregnancy, sexually transmitted diseases, fitness, substance abuse, body piercing, tattoos, firearms, and gangs. Special sections on parenting concerns offer information on communication, driving, education, learning disabilities, college preparation, and other important issues. A list of resources is provided for additional help and information.

How to Use This Book

This book is divided into parts and chapters. Parts focus on broad areas of interest. Chapters are devoted to single topics within a part.

Part I: Emotional and Mental Health Issues Affecting Adolescents discusses emotional and mental development in teens, gives information about various disorders, and describes how to get help for adolescents with mental health issues.

Part II: Physical Health Issues Affecting Adolescents offers information about various physical diseases which are common in teenagers. It also provides answers to questions about cosmetics, tattoos, piercings, medications, loud music and hearing loss, and false medical advertising.

Part III: Adolescent Sexual Health gives information about puberty, general male and female reproductive health, teen pregnancy, sexually transmitted diseases, and sexual crimes against adolescents.

Part IV: Drug Abuse in Adolescents discusses the dangers of alcohol, tobacco, and other drugs, and their effects on teenagers today.

Part V: Social Issues and Other Parenting Concerns Affecting Adolescent Health and Safety provides useful information about peer pressure, teenagers and the media, internet safety, driving safety, and youth violence.

Part VI: Adolescent Education offers advice about helping teens who experience difficulty in school due to social factors or learning disabilities. It also discusses how to prepare your adolescent for college.

Part VII: Additional Help and Information includes a glossary of related terms, a list of references for additional reading, and a directory of resources for additional information.

Bibliographic Note

This volume contains documents and excerpts from publications issued by the following government agencies: Centers for Disease Control and Prevention (CDC), Department of Labor (DOL), Educational Resource Information Center (ERIC), Food and Drug Administration (FDA), FDA's Center for Devices and Radiological Health (CDRH), National Adoption Information Clearinghouse (NAIC), National Cancer Institute (NCI), National Center for Chronic Disease Prevention and Health, National Center for HIV, STD, and TB Prevention, Division of Sexually Transmitted Diseases (DSTD), National Center for Injury Prevention and Control, National Center on Sleep Disorders Research (NCSDR), National Heart, Lung, and Blood Institute (NHLBI), National Institute of Allergy and Infectious Diseases

(NIAID), National Institute of Arthritis and Musculoskeletal and Skin Diseases (NIAMS), National Institute of Neurological Disorders and Stroke (NINDS), National Institute on Alcohol Abuse and Alcoholism (NIAAA), National Institute on Drug Abuse (NIDA), National Institutes of Health (NIH), National Institute of Mental Health (NIMH), U.S. Department of Education, U.S. Department of Health and Human Services (DHHS), and the U.S. Department of Transportation's National Highway Traffic Safety Administration (NHTSA).

In addition, this volume contains copyrighted articles from the American Academy of Child and Adolescent Psychiatry (AACAP), American Academy of Dermatology (AAD), Brain Injury Association, Inc., British Columbia Schizophrenia Society, *Brown University Child and Adolescent Behavior Letter*, Canadian Hockey Association (CHA), Child and Family Canada, Canadian Child Care Federation, Cooperative Extension Institute of Agriculture and Natural Resources, University of Nebraska, Do It Now Foundation, Family Support Network, Florida SAFE Inc., Jim Chandler, MD, Juvenile Diabetes Research Foundation International, *Lubbock Avalanche-Journal*, *Marblehead Reporter*, Medical College of Wisconsin, National Athletic Trainer's Association (NATA), National Campaign to Prevent Teen Pregnancy, National Coalition for Adult Immunization, National Crime Prevention Council (NCPC), National Institute on Media and the Family, National Network for Child Care, National Network for Family Resilience, The National Parenting Center, Not Me, Not Now, PDRnet, Pennsylvania Hospital, John Suler, State of Connecticut, Teenagers Today/iParenting, University of Minnesota, *U.S. News and World Report*, and the Virginia Youth Violence Project.

Full citation information is provided on the first page of each chapter. Every effort has been made to secure all necessary rights to reprint the copyrighted material. If any omissions have been made, please contact Omnigraphics to make corrections for future editions.

Acknowledgements

Thanks go to Karen Bellenir and Carol Munson for their help with the many details involved in the production of this book.

Note from the Editor

This book is part of Omnigraphics' *Health Reference Series*. The *Series* provides basic information about a broad range of medical concerns. It is not intended to serve as a tool for diagnosing illness, in prescribing treatments, or as a substitute for the physician/patient relationship. All persons concerned about medical symptoms or the possibility of disease are encouraged to seek professional care from an appropriate health care provider.

Our Advisory Board

The *Health Reference Series* is reviewed by an Advisory Board comprised of librarians from public, academic, and medical libraries. We would like to thank the following board members for providing guidance to the development of this series:

Dr. Lynda Baker, Associate Professor of Library and Information Science, Wayne State University, Detroit, MI

Nancy Bulgarelli, William Beaumont Hospital Library, Royal Oak, MI

Karen Imarisio, Bloomfield Township Public Library, Bloomfield Township, MI

Karen Morgan, Mardigian Library, University of Michigan-Dearborn, Dearborn, MI

Rosemary Orlando, St. Clair Shores Public Library, St. Clair Shores, MI

Medical Consultant

Medical consultation services are provided to the *Health Reference Series* editors by David A. Cooke, M.D. Dr. Cooke is a graduate of Brandeis University, and he received his M.D. degree from the University of Michigan. He completed residency training at the University of Wisconsin Hospital and Clinics. He is board-certified in Internal Medicine. Dr. Cooke currently works as part of the University of Michigan Health System and practices in Brighton, MI. In his free time, he enjoys writing, science fiction, and spending time with his family.

Health Reference Series *Update Policy*

The inaugural book in the *Health Reference Series* was the first edition of *Cancer Sourcebook* published in 1992. Since then, the *Series* has been enthusiastically received by librarians and in the medical community. In order to maintain the standard of providing high-quality health information for the layperson, the editorial staff at Omnigraphics felt it was necessary to implement a policy of updating volumes when warranted.

Medical researchers have been making tremendous strides, and it is the purpose of the *Health Reference Series* to stay current with the most recent advances. Each decision to update a volume will be made on an individual basis. Some of the considerations will include how much new information is available and the feedback we receive from people who use the books. If there is a topic you would like to see added to the update list, or an area of medical concern you feel has not been adequately addressed, please write to:

Editor
Health Reference Series
Omnigraphics, Inc.
615 Griswold
Detroit, MI 48226

The commitment to providing on-going coverage of important medical developments has also led to some format changes in the *Health Reference Series*. Each new volume on a topic is individually titled and called a "First Edition." Subsequent updates will carry sequential edition numbers. To help avoid confusion and to provide maximum flexibility in our ability to respond to informational needs, the practice of consecutively numbering each volume has been discontinued.

Part One

Emotional and Mental Health Issues Affecting Adolescents

Chapter 1

Normal Adolescent Emotional Development

Normal Adolescent Development, Middle School and Early High School Years

Parents are often worried or confused by changes in their teenagers. The following information should help parents understand this phase of development. Each teenager is an individual with a unique personality and special interests, likes, and dislikes. However, there are also numerous developmental issues that everyone faces during the adolescent years. The normal feelings and behaviors of the middle school and early high school adolescent are described below.

Movement Towards Independence

- Struggle with sense of identity

- Feeling awkward or strange about one's self and one's body

- Focus on self, alternating between high expectations and poor self-concept

- Interests and clothing style influenced by peer group

This chapter contains text from "Normal Adolescent Development, Middle School and Early High School Years," http://www.aacap.org/publications/factsfam/develop.htm, and "Normal Adolescent Development, Late High School Years and Beyond," http://www.aacap.org/publications/factsfam/develop2.htm, from *Facts for Families*, American Academy of Child and Adolescent Psychiatry (AACAP), May, 1997. Reprinted with permission.

- Moodiness
- Improved ability to use speech to express one's self
- Realization that parents are not perfect; identification of their faults
- Less overt affection shown to parents, with occasional rudeness
- Complaints that parents interfere with independence
- Tendency to return to childish behavior, particularly when stressed

Future Interests and Cognitive Changes

- Mostly interested in present, limited thoughts of future
- Intellectual interests expand and gain in importance
- Greater ability to do work (physical, mental, emotional)

Sexuality

- Display shyness, blushing, and modesty
- Girls develop physically sooner than boys
- Increased interest in the opposite sex
- Movement toward heterosexuality with fears of homosexuality
- Concerns regarding physical and sexual attractiveness to others
- Frequently changing relationships
- Worries about being normal

Morals, Values, and Self-Direction

- Rule and limit testing
- Capacity for abstract thought
- Development of ideals and selection of role models
- More consistent evidence of conscience
- Experimentation with sex and drugs (cigarettes, alcohol, and marijuana)

Normal Adolescent Development, Late High School Years and Beyond

Movement Towards Independence

- Increased independent functioning
- Firmer and more cohesive sense of identity
- Examination of inner experiences
- Ability to think ideas through
- Conflict with parents begins to decrease
- Increased ability for delayed gratification and compromise
- Increased emotional stability
- Increased concern for others
- Increased self-reliance
- Peer relationships remain important and take an appropriate place among other interests

Future Interests and Cognitive Changes

- Work habits become more defined
- Increased concern for the future
- More importance is placed on one's role in life

Sexuality

- Feelings of love and passion
- Development of more serious relationships
- Firmer sense of sexual identity
- Increased capacity for tender and sensual love

Morals, Values, and Self-Direction

- Greater capacity for setting goals
- Interest in moral reasoning
- Capacity to use insight

- Increased emphasis on personal dignity and self-esteem

- Social and cultural traditions regain some of their previous importance

Teenagers do vary slightly from the above descriptions, but the feelings and behaviors are, in general, considered normal for each stage of adolescence.

Chapter 2

Self-Esteem and Body Image

Self esteem consists of our own personal view of who we are, developed over time by our successes and failures, positive and negative comments from others, our messages to ourselves, and our interpretation of these via our thoughts and feelings. Some teens (and adults too!) appear very confident to others, but this does not always reflect what is felt inside. Self esteem is our inward picture of ourselves—either positive or negative.

Self esteem varies over time. During the teen years, self esteem, particularly in girls in the early and mid teens, may drop considerably. Girls are bombarded with pictures and images of female perfection and unrealistic thinness portrayed in magazines, videos and TV. Confidence-destroying images of perfection, surging hormones, the physical changes of puberty, together with social and emotional pressures form peer groups combine together to knock down self esteem.

Tips for Enhancing Self Esteem

While self esteem comes from within, parents, teachers, and other family members can help to enhance positive self esteem. Here are a few ideas:

Excerpted from "You and Your Teen: Self Esteem," from an undated document published by Grey Bruce Health Unit, available on the Internet at http://www. publichealthgreybruce.on.ca/FamilyTeens/FamilyYourteenselfesteemFS.html, accessed in November 2001.

- Put critical messages on hold and take note of what your teen does well. Too often parents and other adults notice only what needs correction! Share positive messages (it must be genuine!) with your teen and build on his/her strengths and capabilities. Show that you have confidence in your teen.

- Encourage your teen to try to learn something new, to try a new sport or activity. Involvement in several different sports or activities can provide alternate peer groups and more diverse friendships.

- Help teens learn to see problems as challenges which they can develop the skills to overcome. Encourage problem solving and provide your support.

- Value your teen as an individual. Let him/her know that they are capable and loveable.

- Teens need love and affection. Find ways of showing affection— a hug, a shoulder massage, or backrub. They need to hear that you love and care about them. Don't assume that they know you love them.

- As an adult in their lives, demonstrate your own healthy self esteem.

Your teen is influenced by many people beyond the family unit. If your teen has developed positive self esteem he/she will more effectively cope with peer pressure, problems and challenges in the years ahead.

Chapter 3

Teenagers and Stress

Chapter Contents

Section 3.1

Helping Young Adolescents Cope with Stress

Reprinted with permission from the National Network for Child Care (NNCC). Ebata, A. T. (1994). Helping young adolescents cope with stress. In Todd, C.M. (Ed.), *School-age connections*, 4(2), pp. 1–3. Urbana-Champaign, IL: University of Illinois Cooperative Extension Service. http://www.nncc.org/SACC/sac42_adolesc.stress.html. Reviewed and accepted for publication by a professional journal editorial board, 4-H curriculum review, SOCC review, and North Central Regional Educational Materials Project review, 1996. Despite the age of this document, readers seeking an understanding of adolescent stress will still find this information useful.

Early adolescence can be a stressful time for children, parents, and adults who work with teens. Children are dealing with the challenges of growing. They are going through puberty, meeting the changing expectations of others, and coping with feelings they might not have had before. Many also worry about moving from an elementary to a middle or junior high school. And some kids may have to deal with things that their peers don't have to face, such as the death of a family member or moving to a new town. Most children meet these challenges successfully and grow into healthy adults. Others have a harder time coping with their problems. In this article, we will talk about the kinds of difficulties young adolescents face. We'll learn how they cope with these difficulties and what adults can do to help them deal with stress. The changes of adolescence may begin as early as fourth grade, so it is important for school-age providers to know how to help.

What Stresses Adolescents?

When we talk about stress, most people think about how we react to problems that are difficult to deal with. Sometimes these problems are major "life events" that are unexpected or unusual. Parents may be going through a divorce. Young teens may be breaking up with a boyfriend or girlfriend. Perhaps the adolescent has been hurt in an accident. Other problems are more common day-to-day difficulties. From studies with adolescents, we have learned two important things.

- A "pile-up" of many stressful life events in a small amount of time is more difficult for adolescents than dealing with just one event.

- Ongoing, day-to-day stresses and strains are harder on adolescents than major life events. If a major event causes stress, it is often because it sets off a chain of events that changes the ongoing, day-to-day conditions of their lives.

The most common sources of day-to-day stress for young adolescents in grades six through nine are

- problems with peers (including "romances")
- family issues or problems with parents
- school-related problems or pressures
- their own thoughts, feelings, or behaviors (feeling depressed or lonely, getting into trouble because of their behavior)

Of course, these problems are fairly routine for most adolescents. Kids who live in different places, though, may face different kinds of stressors. Some adolescents live in neighborhoods with high rates of crime and violence. Others live in isolated, rural areas. Obviously, they'll have different kinds of problems.

How Do Adolescents Cope with Stress?

Adolescents react to stress in much the same ways adults do. Common reactions are excitement, fear, anxiety, sadness, and anger. The behavior of an adolescent who is stressed may change, but each adolescent reacts in a different way. Some adolescents withdraw from others, some lash out at others, and some actively seek the comfort of others.

Although adolescents cope with stress in different ways, there are general patterns in their coping behaviors. There are two major ways to cope with stress. One way is problem solving. This involves trying to deal with the problem by changing the situation or getting rid of the problem. Another way of handling stress is managing emotions. This involves handling the thoughts and feelings caused by the problem.

Adolescents use both methods, and both can be effective, depending on what the problem is and when it started. Studies show that people who deal with their problems, see the positive side of difficult

11

situations, and take part in activities they enjoy are more likely to be well-adjusted. Acting to solve problems often requires planning. Sometimes it requires learning new skills. For example, coping with poor grades might require learning study skills and making time to complete homework. Coping with feeling left out might require learning social skills. An example of seeing the positive side would be focusing on your team's good performance even though they lost the game.

Managing emotions can be very helpful when an adolescent is dealing with an uncontrollable problem. It can also be helpful in the early stages of coping with a problem. For example, blowing off steam, avoidance, and distraction can be important ways of getting prepared to cope more directly with difficult situations. Studies show that the most common ways young adolescents cope with stress are listening to music and watching television. Another way of resolving stressful situations is to find meaning in the experience. It helps if teens can see that something good is coming out of the problem. Finally, doing something enjoyable provides time out from stress. It often "recharges batteries" so the person can go back to dealing with stress.

What Can Adults Do to Help Adolescents Cope with Stress?

Adults can help adolescents solve problems and manage their emotions in at least three ways. They can provide help, encouragement, and support during times of stress. They can help them develop the knowledge and skills to cope with future difficulties. And adults can get help for themselves when they need it.

Provide Help, Encouragement, and Support

• Encourage adolescents to talk about what they are going through, and be willing to listen. Ask questions so you can understand the problem. Don't just jump to conclusions and give advice. Depending on the situation, adolescents may not want advice. They may just want to be understood. Even if a problem seems small to you, it may be a major concern for the child. Minimizing a problem or saying "you'll get over it" is not helpful. It gives the message that you don't understand or are not willing to listen. Ask them if they want your advice or if they would like to know what you would do.

- Offer reassurance, encouragement, and support. Be willing to provide verbal or physical comfort, but don't be discouraged if the adolescent rejects your effort or is irritable. These are normal reactions to stress. Be patient and let the child know you're available if he or she needs you.

- Continue to provide structure, stability, and predictability. Within reason, stick to the same rules, roles, and routines.

- Encourage them to participate in activities they normally enjoy.

- Try to build a relationship so that adolescents will feel comfortable coming to you when they need help. It helps if they can just express how they feel or what they are going through.

Help Them Develop Coping Skills

Model effective coping skills. Talk about how you deal with problems in your life. Make it clear that you are willing to talk about difficulties they may be facing.

Help adolescents learn and practice problem-solving skills. Help them develop social skills.

- Suggest ways of coping with difficult situations. Help them understand that they can cope in different ways.

- Teach them specific skills they can use to make decisions or solve problems. Then give them chances to practice these skills. Help them identify their problem, come up with possible solutions, and evaluate the pros and cons of each.

Help them learn and practice ways of managing their emotions.

- Teach them safe ways to blow off steam and relax. They could go for walks, play basketball, listen to music, or talk with someone.

- Help them develop ways to see problems and situations in a different light. Get them to see the positive side of things and to talk to themselves to help manage their emotions.

Help them learn and practice skills that will allow them to participate in and enjoy new activities. Provide opportunities for activities that are fun and enjoyable. This can help adolescents recharge their batteries and blow off steam.

Seek Help Yourself If You Need It

Helping an adolescent can sometimes be discouraging or frustrating. Monitor your own stress levels and take care of yourself. Be willing to seek help or support from others, especially if you feel like you are in over your head and can't deal with the child. A school counselor or social worker can give you information or advice on where to find help. Or you could try a member of the clergy, the local mental health center, or your health-care provider.

Don't lose heart. Helping young adolescents cope with stress is an important task. You are preparing them to face the challenges that lie ahead as they move into the adult world.

Section 3.2

Adolescent Stress and Depression

Excerpted from Joyce Walker, "Adolescent Stress and Depression," 4-H Youth Development, http://www.extension.umn.edu/distribution/youthdevelopment/DA3083.html, copyright 1997 Regents of University of Minnesota, reprinted with permission. Reviewed in June, 2001 by Dr. David A. Cooke, MD, Diplomate, American Board of Internal Medicine.

Adults commonly tell young people that the teenage years are the "best years of your life." The rosy remembrance highlights happy groups of high school students energetically involved at a dance or sporting event, and a bright-eyed couple holding hands or sipping sodas at a local restaurant. This is only part of the picture. Life for many young people is a painful tug of war filled with mixed messages and conflicting demands from parents, teachers, coaches, employers, friends, and oneself. Growing up negotiating a path between independence and reliance on others is a tough business. It creates stress, and it can create serious depression for young people ill-equipped to cope, communicate, and solve problems.

Adults need to be familiar with the family, biological, and personality factors that predispose a young person to depression. They can

14

learn to recognize the kinds of psychological, behavioral, and social events that most often signal trouble. Awareness of the way these risk factors "pile up" helps any adult living and working with adolescents to be sensitive when stress and depression are imminent.

Stress and Depression Are Real

Stress and depression are serious problems for many teenagers, as a study of Minnesota high school students reveals. Although 61 percent of the students are not depressed and seem to handle their problems in constructive ways, 39 percent suffer from mild to severe depression. These young people often rely on passive or negative behaviors in their attempts to deal with problems.

Stress is characterized by feelings of tension, frustration, worry, sadness, and withdrawal that commonly last from a few hours to a few days. Depression is both more severe and longer lasting. Depression is characterized by more extreme feelings of hopelessness, sadness, isolation, worry, withdrawal and worthlessness that last for two weeks or more. The finding that 9 percent of high school students are severely depressed is important since depression is the most important risk factor for suicide. The Minnesota Study found that 88 percent of the youth who reported making suicide attempts were depressed. Approximately 6 percent of the students reported suicide attempts in the previous six months.

Common Causes and Responses to Stress

Young people become stressed for many reasons. The Minnesota study presented students with a list of 47 common life events and asked them to identify those they had experienced in the last six months that they considered to be "bad." The responses indicated that they had experienced an average of two negative life events in the last six months. The most common of these were:

- break up with boy/girl friend

- increased arguments with parents

- trouble with brother or sister

- increased arguments between parents

- change in parents' financial status

- serious illness or injury of family member

- trouble with classmates

- trouble with parents

These events are centered in the two most important domains of a teenager's life: home and school. They relate to issues of conflict and loss. Loss can reflect the real or perceived loss of something concrete such as a friend or money, and it can mean the loss of such intrinsic things as self-worth, respect, friendship, or love.

In a more informal survey of 60 young people, the primary sources of tension and trouble for teens and their friends were: relationships with friends and family; the pressure of expectations from self and others; pressure at school from teachers, coaches, grades, and homework; financial pressures; and tragedy in the lives of family and friends (described as death, divorce, cancer).

Most teenagers respond to stressful events in their lives by doing something relaxing, trying positive and self-reliant problem-solving, or seeking friendship and support from others. Common examples include listening to music, trying to make their own decisions, daydreaming, trying to figure out solutions, keeping up friendships, watching television, and being close to people they care about. These behaviors are appropriate for adolescents who are trying to become independent, take responsibility for themselves, and draw on friends and family for support.

Troubled Youth Respond Differently

The majority of young people face the stress of negative life events, find internal or external resources to cope, and move on. But for others, the events pile up and the stressors are too great. In the Minnesota study teens who reported that they had made a suicide attempt had five additional "bad" events on their list: parents' divorce, loss of a close friend, change to a new school, failing grades, and personal illness or injury. It is significant that the young people who showed high degrees of depression and who had made suicide attempts reported over five of these "bad" events in the past six months, more than twice as many as the rest of the group.

The actions in response to stress were also different for those who reported serious depression or a suicide attempt. Young people who are depressed are at much greater risk of attempting suicide than non-depressed youth although not all youth who attempt suicide are depressed. These young people report exhibiting much more anger and ventilation; avoidance and passivity; and aggressive, antisocial behavior. They describe yelling, fighting, and complaining; drinking, smoking and using doctor-prescribed drugs more frequently; and sleeping, riding around in cars, and crying more often. They are less inclined to do things with their family or to go along with parents' rules and requests.

A Closer Look at High Risk Youth

It is important not to overreact to isolated incidents. Young people will have problems and will learn, at their own rate, to struggle and deal with them. But it is critical for parents and helping adults to be aware of the factors that put a youth at particular risk, especially when stressful events begin to accumulate for these vulnerable individuals. A good starting point for identifying and intervening with highly troubled and depressed young people is the careful study of suicidal adolescents.

Family history and biology can create a predisposition for dealing poorly with stress. These factors make a person susceptible to depression and self-destructive behavior.

- history of depression and/or suicide in the family
- alcoholism or drug use in the family
- sexual or physical abuse patterns in the family
- chronic illness in oneself or family
- family or individual history of psychiatric disorders such as eating disorders, schizophrenia, manic-depressive disorder, conduct disorders, delinquency
- death or serious loss in the family
- learning disabilities or mental/physical disabilities
- absent or divorced parents; inadequate bonding in adoptive families
- family conflict; poor parent/child relationships

Personality traits, especially when they change dramatically, can signal serious trouble. These traits include:

- impulsive behaviors, obsessions and unreal fears

- aggressive and antisocial behavior

- withdrawal and isolation; detachment

- poor social skills resulting in feelings of humiliation, poor self-worth, blame and feeling ugly

- over-achieving and extreme pressure to perform

- problems with sleeping and/or eating

Psychological and social events contribute to the accumulation of problems and stressors.

- loss experience such as a death or suicide of a friend or family member; broken romance, loss of a close friendship or a family move

- unmet personal or parental expectation such as failure to achieve a goal, poor grades, social rejection

- unresolved conflict with family members, peers, teachers, coaches that results in anger, frustration, rejection

- humiliating experience resulting in loss of self-esteem or rejection

- unexpected events such as pregnancy or financial problems

Predispositions, stressors and behaviors weave together to form a composite picture of a youth at high risk for depression and self-destructive behavior. Symptoms such as personal drug and alcohol use, running away from home, prolonged sadness and crying, unusual impulsiveness or recklessness, or dramatic changes in personal habits are intertwined with the family and personal history, the individual personality, and the emotional/social events taking place in a person's life.

It is not always easy for one person to see the "whole picture." That's why it is essential that people who have "hunches" that something is wrong take the lead to gather perspectives from other friends, family members and professionals who know the young person. It is all too often true that the survivors of an adolescent suicide only "put the pieces together" after the fact, when they sit together and try to figure out what happened. How fortunate a troubled young person is to have a caring adult take the initiative to look more closely before something serious happens!

How Youth Can Manage Problems

- First, young people must learn and practice coping skills to get them through an immediate conflict or problem. Coping strategies must emphasize self-responsibility to find positive, nondestructive ways to find relief.

- Second, communication skills are important. This involves being able to talk and selecting a good listener. It is important to express feelings, vent emotions, and talk about the problems and issues. Peers are good sympathizers, but it often takes an adult perspective to begin to plan how to make changes for the better.

- Third, young people need help to learn problem-solving skills. Sorting out the issues, setting goals, and making plans to move forward are skills that can be taught and practiced.

- Ultimately, most young people will develop and assume the responsibility for their own protection and peace of mind. But during the years of learning and practice, parents, teachers, and helping adults need to be aware of the signs and patterns that signal danger. Awareness of adolescent stress and depression opens the door for adults to begin constructive interventions and stimulate emotional development.

Chapter 4

Eating Disorders in Adolescents

For reasons that are unclear, some people—mainly young women—develop potentially life-threatening eating disorders called bulimia nervosa and anorexia nervosa. People with bulimia, known as bulimics, indulge in binge eating (episodes of eating large amounts of food) and purging (getting rid of the food by vomiting or using laxatives). People with anorexia, whom doctors sometimes call anorectics, severely limit their food intake. About half of them also have bulimia symptoms.

The National Center for Health Statistics estimates that about 9,000 people admitted to hospitals were diagnosed with bulimia in 1994, the latest year for which statistics are available, and about 8,000 were diagnosed with anorexia. Studies indicate that by their first year of college, 4.5 to 18 percent of women and 0.4 percent of men have a history of bulimia and that as many as 1 in 100 females between the ages of 12 and 18 have anorexia.

Males account for only 5 to 10 percent of bulimia and anorexia cases. While people of all races develop the disorders, the vast majority of those diagnosed are white.

Most people find it difficult to stop their bulimic or anorectic behavior without professional help. If untreated, the disorders may become chronic and lead to severe health problems, even death. Antidepressants

Dixie Farley, "On the Teen Scene: Eating Disorders Require Medical Attention," *FDA Consumer*, March 1992, Food and Drug Administration (FDA) Pub. No. 96-1194, http://www.fda.gov/opacom/catalog/eatdis.html. The version below is from a reprint of the original article that was printed in November 1993 and contains revisions made in September 1997.

are sometimes prescribed for people with these eating disorders, and, in November 1996, the Food and Drug Administration (FDA) added the treatment of bulimia to the indications for the antidepressant Prozac (fluoxetine).

About 1,000 women die of anorexia each year, according to the American Anorexia/Bulimia Association. More specific statistics from the National Center for Health Statistics show that "anorexia" or "anorexia nervosa" was the underlying cause of death noted on 101 death certificates in 1994, and was mentioned as one of multiple causes of death on another 2,657 death certificates. In the same year, bulimia was the underlying cause of death on two death certificates and mentioned as one of several causes on 64 others.

As to the causes of bulimia and anorexia, there are many theories. One is that some young women feel abnormally pressured to be as thin as the "ideal" portrayed by magazines, movies and television. Another is that defects in key chemical messengers in the brain may contribute to the disorders' development or persistence.

The Bulimia Secret

Once people begin binge eating and purging, usually in conjunction with a diet, the cycle easily gets out of control. While cases tend to develop during the teens or early 20s, many bulimics successfully hide their symptoms, thereby delaying help until they reach their 30s or 40s. Several years ago, actress Jane Fonda revealed she had been a secret bulimic from age 12 until her recovery at 35. She told of binge eating and purging up to 20 times a day.

Many people with bulimia maintain a nearly normal weight. Though they appear healthy and successful—"perfectionists" at whatever they do—in reality, they have low self-esteem and are often depressed. They may exhibit other compulsive behaviors. For example, one physician reports that a third of his bulimia patients regularly engage in shoplifting and that a quarter of the patients have suffered from alcohol abuse or addiction at some point in their lives.

While normal food intake for women and teenagers is 2,000 to 3,000 calories in a day, bulimic binges average about 3,400 calories in 1 1/4 hours, according to one study. Some bulimics consume up to 20,000 calories in binges lasting as long as eight hours. Some spend $50 or more a day on food and may resort to stealing food or money to support their obsession.

To lose the weight gained during a binge, bulimics begin purging by vomiting (by self-induced gagging or with an emetic, a substance that causes vomiting) or by using laxatives (50 to 100 tablets at a time), diuretics (drugs that increase urination), or enemas. Between binges, they may fast or exercise excessively.

Extreme purging rapidly upsets the body's balance of sodium, potassium, and other chemicals. This can cause fatigue, seizures, irregular heartbeat, and thinner bones. Repeated vomiting can damage the stomach and esophagus (the tube that carries food to the stomach), make the gums recede, and erode tooth enamel (some patients need all their teeth pulled prematurely). Other effects include various skin rashes, broken blood vessels in the face, and irregular menstrual cycles.

Complexities of Anorexia

While anorexia most commonly begins in the teens, it can start at any age and has been reported from age 5 to 60. Incidence among 8- to 11-year-olds is said to be increasing.

Anorexia may be a single, limited episode with large weight loss within a few months followed by recovery. Or it may develop gradually and persist for years. The illness may go back and forth between getting better and getting worse. Or it may steadily get more severe.

Anorectics may exercise excessively. Their preoccupation with food usually prompts habits such as moving food about on the plate and cutting it into tiny pieces to prolong eating, and not eating with the family.

Obsessed with weight loss and fear of becoming fat, anorectics see normal folds of flesh as "fat" that must be eliminated. When the normal fat padding is lost, sitting or lying down brings discomfort not rest, making sleep difficult. As the disorder continues, victims may become isolated and withdraw from friends and family.

The body responds to starvation by slowing or stopping certain bodily processes. Blood pressure falls, breathing rate slows, menstruation ceases (or, in girls in their early teens, never begins), and activity of the thyroid gland (which regulates growth) diminishes. Skin becomes dry, and hair and nails become brittle. Lightheadedness, cold intolerance, constipation, and joint swelling are other symptoms. Reduced fat causes the body temperature to fall. Soft hair called lanugo forms on the skin for warmth. Body chemicals may get so imbalanced that heart failure occurs.

Anorectics who additionally binge and purge impair their health even further. The late recording artist Karen Carpenter, an anorectic who used syrup of ipecac to induce vomiting, died after buildup of the drug irreversibly damaged her heart.

Getting Help

Early treatment is vital. As either disorder becomes more entrenched, its damage becomes less reversible.

Usually, the family is asked to help in the treatment, which may include psychotherapy, nutrition counseling, behavior modification, and self-help groups. Therapy often lasts a year or more—on an outpatient basis unless life-threatening physical symptoms or severe psychological problems require hospitalization. If there is deterioration or no response to therapy, the patient (or parent or other advocate) may want to talk to the health professional about the plan of treatment.

There are no drugs approved specifically for bulimia or anorexia, but several, including some antidepressants, are being investigated for this use.

If you think a friend or family member has bulimia or anorexia, point out in a caring, nonjudgmental way the behavior you have observed and encourage the person to get medical help. If you think you have bulimia or anorexia, remember that you are not alone and that this is a health problem that requires professional help. As a first step, talk to your parents, family doctor, religious counselor, or school counselor or nurse.

Disorders' Definitions

According to the American Psychiatric Association, a person diagnosed as bulimic or anorectic must have all of that disorder's specific symptoms:

Bulimia Nervosa

- recurrent episodes of binge eating (minimum average of two binge-eating episodes a week for at least three months)

- a feeling of lack of control over eating during the binges

- regular use of one or more of the following to prevent weight gain: self-induced vomiting, use of laxatives or diuretics, strict dieting or fasting, or vigorous exercise

- persistent over-concern with body shape and weight.

Anorexia Nervosa

- refusal to maintain weight that's over the lowest weight considered normal for age and height

- intense fear of gaining weight or becoming fat, even though underweight

- distorted body image

- in women, three consecutive missed menstrual periods without pregnancy.

— by Dixie Farley

Dixie Farley is a staff writer for *FDA Consumer*.

Chapter 5

Understanding Depression in Adolescents

Introduction

You know that the school years can be complicated and demanding. Deep down, you are not quite sure of who you are, what you want to be, or whether the choices you make from day to day are the best decisions. Sometimes the many changes and pressures you are facing threaten to overwhelm you. So, it isn't surprising that from time to time you feel "down" or discouraged.

But what about those times when activity and outlook on life stay "down" for weeks? If you know someone like this, they might be suffering from depression. As a friend or care giver, you can help.

Find out More about Depression

What Is Depression?

Depression is more than the blues or the blahs; it is more than the normal, everyday ups and downs.

When that "down" mood, along with other symptoms, lasts for more than a couple of weeks, the condition may be clinical depression. Clinical depression is a serious health problem that affects the total person. In addition to feelings, it can change behavior, physical health

Excerpted from "What to Do When a Friend Is Depressed," National Institutes of Mental Health (NIMH), National Institutes of Health (NIH), NIH Pub. No. 00-3824, http://www.nimh.nih.gov/publicat/friend.cfm, April 2000.

and appearance, academic performance, social activity, and the ability to handle everyday decisions and pressures.

What Causes Clinical Depression?

We do not yet know all the causes of depression, but there seem to be biological and emotional factors that may increase the likelihood that an individual will develop a depressive disorder.

Research over the past decade strongly suggests a genetic link to depressive disorders; depression can run in families. Difficult life experiences and certain personal patterns such as difficulty handling stress, low self-esteem, or extreme pessimism about the future can increase the chances of becoming depressed.

How Common Is It?

Clinical depression is a lot more common than most people think. It will affect more than 19 million Americans this year.

One-fourth of all women and one-eighth of all men will suffer at least one episode or occurrence of depression during their lifetimes. Depression affects people of all ages but is less common for teenagers than for adults. Approximately 3 to 5 percent of the teen population experiences clinical depression every year. That means among 25 friends, 1 could be clinically depressed.

Is It Serious?

Depression can be very serious.

It has been linked to poor school performance, truancy, alcohol and drug abuse, running away, and feelings of worthlessness and hopelessness. In the past 25 years, the rate of suicide among teenagers and young adults has increased dramatically. Suicide is often linked to depression.

Are All Depressive Disorders Alike?

There are various forms or types of depression.

Some people experience only one episode of depression in their whole life, but many have several recurrences. Some depressive episodes begin suddenly for no apparent reason, while others can be associated with a life situation or stress. Sometimes people who are depressed cannot perform even the simplest daily activities—like getting out of bed or getting dressed; others go through the motions, but it is clear they are not acting or thinking as usual. Some people suffer from bipolar depression in which their moods cycle between two extremes—from the depths of desperation to frenzied talking or activity or grandiose ideas about their own competence.

Can It Be Treated?

Yes, depression is treatable. Between 80 and 90 percent of people with depression—even the most serious forms—can be helped.

There are a variety of antidepressant medications and psychotherapies that can be used to treat depressive disorders. Some people with milder forms may do well with psychotherapy alone. People with moderate to severe depression most often benefit from antidepressants. Most do best with combined treatment: medication to gain relatively quick symptom relief and psychotherapy to learn more effective ways to deal with life's problems, including depression.

The most important step toward overcoming depression—and sometimes the most difficult—is asking for help.

Why Don't People Get the Help they Need?

Often people don't know they are depressed, so they don't ask for or get the right help. Teenagers and adults share a problem—they often fail to recognize the symptoms of depression in themselves or in other people.

Be Able to Tell Fact from Fiction

Myths about depression often separate people from the effective treatments now available. Friends need to know the facts. Some of the most common myths are these:

Myth: Young people who claim to be depressed are weak and just need to pull themselves together. There's nothing anyone else can do to help.

Fact: Depression is not a weakness, but a serious health disorder. Both young people and adults who are depressed need professional treatment. A trained therapist or counselor can help them learn more positive ways to think about themselves, change behavior, cope with problems, or handle relationships. A physician can prescribe medications to help relieve the symptoms of depression. For many people, a combination of psychotherapy and medication is beneficial.

29

Myth: Talking about depression only makes it worse.

Fact: Talking through feelings may help someone recognize the need for professional help. By showing friendship and concern and giving uncritical support, you can encourage someone to get treatment.

Myth: Telling an adult that a friend might be depressed is betraying a trust. If someone wants help, he or she will get it.

Fact: Depression, which saps energy and self-esteem, interferes with a person's ability or wish to get help. And many parents may not understand the seriousness of depression or of thoughts of death or suicide. It is an act of true friendship to share your concerns with a school guidance counselor, a favorite teacher, your own parents, or another trusted adult.

Know the Symptoms

The first step toward defeating depression is to define it. But people who are depressed often have a hard time thinking clearly or recognizing their own symptoms. They may need help. Check the following to see if the person has had any of these symptoms persisting longer than two weeks.

Do they express feelings of

- sadness or "emptiness"?
- hopelessness, pessimism, or guilt?
- helplessness or worthlessness?

Do they seem

- unable to make decisions?
- unable to concentrate and remember?
- to have lost interest or pleasure in ordinary activities—like sports or band or talking on the phone?
- to have more problems with school and family?

Do they complain of

- loss of energy and drive—so they seem "slowed down"?

- trouble falling asleep, staying asleep, or getting up?

- appetite problems; are they losing or gaining weight?

- headaches, stomach aches, or backaches?

- chronic aches and pains in joints and muscles?

Has their behavior changed suddenly so that

- they are restless or more irritable?

- they want to be alone most of the time?

- they've started cutting classes or dropped hobbies and activities?

- you think they may be drinking heavily or taking drugs?

Have they talked about

- death?

- suicide—or have they attempted suicide?

Find Someone Who Can Help

If you answered yes to several of the items, this young person may need help. Don't assume that someone else is taking care of the problem. Negative thinking, inappropriate behavior or physical changes need to be reversed as quickly as possible. Not only does treatment lessen the severity of depression, treatment also may reduce the length of time (duration) the young person is depressed and may prevent additional bouts of depression.

If a young person shows many symptoms of depression, you can listen and encourage him or her to ask a parent or teacher about treatments.

There are many places in the community where people with depressive disorders can be diagnosed and treated. Help is available from family doctors, mental health specialists in community mental health centers or private clinics, and from other health professionals. See the "Resources" section of this *Sourcebook* for contact information.

Chapter 6

Bipolar Disorder in Children and Adolescents

What Is Bipolar Illness?

The bipolar disorders are mood disorders. That means that amongst other things, there is a major change in mood. In bipolar disorders, this change in mood can be down, as in depression, or the opposite, mania. That is, a person can be inappropriately up. Some types of bipolar disorder have a lot of depression and only a little mania. Others have half and half. Still others seem to be both manic and depressed at the same time. Some people with bipolar disorders only have a few cycles of depression and mania. Others have many cycles a year. When bipolar illness is present in children and adolescents, it is more severe and harder to treat than when it occurs in adults. Pediatric bipolar illness is one of the most severe conditions in pediatrics. In the milder forms, it can be disabling. In the severe forms, it can be lethal.

All bipolar disorders are a combination of mania with or without depression. So what is mania? Here are the official criteria:

Mania

An elevated, expansive, or irritable mood, lasting at least 1 week. This mood is also accompanied by at least three (four if mood is only irritable) of the following:

Jim Chandler, MD, FRCPC, "Bipolar Affective Disorder (Manic Depressive disorder) in Children and Adolescents," http://www.klis.com/chandler/pamphlet/bipolar/bipolarpamphlet.htm, June 8, 2000, downloaded June 27, 2001. Reprinted with permission.

1. Inflated self-esteem or grandiosity

2. Decreased need for sleep

3. Increased talkativeness or pressure to keep talking

4. Racing thoughts or flight of ideas

5. Distractibility

6. Increased activity or psychomotor agitation

7. Excessive involvement in pleasurable activities that have a high potential for painful consequences

The mood disturbance should be so severe that hospitalization is required to avoid harming themselves or others. Hypomania is severe enough to cause a marked disability, can last only four days, but is not so severe as to require hospitalization.

In pediatric mania and hypomania, the mood is more likely irritability. These features come and go throughout the day and are not as persistent as in adults.

Bipolar Depression

Usually a child will show episodes of depression before he or she shows episodes of mania. Sometimes the depression comes 3–4 years earlier. One common question is whether or not you can tell depression that is going to turn into bipolar disorder from the kind of depression that will never result in mania.

There are some signs and symptoms that suggest that depression may be the beginning of bipolar disorder. If a child has all of them, I would probably not give an antidepressant (they can make you manic). If they had a few I would watch very closely.

Signs of bipolar depression:

- Very slowed down movements

- Feeling like you are made of lead

- Too much sleeping

- Hallucinations or strange beliefs in the past

- Severe worthlessness

- Family history of bipolar disorder

Types of Bipolar Illness

The type of bipolar illness is determined by the combination of mania or hypomania and either mild or severe depression. It is also determined by how fast the cycling is. That is, how often do they have an episode in a year?

Bipolar I disorder. Children with this disorder have episodes of mania and episodes of depression. Sometimes there are fairly longer periods of normality between the episodes. Usually people spend much more time depressed than manic. However, some children will have chronic mania and rarely get depressed.

Bipolar II disorder. Here people mostly have depression and occasionally have an episode of hypomania, but not mania. Most people with this have long episodes of depression and virtually no time of wellness.

Cyclothymia. This variant is characterized by many episodes of hypomania and occasional episodes of mild depression only. A child may have quite a few episodes of hypomania over the span of a year.

Mixed states. In these conditions, a child will show signs of depression and mania at the same time. Most often, the mood is depressed and there are thoughts of suicide and hopelessness. The rest of the picture is, however, mania.

Rapid cycling bipolar illness. This means there are many cycles of mania and depression each year.

The above types are incredibly rare in children under age 15. In the space of a year I might see one or two children like the above. What is common in children is something which has no formal name but what is usually called childhood onset bipolar disorder.

Childhood Onset Bipolar Disorder

This is a new concept and there are no formal criteria. Children with this picture have episodes of mania and depression just like adult bipolar disorder but there are three differences.

- The cycling is fast. Often a person will cycle between mania (or hypomania) and depression many times a day

- The episodes are short. Rarely will they have days of any one state.

- Often mania and depression are mixed up together at the same time.

Prevalence of Bipolar Illness

About 1% of adults have a type of bipolar illness. As a person's age goes down, the smaller the chance of bipolar illness. It is currently very unclear how common it is in children. In adults, bipolar illness is more common in females. In children and adolescents, it is more common in males.

Causes of Bipolar Illness

Genetic. This is a strongly genetic condition. If a child has two parents who have had mood disorders, nearly every child will have a mood disorder (either a type of depression or a type of mania). If one parent has a mood disorder, about a quarter of the children will get a mood disorder.

Drugs. A number of drugs can make a person manic or look like mania. Steroids (by mouth, not just inhalers) are the most common prescription cause. Street drugs can mimic mania. A few other rarely used medications can, too.

However, the most important one to be aware of are the antidepressant medications. The drugs used for depression can make some people manic or hypomanic. In a recent study of Prozac in children for depression, about 5–10% switched to mania. These were children who had not had mania before.

Infections. In rare cases, infections of the brain, AIDS (Acquired Immune Deficiency Syndrome), and a few other rare diseases can cause mania. This is very rare in otherwise well children.

Hormones. Too much thyroid hormone can make you manic. This is also very, very rare in children.

Other rare neurologic conditions. Strokes, multiple sclerosis, tumors, epilepsy, and a few other rare causes can cause mania in children.

Diagnosing Mania in Children

There are two types of mistakes you can make in diagnosing any disease. You can think something is mania when it really is something else, for example, street drugs. Or you can think a disorder is something else when it is really mania. In children, the mistakes are almost always the second kind.

Making Sure You Don't Diagnose Something as Mania When It Really Isn't

Besides a complete history and physical and talking to everyone involved, it is often times necessary to do other tests. Urine drug screens, CAT (computed tomography scan) scans of the head, and blood tests are often used. If there is no family history of a mood disorder, then I am more aggressive in finding other causes.

Making Sure You Don't Diagnose Something Else When Really It Is Mania

This is the hard part. Mania can look a lot like a few other psychiatric disorders. It can look like a oppositional defiant disorder or conduct disorder (personality characterized by persistent violation of the rights of others and their property). It can look like attention deficit hyperactivity disorder (ADHD). Almost 90% of children who get mania will also have ADHD. It can look like "stress." Mania can also look like schizophrenia. Pediatric mania is more often accompanied by psychosis than in adults. Also mixed states and a rapid cycling are more common. These atypical features (for adults) can remind people of adult schizophrenia.

Usually by keeping two things in mind you can keep from missing mania. First, conduct disorders usually do not get suddenly ten times worse. Nor do they appear out of the blue over age 7. Second, mania is usually genetic. A strong family history of mood disorders, especially mania, makes me wonder about mania in any episode of wild and out of character behavior.

Medical Treatments

The aims of treatment are fourfold.

1. Treating acute symptoms
2. Prevention of relapse

3. Reduction of long-term morbidity

4. Promotion of long-term development and growth

Each of these goals is achieved with a combination of different treatments. Here are the different types of treatments. Nearly every person with bipolar illness will need a number of different types of treatments.

Older Mood Stabilizers (Epival, Lithium, Tegretol)

These drugs change the chemical balance in the brain. When they are effective, hypomania or mania goes away. They also will reduce cycling and make a person less likely to become manic again. In some people they are also effective for depression. However, they are much more effective for mania than depression. So, you could easily see the cycling stop and see the mania end, and have a child end up depressed.

We know these agents are effective in many adults with bipolar illness. They are less effective in pediatric bipolar illness. For example, adolescents who have bipolar illness and are prescribed lithium (and take it) will have a 37% chance of relapsing over the next 18 months. If they don't take the lithium, they have a 90% chance of relapsing. In severe cases of rapid cycling bipolar illness, these drugs are often used in combination.

Atypical Antipsychotics

Risperidone (Risperidal)

This drug has been studied the most for pediatric patients. It has been found to be effective in pediatric bipolar disorder using about 1–2 mg a day. About 85% responded. Risperidone is called Risperidal and comes in a variety of sizes; .25mg, .5 mg, 1mg, 2mg and liquid. It also helps Tourette's and conduct disorder and psychosis. Usually this is given once or twice a day.

Olanzapine (Zyprexa)

This drug was recently approved for mania in adults. It has been studied less in children. However the early reports are positive. The usual dose is about 5–15 mg a day. It comes in 2.5 mg, 5mg and 10 mg. It is also called Zyprexa. It is more expensive than Risperidone and in adults is associated with more weight gain. This can be given once a day.

Quetiapine (Seroquel)

This drug is a little different than the above ones as it seems to cause very little problems with things like tremor and stiffness. In adolescents it can lower the blood pressure so the dose has to be increased slower. The dosage range is 200–800 mg a day. It has been found to cause the least amount of weight gain in children. There are only a few articles on its use in children and adolescents, but these have been quite positive. It comes in a 25mg and 100 mg size and has to be given twice a day. It is called Seroquel.

New Mood Stabilizers

This includes three drugs at present, Lamictal (Lamotrigine), Neurontin (gabapentin) and Topamax (Toprimate).

They are being used a fair amount in children as they have been tested for epilepsy in children. There is evidence that they are effective in adults with bipolar disorder but there are still no reports in the literature of careful trials of these drugs in children and adolescents.

Psychological Treatments

There is unfortunately no specific treatment of this type for bipolar illness. There are a few types of counseling used in bipolar children.

Psychoeducational

If you have bipolar illness, it is a terrifying experience. Children need to learn all about it from doctors, nurses, families, and other people with bipolar illness.

Relapse Prevention

This involves teaching families and children about the impact of noncompliance, how to tell if you are relapsing, and what to do to avoid getting sick. In this category are things like avoiding substance abuse and not getting sleep deprived.

Working with Families

If a child has been ill with bipolar illness, it has, by definition, been rough on some of the other people in the family. Other sibs have often been ignored. Some members are scared of being alone with the person. Others might think it is someone's fault (or theirs). Often pediatric psychiatrists and other professionals need to meet with families to work this out.

Integration into the Community

If a person has or had bipolar illness, they need help getting back into the community. The same concerns that family members have are often found in the community and school. Pediatric psychiatrists and other professionals often need to work with teachers, community groups, and churches to help victims of bipolar illness get back into the mainstream of life.

Treating Substance Abuse

Whether children abuse drugs or not makes a bigger difference than if they take medications or not. It is just as important to keep teens with bipolar disorder street drug free as it is to make sure they take their medication. In the long term, staying free of street drugs is one of the biggest factors in preventing relapses.

Chapter 7

Anxiety in Adolescents

Chapter Contents

Section 7.1

Panic Disorder

Excerpted from Jim Chandler, MD, "Panic Disorder, Separation Anxiety Disorder, and Agoraphobia in Children and Adolescents," http://www.klis.com/ chandler/pamphlet/panic/panicpamphlet.htm, updated January 23, 2000, downloaded September 10, 2001. Reprinted with permission of the author.

Introduction

Up to 12% of ninth graders have had a panic attack. About 1–2% of all adults have multiple panic attacks. If you look at adults with panic disorder, 20% had their first panic attack before age 10. The first question is, What is a Panic attack? Here are the official criteria:

Panic Attack

A discrete period of intense fear or discomfort, in which four (or more) of the following symptoms develop abruptly and reach a peak within 10 minutes:

1. palpitations, pounding heart, or accelerated heart rate
2. sweating
3. trembling or shaking
4. sensations of shortness of breath or smothering
5. feeling of choking
6. chest pain or discomfort
7. nausea or abdominal distress
8. feeling dizzy, unsteady, lightheaded, or faint
9. derealization (feelings of unreality) or depersonalization (being detached from oneself)
10. fear of losing control or going crazy
11. fear of dying

12. parasthesia (numbness or tingling sensation)

13. chills or hot flushes

What Causes Panic Attacks?

Most researchers have found that they are caused by an abnormality in the part of the brain which tells the brain how much carbon dioxide (CO_2) is in the blood. If your brain finds there is too much CO_2, it usually means that you are not breathing fast enough, or there is too much CO_2 in the air (for example, in a room with no ventilation or a cave). So your body sends all sorts of signals to increase breathing and a rush of adrenaline to help you get out of wherever you are in a hurry. This is a great thing if you are in a fire, for example.

It is thought that in panic attacks this carbon dioxide sensor is too sensitive, and tells the brain there is not enough oxygen when there is just plenty. So a person could be just sitting quietly and then BOOM, this rush of adrenaline and fast breathing appears out of nowhere. Since there is no reason outside the body to be worried, most people will start thinking there is something horribly wrong with their own body.

Beyond this brain problem, panic attacks are inherited. If a parent has an anxiety disorder, their children are much more likely to have an anxiety disorder, too. Part of this heredity is expressed through something called behavioral inhibition.

Behavioral inhibition is a tendency to react negatively to new situations or things. Some infants and children will be very happy and curious about new people and things. However, roughly 15% of children will be shy, withdrawn, and irritable when they are in a new situation or with new people or things. Often these children and irritable as infants, shy and fearful as toddlers, and cautious, quiet, and introverted at school age. Children who are consistently this way are much more likely to have biological parents with anxiety disorders. The children themselves are much more likely to develop anxiety disorders. On the other hand 5–10 percent of children with behavioral inhibition will never develop anxiety disorders. At the moment it is thought that the majority of the genetic predisposition to anxiety disorders is expressed through behavioral inhibition. Often there is a combination of an inherited predisposition plus stress in the environment. Deaths in the family, divorce, and abuse will make panic attacks much more likely.

How Can You Be Sure That What Happened Was a Panic Attack and Not Some Other Medical Problem?

Panic attacks in children can be confused with many things. Common imitators are ulcers, irritable bowel syndrome, thyroid disease, some prescription drugs, migraines, epilepsy, diabetes, drug abuse, and other psychiatric disorders. There are some research tests which look at the brain which will show certain abnormalities in panic attacks. However, for a variety of reasons these are not in regular clinical use. The main principle is to rule out other problems using a careful medical history, a physical exam, and often certain lab or x-ray examinations. If the history and exam looks like panic attacks and no other cause is found, then a physician assumes it is a panic attack.

In females, stomach aches and headaches together are very, very common. In fact, recent studies have shown that when these two are found together in the same child, 69% had an anxiety disorder.

Panic Disorder

One panic attack is bad enough, but recurrent panic attacks can be devastating. If a child or adolescent has recurrent panic attacks and the following, it is called panic disorder.

1. recurrent unexpected panic attacks

2. at least one of the attacks has been followed by 1 month (or more) of one (or more) of the following:

   a. persistent concern about having additional attacks

   b. worry about the implications of the attack or its consequences (e.g., losing control, having a heart attack, "going crazy")

   c. a significant change in behavior related to the attacks.

Panic disorder in children is a very disabling condition. It will often affect a child's school performance. It almost always impairs them socially, and can lead to a lot of other problems. It is not a common illness in children. While perhaps 10% of children will have a panic attack, about 1–2% will develop panic disorder. Of those that do develop panic disorder, 10–35% will recover and remain well the rest of their lives. At least 50% will be mildly affected years later, and the rest will have chronic panic disorder for years. If you follow-up children with panic disorder, about 25% will still have it years later. Of those who continue to have panic disorder as they go into adulthood, many will develop other psychiatric difficulties. About 50% will develop agoraphobia, 20% will make suicide attempts, 27% will develop alcohol abuse, 60% will develop depression, 35% will believe they are unhealthy, 27% will not be financially independent, 28% will make frequent outpatients visits, and 50% will show significant social impairment.

Comorbidity

"My daughter has panic attacks, but it is her other nervous problems which are causing her the most trouble. What is going on?"

Panic disorder with agoraphobia often does not exist alone. Many children will also have another disorder. Here is a list of the other common childhood disorders.

- separation anxiety disorder
- obsessive-compulsive disorder
- generalized anxiety disorder
- social phobia
- selective mutism
- post-traumatic stress disorder
- tic disorders
- specific phobias
- attention deficit hyperactivity disorder (ADHD)
- depression

What Can Be Done?

If panic disorder with or without agoraphobia persists into adolescence, often the teenager will have become depressed, become involved with drugs and alcohol, fail or drop out of school, become socially isolated and almost house bound, or all of the above. The same is true for separation anxiety disorder.

The treatment of these conditions revolves around two things, medications and psychological treatments. I will start with psychological treatments. There are three elements to the psychological treatment of anxiety disorders.

Behavioral Treatments

Graduated exposure. It has been found that children, like adults, will be able to overcome phobias with this technique. What you do is gradually expose yourself to the thing that makes you so panicky.

Response prevention. The key to this technique is to keep yourself from doing the thing you want to when you get panicky. For example, if a child is in class and wants desperately to raise his hand so that he can go home and call his mother to come and get him, teach the child to wait 5 minutes before calling.

Relaxation techniques. When people start having panic symptoms, or if they are having to tolerate separation in separation anxiety disorder, if they have learned some specific techniques they can often ride out the panic much easier. These involve 1) slow, regulated breathing 2) saying a little memorized phrase like, "Everyone's stomachs gurgle. My stomach gurgles many times a day. I do not need to leave and go to the bathroom."

Cognitive therapy. This consists of learning about how certain thought patterns are leading to worsening of the anxiety disorder.

Medical Treatments

Often the idea of taking medicines for anxiety disorders makes either the parents or the child very nervous. Before discussing the individual drugs, I will discuss the general approach to pediatric psychopharmacology that I use.

Why Would Anyone Want to Give Drugs That Affect the Brain to Children?

The main reason would be if the non-medical interventions are not working. No one would suggest trying medical treatments before the non-medical interventions are used. It is similar to diabetes in that way. If you have diabetes which is not severe, your doctor will first suggest you try diet control. If that doesn't work, only then will the doctor consider medical treatment. In some situations, a child is very ill, has numerous disorders or there is some urgency. For example, a child has multiple anxiety disorders and depression and is either in the hospital or unable to go to school. Then I consider medications as a first line approach along with other interventions.

If the Drug Works, How Will My Child Be Different?

In cases where the drugs work very well, a child will be able to face situations in which they usually panic with little or no anxiety. Panic attacks should be basically eliminated. Children are usually more carefree, enthusiastic, and less depressed. Each drug works in a different way on the chemical transmitters in the brain.

What If It Doesn't Work?

Sometimes a medication won't work because the dose is too high or too low. Some people will not respond to one medication for the treatment of this problem but they will respond to another. If the drug doesn't work, of course, it is discontinued, and then you and your child's doctor decide what do next. Try something else? Abandon medical treatment? Both are sometimes reasonable options.

I Have Heard That These Drugs Can Do a Lot of Bad Things. Is This True?

Yes, it is. Like all medical treatments, there are side effects and sometimes people can have pretty bad side effects. There are two types of side effects. One type are the kind that disappear when you stop the drug. The other kind can last long after the drug is discontinued. I do not use any of the drugs which can cause permanent side effects after the drug is stopped.

Are They That Dangerous?

Yes, when used improperly they can be quite dangerous. However, when used carefully they can be almost 100% safe.

Here Are the Specific Drugs

Serotonin reuptake inhibitors (SRIs). In most cases, these are the first choice drugs for anxiety disorders in pediatrics. They are well tolerated, cause few side effects, and have been found to be quite effective in multiple studies. While there are fewer studies involving their use in separation anxiety disorder, researchers have found these drugs to work as well as in panic disorder. Common brands are Prozac, Paxil, Celexa, Zoloft, and Luvox.

Benzodiazepines. This is a group of drugs which are commonly called "minor tranquilizers." They work on a certain chemical in the brain called GABA and basically slow down many brain functions. The primary use in children is anxiety disorders or to help with anesthesia. Two are used for seizures. Commonly used ones are Xanax, Ativan, Serax, Valium, Dalmane, Librium, and Rivotril.

Other drugs. Venlafaxine (Effexor XR) has been found to be very useful for the treatment of anxiety disorders in adults. It is mostly used for depression in adults. There have been recent studies of this drug for anxiety disorders in children. Nevertheless, if a child, especially a teenager, had failed two trials of an SRI, it is the next choice.

In summary, anxiety disorders can be very disabling in children and should be treated. You need to make sure it is not some other medical problem and also see if other psychiatric problems are present, too. Most studies have found the best results when medical and non-medical treatments are combined. Most children with anxiety disorder should benefit significantly from treatment.

Section 7.2

Agoraphobia

Excerpted from Jim Chandler, MD, "Panic Disorder, Separation Anxiety Disorder, and Agoraphobia in Children and Adolescents," http://www.klis.com/chandler/pamphlet/panic/panicpamphlet.htm, updated January 23, 2000, downloaded September 10, 2001. Reprinted with permission of the author.

The most common fear or phobia in the context of panic disorder is agoraphobia. Here is the official definition of agoraphobia.

1. Anxiety about being in places or situations from which escape might be difficult (or embarrassing) or in which help might not be available in the event of having an unexpected panic attack or panic-like symptoms. Agoraphobic fears typically involve characteristic clusters of situations that include being outside the home alone, being in a crowd or standing in line, being on a bridge, and traveling in a bus, train, automobile, or plane.

2. The situations are avoided (e.g., travel is restricted) or else are endured with marked distress or with anxiety about having a panic attack or panic-like symptoms, or require the presence of a companion.

3. This is not due to social phobia, obsessive-compulsive disorder, post traumatic stress disorder, or separation anxiety disorder.

The usual pattern I find with children is not that different than with adults. Panic attacks will set in process a slow restricting of peoples lives. Slowly they stop doing all sorts of things they used to and stop going all sorts of places. Lots of times, especially with children, they have some excuse (other than fear of panic) for not going which seems fairly reasonable at first. Often they play at their home without problems, but if they have to go there is always a reason they aren't going. Sometimes it is because the child says he doesn't want to (even though you know he would love to do this before) other times it is because all of a sudden her stomach is hurting, she feels weak and tired, her eyes hurt, or she needs to go use the bathroom.

Agoraphobia and School

This is of only minor concern compared with agoraphobia that revolves around school. There are many parts of school which are the cause of problems in agoraphobics. I have never seen an agoraphobic child or adolescent who did not have problems with school. I will start from the beginning.

Wake up—Many children with agoraphobia will awaken on school days with horrible abdominal pain, diarrhea, nausea, headache, or many other signs of physical illness which all disappear as soon as there is no chance they are going to school. This is real, not made up. The anxiety is making their body react this way.

Bus rides—It is common that children with agoraphobia will be afraid that something horrible or embarrassing will happen on the bus such as diarrhea, vomiting, going crazy, and getting sick with no one to help. Often this results in parents driving the child to school.

Going in the school—Other children are fine until they see the school and they know they have to go in. The idea of going and sitting in their classrooms leads to all sorts of anxiety about what could go wrong (as in the bus ride). Some children will just refuse to go to school.

Leaving class—For some agoraphobic children, they get into school, but they can not stay the whole day. Their physical signs of anxiety are enough to get most teachers to call home and have a parent come and get the child. As a result, the parent is basically "on-call" throughout the school day.

Special events—Some agoraphobic children can handle the usual school day but not field trips (without their mother), performances, and changes in teachers.

All of these can lead to school refusal. There are other reasons besides agoraphobia that children will refuse to go to school. However, it is usually what will bring a child to my attention. Any of the other anxiety disorders of children can lead to school refusal. The most important thing is to get them back in school as soon as possible and find out what the problem(s) is.

My Son Says He Is Fine As Long As We Don't Do Anything to Make Him Worse

Many children with agoraphobia and panic disorder will have come up with their own "treatment." This consists of getting everyone else on the planet to live their lives such that it minimizes the anxiety for this child. When people (usually family members) forget or refuse to follow one of these many rules, then the child with the anxiety disorder blames the family member for his or her anxiety. Common rules are:

- I don't ride in other people's cars.
- I don't go to birthday parties.
- I don't go to the mall.
- I am driven to school.
- I don't wait in lines.
- I don't go on the 101 or 103.

This "treatment" drives caregivers nuts. Any worsening of anxiety is now the parents fault. Obviously, this is not the way to go. However, most children prefer this as they have no responsibility, and the focus is not on them.

Section 7.3

Separation Anxiety Disorder in Teens

Excerpted from Jim Chandler, MD, "Panic Disorder, Separation Anxiety Disorder, and Agoraphobia in Children and Adolescents," http://www.klis.com/chandler/pamphlet/panic/panicpamphlet.htm, updated January 23, 2000, downloaded September 10, 2001. Reprinted with permission of the author.

Agoraphobia and panic attacks often go together. More recently it has been discovered that panic attacks and agoraphobia are much more common in children who currently have separation anxiety disorder or had it in the past.

What Is Separation Anxiety Disorder?

It is a worry about being away from home or about being away from parents which is way out of line for that child's age, culture, and life.

Signs of Separation Anxiety Disorder

- getting nervous if the parent is going to leave, even if they haven't left yet

- worrying that something bad is going to happen to a parent

- worrying that a they will be lost or kidnaped

- being afraid to go places without parents

- can't be alone at home without parents

- can't sleep alone

- nightmares about being separated

- all the signs of Panic Attacks occurring when parent is leaving or child is forced to leave

Separation anxiety disorder can persist into adulthood. As mentioned above, it is very common for a child to start with this and later develop panic disorder or agoraphobia or all three! As far as causes go, the same things cause separation anxiety disorder that cause panic and agoraphobia. However, some research now suggests that having a parent with alcoholism significantly increases a child's risk of having separation anxiety disorder. About 14% of children of alcoholic parents will have separation anxiety disorder.

Chapter 8

Obsessive-Compulsive Disorder in Youth

Introduction

Up until about 20 years ago, obsessive-compulsive disorder (OCD) was thought to be a very, very, rare disorder. I only saw two cases in my training in the mid 1980s, and neither were children. It wasn't important to find OCD anyway—little was known about it and there were no effective treatments. Over the last decade, everything has changed. We now know that OCD is one of the most common neuropsychiatric disorders. It is also one of the most treatable ones. In pediatric psychiatry I am always on the lookout for OCD because it is common and often very treatable.

What Is OCD?

To be diagnosed with OCD, a person must have obsessions or compulsions or both. Besides this, the obsessions and/or compulsions must be disabling.

Obsessions

These are thoughts which are invisible to anyone else. The thoughts bring some distress to the person. The person wishes they

Jim Chandler, MD, FRCPC, "Obsessive-Compulsive Disorder (OCD)," http://www.klis.com/chandler/pamphlet/ocd/ocdpamphlet.htm, last updated February 14, 2001, downloaded June 28, 2001. Reprinted with permission.

did not have these thoughts. They are not based on what is realistically worrisome in that person's life. These thoughts occur over and over, usually hundreds of times a day. A person spends so much time thinking about these things they have a hard time doing their work, taking care of themselves, or relating to others in a normal way.

Common obsessions in children are fears of bad things happening to family members, exactness and symmetry, bodily functions, lucky numbers, and less likely, sexual and aggressive thoughts. Religious obsessions are less common. Here is the official definition.

Obsessions are:

1. Recurrent and persistent ideas, thoughts, impulses, or images that are experienced at some time during the disturbance as intrusive and inappropriate and cause marked anxiety or distress.

2. The thoughts, impulses, or images are not simply excessive worries about real-life problems.

3. The person attempts to ignore or suppress such thoughts, impulses, or images to neutralize them with some other thought or action.

4. The person recognizes that the obsessional thoughts are the product of his or her own mind (They are not hallucinations. They are not felt to be inserted into your mind by someone or something else)

Obsessions are usually in some way extremely private, embarrassing, or disgusting. Rarely will an adult or child with OCD tell me all of their obsessions. Rarely are obsessions present alone. Usually there are also related compulsions.

Examples of Obsessions

Reading about descriptions of obsessions doesn't give you much feeling for what they really are like. Examples do. Here are some.

Jonathan — Unlucky Numbers

This 11 year old boy started doing badly in school. This was pretty surprising as he had always been a good student. Jonathan knew why, but he was afraid to tell anyone. He was worrying that he might loose his temper and hurt someone. He never had, but he felt like he might just do it some day. For some reason that he cannot explain, if he does anything with the number "9" he thinks he will loose control and attack someone. So the more number "9" he sees, the more he worries about losing control and attacking someone. He wishes he didn't have to think about this all the time, but he can't help it. It takes a lot of energy out of a person to avoid reading or saying the number "9." It means that he is very slow to do his homework (especially math) and has a hard time playing games with his friends. His parents are about to kill him. He will not go to bed at the usual time (9:00 O'clock!). He refuses to ride the bus, is slow to get ready, and never seems to listen. He is in a world of his own.

Ashley — Disease

Ashley once was walking along the sidewalk with her friends. She stepped on something yucky, but didn't think much about it until they got to the hotel. The idea came to her that it was a condom, and probably she would now get AIDS (acquired immune deficiency syndrome) from it. She asked her friends what they thought. She asked her mom. Ashley was 15 and had never even kissed someone and was at zero risk for AIDS. She called the AIDS Hotline at least twice a day for assurance. She begged to go to the doctor for more tests. She read every book she could about AIDS. When she started talking about her funeral arrangements, her mother took her to the doctor who sent her to the psychiatrist.

Compulsions

Compulsions are things that people do or acts they perform in their heads. They are repetitive and senseless, just like obsessions. In many people, the compulsion is linked to an obsession. Here is the official definition.

1. Repetitive behaviors are mental acts that the person feels driven to perform in response to an obsession.

2. The behaviors or mental acts are aimed at preventing or reducing distress or preventing some dreaded event or situation; however, these behaviors or mental acts either are not connected in a realistic way with what they are designed to neutralize or prevent or are clearly excessive.

Common compulsions in pediatric OCD are: washing, repeating, checking and ordering. Less common ones are rituals to protect themselves from bad things, counting, hoarding and slowness.

The pain of OCD is hidden from most people in a child's life. While many neuropsychiatric disorders of children are partly private, a lot of the signs and symptoms are quite obvious to parents, teachers, friends, and family. If you spend a fair amount of time with a child with a mood disorder, tics, ADHD (attention deficit hyperactivity disorder), learning disorders, ODD (oppositional defiant disorder), or conduct disorder, you will get to see plenty of signs of the disorder.

Why is this? All of us have little habits that we are far less likely to engage in out of our homes. Things like picking sores, scratching your groin, and farting are common examples. Although we might have the urge to do these in public, we can usually control it, at least until we get home. The same applies to OCD. A child who is really bugged by things being out of order at school may be able to control it at school.

Another reason is that things that family members do or do not do always bug us more than what total strangers do. Likewise a mess in my neighbors house is far less bothersome than one in my own home. So with OCD, the biggest problem is when a person is with those she loves and in her own home.

1. OCD is a very private type of suffering. Most compulsions and obsessions are not noticed by anyone other than the person who has the disorder. What I, as the physician, see and hear about is usually just the tip of the iceberg. Often parents and teachers notice almost nothing at all.

2. It is usually depression or a crisis that brings pediatric OCD "out of the closet."

3. OCD is probably the most embarrassing neuropsychiatric disorder. The thoughts which go through the person's mind are often very embarrassing, and so are the compulsions.

Long Term Course

When researchers follow children with OCD for years, many children still show signs of OCD 2–7 years later. About 43% of children still have the diagnosis of OCD, which means disabling obsessions and/or compulsions. About 11% had no sign of OCD whatsoever. The remaining 46% showed some signs of OCD, but not enough to make a diagnosis. It is very hard to predict who will be the lucky ones who get rid of it forever, and who will not. No factor, including age, sex, type of OCD, or insight into the illness has been proven to be a good predictor. Most researchers think, however, that comorbidity and family problems make a bad outcome more likely.

Does OCD Turn into Something Worse?

Many people are afraid that they will go crazy when they have OCD. If being crazy means schizophrenia, then they shouldn't worry. It is extremely unlikely that routine OCD will turn into an illness like that.

How Common Is OCD?

Pediatric OCD usually comes on between age 7 and 12, but can come much earlier. Between two and four percent of all children have OCD. It is a little more common in males than females. This wouldn't be so bad if those children were identified with OCD and then treated for it. The problem is it is not picked up. In most surveys children or adolescents, most of the children who are found to have OCD have never gone for professional help, even though the disorder is quite disabling. Sadder yet, of the few who get professional help, almost none are correctly identified as having OCD. Most are thought to have some sort of family problem. Sadder still is the fact that even when OCD is identified, most children are not given appropriate treatment.

Co-Morbidity

Co-morbidity is the tendency of certain diseases and disorders to run together. For example, high blood pressure and diabetes occur more often together than one would expect. OCD that comes to the attention of professionals is usually accompanied by some other neuropsychiatric disorder. When I initially see a child with OCD, I spend a lot of time trying to figure what else they might have. Over 75% of children with OCD will have had at least one other psychiatric disorder in their lives. The most common co-morbid conditions are depression, disruptive behavior disorders, anxiety disorders, learning disorders, tic disorders, and OCD spectrum disorders (psychiatric disorders that are like OCD, but not exactly).

What Is the Cause of OCD?

Until the last 15 years or so, many people thought that there was some deep and dark secret in the minds of people who had OCD. When it did occur in children, it was assumed to be due to some family problem or difficulty in growing up. We now know that while these can affect OCD, OCD is not caused by this sort of thing. OCD is about as physical as diabetes, asthma, and other common pediatric illnesses. In fact, there is more known about the physical causes of OCD than most other neuropsychiatric disorders. At this point, most of the evidence points to two causes of OCD, genetics and infections.

Genetics

OCD runs in families. About 30% of teenagers with OCD have a relative in their immediate family with OCD or some signs of OCD. When OCD appears early in childhood, it is even more likely that there will be family members with the disorder. Other studies have not found as much OCD as this in relatives, but have found lots of other anxiety disorders besides OCD in the relatives. In families where OCD seems to be inherited, often times tic disorders are found, too. The usual pattern is for the males in the family to be more likely to have tic disorders and the females to be more likely to have OCD. However, the opposite is not uncommon. These studies show that OCD runs in families, but it doesn't point to an exact cause. Other studies do point to certain problems in the brain.

Imaging

Many people have heard of CT (computed tomography) scans. They are very fancy x-rays of the brain. There are some other tests which can be used to investigate the brain which are like CT scans. These include MRI, PET, and MRS. These pictures of the brain show that children and adults with OCD have some abnormalities in the brain. They involve the part of the brain above the eyes (orbital area), and some of the structures that are deep down in the brain (basal ganglia and thalmus). This research suggests that somehow the communication between these areas is not right in OCD.

Chemistry

It is not uncommon to hear people say that someone has a "chemical imbalance" in their brain. A lot of work has been put into trying to determine if there is a chemical imbalance in OCD. There is quite a bit of evidence to suggest that one chemical messenger, Serotonin, is very involved. All the drugs which help OCD affect this chemical messenger in one way or another. Tests of the spinal fluid also suggest that this chemical is involved. Unfortunately, the more scientists find out about the chemistry of OCD in the brain, the more confusing and complicated it gets. Five years ago, we didn't know that serotonin can attach to nerve cells in the brain in many different ways and cause a host of different things. Although we know serotonin is involved, now the question is which part? Is the problem one of the ten or so plugs or receptors that serotonin attaches to? Is the real problem another chemical? Where in the brain are these serotonin receptors messed up, if they are? Although a lot more is now known about what causes OCD, scientists are still a long way from having the final answer.

Infections

One way of learning about what causes OCD may easily come from some research in the last couple of years on how infections can cause OCD. Many people have heard of rheumatic fever. This is a heart disease that is caused by a person getting strep throat and then in the process of fighting off the infection, the person's body starts confusing the cells on the heart valves with the strep bacteria. So the person's body attacks the strep bacteria and the heart valves. As a result, the heart valves are damaged. It has been known for years that the same thing can happen in the brain. During the course of a strep infection, a person's infection fighting system confuses strep and the outside of nerve cells in the brain. As a result, the person's infection fighting system attacks the strep and also certain cells of the brain. This is the same part of the brain, basal ganglia, which has been found to be part of the problem in OCD. People who acquire this have something called "Sydenham's chorea." They have a movement disorder which is sort of like tics. Then researchers found out that they had a lot of OCD symptoms, too. Now it has been discovered that some people who have this problem with their infection fighting system attacking their brain will not get a movement disorder at all but just very severe OCD. The signs and symptoms can be just the same as the genetic variety. It usually comes on very suddenly. Usually it goes away after awhile. Sometimes it happens in a person who already has mild OCD. It has a strange name. It is called PANDAS. This stands for pediatric autoimmune neuropsychiatric disorder associated with streptococcal infections. No one knows how often it occurs, but everyone agrees it is quite rare. The big question right now is what to do about it and how to diagnosis it. On one extreme, some doctors give something like kidney dialysis if they think a person has this. Others give penicillin. At the moment, if I see someone who has signs of this,

I do some lab tests. If they were positive, I would get a few more opinions. What is reasonable to do for this seems to change every few months right now.

Diagnosing OCD

Like all neuropsychiatric disorders, OCD is diagnosed based on the history, physical signs, and lab tests. There is no lab test that will show that a person has OCD. There are some that are highly suggestive of PANDAS.

History

When I talk to children or teenagers or their parents about OCD, I want to ask them about all the different obsessions and compulsions. I also want to ask them about all of the co-morbid disorders, especially other anxiety disorders, depression, and tics. I want to know how the disorder started and what has been done to treat it.

Exam

The only part of the physical examination that is useful is the part which is done to look for tics. Other wise I am looking for signs of OCD—trouble managing the disorder in my office, touching things, having to enter a certain way, and preoccupations with certain themes. I also want to see how depressed they are.

Lab

I only get lab tests done if there are some unusual features to the history and examination. I also get lab tests if I suspect PANDAS.

Treatment

These are three categories of treatments for OCD.

1. Treatments which have been carefully researched and have been found to be effective. This includes cognitive-behavior therapy and medications.

2. Treatments which have been studied some and are useful in certain circumstances. This includes family therapy, relaxation techniques, and surgery. These are not of interest to the general reader and I have not included information about them.

3. Treatments that have not been carefully researched but are still used by people anyway. This includes diet and nutrition therapy, psychoanalysis, all sorts of other psychotherapies, group therapy, and many, many more. Many of these treatments in this third group may be effective and they may be safe, but I don't know. Usually I don't know because there isn't enough careful scientific research on the treatment. The fact that something worked for OCD in 10 people in one clinic doesn't mean it is time to try it on others outside of a research setting. Sometimes I don't know about the treatment because it is just too new. Then my approach is to find out, or find someone who I respect who knows.

That leaves us with the first and main category: treatments which have been carefully researched and have been found to be effective.

Cognitive Behavioral Treatment

Cognitive behavioral treatment of OCD is based on two principles, exposure and response prevention. It is a "doing" treatment, not an understanding and counseling treatment. It involves a lot of homework.

Graduated Exposure

These means exposing yourself to the thing that makes you anxious. For example, if a person is having disabling compulsions to order things, they might expose themselves to clutter for five minutes without touching anything. A fear of germs might be treated by touching a sink in a public washroom. In a sense, it is facing the thing you fear a little bit at a time until you have finally conquered it. Sometimes, people start by just imagining they have exposed themselves to something.

Response Prevention

These is preventing a person from doing a compulsion or mental act. If you are a checker, it means preventing yourself from checking things by having someone with you or a physical barrier. It may mean at first just preventing yourself from checking for a short amount of time.

Cognitive Treatment

These works on what a person is thinking, not what they are doing. When you are doing cognitive therapy, you are learning what thoughts you are thinking and then learning techniques to control these thoughts. A common one in the treatment of OCD in children is labeling these OCD thoughts as not your own. This technique is used to encourage children to talk to their OCD as if it were a bad guy. For example, a girl who kept obsessing about getting AIDS would be taught to label these thoughts as from the OCD, and not her. Then she would learn some ways to tell these thoughts to "get out of town." Other techniques involve thought stopping, where you do something physical to stop obsessing which you have learned in therapy, like snapping a rubber band on your wrist ever time you start obsessing.

Like most things, the best way to understand cognitive behavioral treatment is to see how it works with examples. Here are those same ill children from the first section and how they could be treated with a combination of exposure and response prevention and cognitive therapy.

In Summary

These gives you an idea of how cognitive behavioral treatment works and doesn't work in OCD. Overall, about 60–70% of children will improve with this treatment. To do this type of treatment, a child has to be motivated to do the homework, believe that she or he really needs help, and be patient enough to wait a while. In children, the behavioral techniques are used more frequently than the cognitive ones. However, making the OCD into something that the child is fighting sometimes works well. The other good thing about behavioral treatments is that people have a great sense of accomplishment if they can get better without medications.

To do behavioral treatment you need:

- a motivated person who wants to get better
- a family which is willing to help
- dedication to work on homework even though it is hard and slow going
- a professional who knows how to do the therapy

Medications

Introduction

The medications used for OCD are the same ones that are used for severe depression and other anxiety disorders in children and adolescents. These drugs all affect serotonin, a chemical in the brain which is used to communicate between the different parts of the brain. We don't know exactly how this works yet. We do know one thing for certain: if a drug has no effect on the serotonin system, it won't be effective alone in OCD. At present, there are five drugs in this group. The are Prozac (fluoxetine), Paxil (paroxetine), Zoloft (sertraline), Luvox (fluvoxamine), and Anafranil (clomipramine). All of these drugs have been used in pediatric OCD. Clomipramine has been used the longest.

What Are These Drugs Supposed to Do and How Fast Do They Work?

In adults, when these drugs work, which is 60–80% of the time, they do not work overnight. Usually a person will see a change in the first month, but sometimes a person can have no change for 6–8 weeks and then start to improve. However, some recent work suggests that they may work faster in children. A very large study of Fluvoxamine (Luvox) in children with OCD showed after only one week there were signs of improvement and most of the improvement was seen within the first three weeks. In some people, the obsessions and compulsions just start to drop away. In other cases, the obsessive thoughts still go through their mind, but only to a mild degree. In other cases, the medicines just make it easier to do the behavior treatment. Sometimes they help certain parts of OCD and not others. Sometimes, of course, they don't do anything at all for OCD.

How Long Does a Person Take Them?

At a minimum, six months. If a person has been very ill and it has been a real battle to get them better, I usually advise they take medications for 12–18 months. Either way, we try to discontinue medications in the summer when school is out. When we discontinue medications a couple of things can happen:

Nothing. The person does just as well off medications as on. That is the best sign. Overall, about 50% of people will be able to do that.

Worsening right away. The child gets worse over the next few weeks. In this case we put the child back on medications for at least another year.

Worsening later on. Sometimes a child will do well off medications for a few months, and then have a worsening of OCD again. We then restart the medications for another year or so and then try discontinuing again.

Of the children I see that are more severely ill, at least 50% cannot get off the medications without relapsing. There is no danger in this, as these drugs do not have any long term side effects.

What Are the Drugs and Their Side Effects?

These drugs are really in two families that are quite different. Clomipramine is one family and all the others are in another.

Clomipramine (Anafranil). This drug can have a lot of side effects. It was for this reason, in part, that researchers started using the other drugs mentioned above. The side effects can be either nuisance or serious.

Other serotonin reuptake inhibitors (SRI) [see Table 8.1]. All of these drugs have been tested in OCD in children. However since Celexa is new, there is only one study of this medication in the literature. These drugs all have the same side effects. However one person might tolerate one drug very well but not another. Likewise one might work, but not another.

In Summary

Medications can be very effective in OCD. They also can cause problems. As long as the patient, family and doctor understand what they are doing, they are quite safe.

Table 8.1. Serotonin Reuptake Inhibitors (SRI)

Drug	Brand Name	Usual Dosage	Sizes	Comments
Fluoxetine	Prozac	about 1mg/kg	10, 20, liquid	long acting
Paroxetine	Paxil	20–60mg a day	10, 20, 30	worse withdrawal symptoms
Citalopram	Celexa	20–40mg a day	20	new in 1999
Sertraline	Zoloft	3mg/kg max	25, 50	capsules
Fluvoxamine	Luvox	3mg/kg max	50, 100	pills are scored

Chapter 9

Tic Disorders and Tourette's Syndrome in Adolescents

Tic Disorders

A tic is a problem in which a part of the body moves repeatedly, quickly, suddenly, and uncontrollably. Tics can occur in any body part, such as the face, shoulders, hands, or legs. They can be stopped voluntarily for brief periods. Sounds that are made involuntarily (such as throat clearing) are called vocal tics. Most tics are mild and hardly noticeable. However, in some cases they are frequent and severe, and can affect many areas of a child's life.

The most common tic disorder is called "transient tic disorder," which may affect up to 10 percent of children during the early school years. Teachers or others may notice the tics and wonder if the youth is under stress or "nervous." Transient tics go away by themselves. Some may get worse with anxiety, tiredness, and some medications.

Some tics do not go away. Tics which last one year or more are called "chronic tics." Chronic tics affect less than one percent of youth and may be related to a special, more unusual tic disorder called Tourette's syndrome.

This chapter contains text from "Tic Disorders," American Academy of Child and Adolescent Psychiatry (AACAP), Facts for Families #35, http://www.aacap.org/publications/factsfam/tics.htm, updated January 2000, reprinted with permission, and "Tourette Syndrome Fact Sheet," National Institute of Neurological Disorders and Stroke (NINDS), National Institutes of Health (NIH), http://www.ninds.nih.gov/health_and_medical/pubs/tourette_syndrome.htm, reviewed July 1, 2001.

Children with Tourette's syndrome have both body and vocal tics (throat clearing). Some tics disappear by early adulthood, and some continue. Children with Tourette's syndrome may have problems with attention, concentration, and may have learning disabilities as well. They may act impulsively, or develop obsessions and compulsions.

Sometimes people with Tourette's syndrome may blurt out obscene words, insult others, or make obscene gestures or movements. They cannot control these sounds and movements and should not be blamed for them. Punishment by parents, teasing by classmates, and scolding by teachers will not help the youth to control the tics but will hurt the youth's self-esteem.

Through a comprehensive medical evaluation, often involving pediatric and/or neurologic consultation, a child and adolescent psychiatrist can determine whether the youth has Tourette's syndrome or another tic disorder. Treatment for the youth with a tic disorder may include medication to help control the symptoms. The child and adolescent psychiatrist can also advise the family about how to provide emotional support and the appropriate educational environment for the youngster.

Tourette's Syndrome Fact Sheet

What Is Tourette's Syndrome?

Tourette's syndrome (TS) is an inherited, neurological disorder characterized by multiple involuntary movements and uncontrollable vocalizations called tics that come and go over years.

The disorder is named for Dr. Georges Gilles de la Tourette, the pioneering French neurologist who first described an 86-year-old French noblewoman with the condition in 1885.

The symptoms of TS generally appear before the individual is 18 years old. TS can affect people of all ethnic groups; males are affected 3 to 4 times more often than females. It is estimated that 100,000 Americans have full-blown TS, and that perhaps as many as 1 in 200 show a partial expression of the disorder, such as chronic multiple tics or transient childhood tics.

The natural course of TS varies from patient to patient. Although TS symptoms range from very mild to quite severe, the majority of cases fall in the mild category.

What Are the Symptoms?

The first symptoms of TS are usually facial tics—commonly eye blinking. However, facial tics can also include nose twitching or grimaces. With time, other motor tics may appear such as head jerking, neck stretching, foot stamping, or body twisting and bending.

TS patients may utter strange and unacceptable sounds, words, or phrases. It is not uncommon for a person with TS to continuously clear his or her throat, cough, sniff, grunt, yelp, bark, or shout.

People with TS may involuntarily shout obscenities (coprolalia) or constantly repeat the words of other people (echolalia). They may touch other people excessively or repeat actions obsessively and unnecessarily. A few patients with severe TS demonstrate self-harming behaviors such as lip and cheek biting and head banging against hard objects. However, these behaviors are extremely rare.

Tics alternately increase and decrease in severity, and periodically change in number, frequency, type, and location. Symptoms may subside for weeks or months at a time and later recur.

How Are Tics Classified?

There are two categories of tics: simple and complex. Simple tics are sudden, brief movements that involve a limited number of muscle groups. They occur in a single or isolated fashion and are often repetitive. Some of the more common examples of simple tics include eye blinking, shoulder shrugging, facial grimacing, head jerking, yelping, and sniffing. Complex tics are distinct, coordinated patterns of successive movements involving several muscle groups. Complex tics might include jumping, smelling objects, touching the nose, touching other people, coprolalia, echolalia, or self-harming behaviors.

Can People with TS Control Their Tics?

People with TS can sometimes suppress their tics for a short time, but the effort is similar to that of holding back a sneeze. Eventually tension mounts to the point where the tic escapes. Tics worsen in stressful situations; however they improve when the person is relaxed or absorbed in an activity. In most cases tics decrease markedly during sleep.

What Causes TS?

Although the basic cause of TS is unknown, current research suggests that there is an abnormality in the gene(s) affecting the brain's metabolism of neurotransmitters such as dopamine, serotonin, and norepinephrine. Neurotransmitters are chemicals in the brain that carry signals from one nerve cell to another.

How Is TS Diagnosed?

Generally, TS is diagnosed by obtaining a description of the tics and evaluating family history. For a diagnosis of TS to be made, both motor and phonic tics must be present for at least 1 year. Neuroimaging studies, such as magnetic resonance imaging (MRI), computerized tomography (CT), and electroencephalogram (EEG) scans, or certain blood tests may be used to rule out other conditions that might be confused with TS. However, TS is a clinical diagnosis. There are no blood tests or other laboratory tests that definitively diagnose the disorder.

Studies show that correct diagnosis of TS is frequently delayed after the start of symptoms because many physicians may not be familiar with the disorder. The behavioral symptoms and tics are easily misinterpreted, often causing children with TS to be misunderstood at school, at home, and even in the doctor's office. Parents, relatives, and peers who are unfamiliar with the disorder may incorrectly attribute the tics and other symptoms to psychological problems, thereby increasing the social isolation of those with the disorder. And because tics can wax and wane in severity and can also be suppressed, they are often absent during doctor visits, which further complicates making a diagnosis.

In many cases, parents, relatives, friends, or even the patients themselves become aware of the disorder based on information they have heard or read in the popular media.

How Is TS Treated?

Because symptoms do not impair most patients and development usually proceeds normally, the majority of people with TS require no medication. However, medications are available to help when symptoms interfere with functioning. Unfortunately, there is no one medication that is helpful to all persons with TS, nor does any medication completely eliminate symptoms; in addition, all medications have side effects. Instead, the available TS medications are only able to help reduce specific symptoms.

Some patients who require medication to reduce the frequency and intensity of the tic symptoms may be treated with neuroleptic drugs such as haloperidol and pimozide. These medications are usually given in very small doses that are increased slowly until the best possible balance between symptoms and side effects is achieved.

Recently scientists have discovered that long-term use of neuroleptic drugs may cause an involuntary movement disorder called tardive dyskinesia. However, this condition usually disappears when medication is discontinued. Short-term side effects of haloperidol and pimozide include muscular rigidity, drooling, tremor, lack of facial expression, slow movement, and restlessness. These side effects can be reduced by drugs commonly used to treat Parkinson's disease. Other side effects such as fatigue, depression, anxiety, weight gain, and difficulties in thinking clearly may be more troublesome.

Clonidine, an antihypertensive drug, is also used in the treatment of tics. Studies show that it is more effective in reducing motor tics than reducing vocal tics. Fatigue, dry mouth, irritability, dizziness, headache, and insomnia are common side effects associated with clonidine use. Fluphenazine and clonazepam may also be prescribed to help control tic symptoms.

Other types of therapy may also be helpful. Although psychological problems do not cause TS, psychotherapy may help the person better cope with the disorder and deal with the secondary social and emotional problems that sometimes occur. Psychotherapy does not help suppress the patient's tics.

Relaxation techniques and biofeedback may be useful in alleviating stress which can lead to an increase in tic symptoms.

Is TS Inherited?

Evidence from genetic studies suggests that TS is inherited in a dominant mode and the gene(s) involved can cause a variable range of symptoms in different family members. A person with TS has about a 50-50 chance of passing on the gene(s) to one of his or her offspring. However, that genetic predisposition may not necessarily result in full-blown TS; instead, it may express itself as a milder tic disorder or as obsessive compulsive behaviors or possibly attention deficit-hyperactivity disorder with few or no tics at all. It is also possible that the gene-carrying offspring will not develop any TS symptoms. A higher than normal incidence of milder tic disorders and obsessive compulsive behaviors has been found in families of individuals with TS.

Gender also plays an important role in TS gene expression. If the gene-carrying offspring of a TS patient is male, then the risk of developing symptoms is 3 to 4 times higher. However, most people who inherit the gene(s) will not develop symptoms severe enough to warrant medical attention. In some cases of TS, inheritance cannot be determined. These cases are called sporadic and their cause is unknown.

What Is the Prognosis?

There is no cure for TS; however, the condition in many individuals improves as they mature. Individuals with TS can expect to live a normal life span. Although the disorder is generally lifelong and chronic, it is not a degenerative condition. TS does not impair intelligence. Tics tend to decrease with age, enabling some patients to discontinue using medication. In a few cases, complete remission occurs after adolescence. Although tic symptoms tend to decrease with age, it is possible that neuropsychiatric disorders such as depression, panic attacks, mood swings, and antisocial behaviors may increase.

What Is the Best Educational Setting for Children with TS?

Although students with TS often function well in the regular classroom, it is estimated that many may have some kind of learning disability. When attention deficit-hyperactivity disorder, obsessive compulsive disorder, and frequent tics greatly interfere with academic performance or social adjustment, students should be placed in an educational setting that meets their individual needs. These students may require tutoring, smaller or special classes, and in some cases special schools.

All students with TS need a tolerant and compassionate setting that both encourages them to work to their full potential and is flexible enough to accommodate their special needs. This setting may include a private study area, exams outside the regular classroom, or even oral exams when the child's symptoms interfere with his or her ability to write. Untimed testing reduces stress for students with TS.

What Research Is Being Done?

Recent research has led to several notable advances in the understanding of TS. Already scientists have learned that TS is inherited from a dominant gene(s) that causes different symptoms from patient to patient, and that the disorder is more common than was previously thought.

Genetic studies. Currently, investigators are conducting genetic linkage studies in large multigenerational families affected with TS in an effort to find the chromosomal location of the TS gene(s). Finding a genetic marker (a biochemical abnormality that all TS patients might share) for TS would be a major step toward understanding the genetic risk factors for TS. Once the marker is found, research efforts would then focus on locating the TS gene(s). Understanding the genetics of TS will directly benefit patients who are concerned about recurrence in their families and will ultimately help to clarify the development of the disorder. Localization of the TS gene will strengthen clinical diagnosis, improve genetic counseling, lead to the clarification of pathophysiology, and provide clues for more effective therapies.

Neurotransmitter studies. Investigators continue to study certain neurotransmitters to increase our understanding of the syndrome, explore the role they play in the disease process, and provide more effective therapies.

Environmental studies. Other research projects currently under way include analyzing young unaffected children at high risk for TS in order to identify environmental factors such as life stresses or exposure to certain medications that may influence the expression of the disorder.

Scientists are also conducting neuropsychological tests and neuroimaging studies of brain activity and structure to determine the extent to which specific environmental exposures may affect the emergence of tics and/or obsessive compulsive symptoms.

Chapter 10

Schizophrenia in Adolescents

Schizophrenia: Get the Facts

- Schizophrenia is a disease that strikes young people in their prime.

- The disease distorts the senses, making it very difficult for the individual to tell what is real from what is not real.

- Usual age of onset is between 16 and 25.

- Schizophrenia is a medical illness. Period.

- Treatment works!

- Early diagnosis and stabilization on modern treatment can greatly improve prognosis for the illness.

Schizophrenia Is Not Rare: No One Is Immune

- Schizophrenia is found all over the world—in all races, in all cultures and in all social classes.

- It affects 1 in 100 people worldwide.

Excerpted from "Basic Facts about Schizophrenia," 9th edition, http://www.mentalhealth.com/book/p40-sc02.html, British Columbia Schizophrenia Society, April 2001. Reprinted with permission.

Men and Women Are Affected with Equal Frequency

- For men, the age of onset for schizophrenia is often ages 16 to 20.

- For women, the age of onset is sometimes later—ages 20 to 30.

What Causes Schizophrenia?

Researchers now agree that, while we do not yet know what "causes" schizophrenia, many pieces of the puzzle are becoming clearer. Areas of study and interest are:

Biochemistry. People with schizophrenia appear to have a neurochemical imbalance. Thus, some researchers study the neurotransmitters that allow communication between brain cells. Modern antipsychotic medications now target three different neurotransmitter systems (dopamine, serotonin, and norepinephrine).

Cerebral blood flow. With modern brain imaging techniques (PET scans), researchers can identify areas that are activated when the brain is engaged in processing information. People with schizophrenia appear to have difficulty "coordinating" activity between different areas of the brain. For example, when thinking or speaking, most people show increased activity in their frontal lobes, and a lessening of activity in the area of the brain used for listening. People with schizophrenia show the same increase in frontal lobe activity—but there is no decrease of activity ("dampening" or "filtering") in the other area. Researchers have also been able to identify specific areas of unusual activity during hallucinations.

Molecular biology. People with schizophrenia have an irregular pattern of certain brain cells. Since these cells are formed long before a baby is born, there is speculation that this irregular pattern may point towards a possible "cause" of schizophrenia in the prenatal period; or the pattern indicates a predisposition to acquire the disease at a later date.

Genetic predisposition. Genetic research continues, but has not yet identified a hereditary gene for schizophrenia. Schizophrenia does appear more regularly in some families. Then again, many people with schizophrenia have no family history of the illness.

Stress. Stress does not cause schizophrenia. However, it has been proven that stress makes symptoms worse when the illness is already present.

Drug abuse. Drugs (including alcohol, tobacco, and street drugs) themselves do not cause schizophrenia. However, certain drugs can make symptoms worse or trigger a psychotic episode if a person already has schizophrenia. Drugs can also create schizophrenia-like symptoms in otherwise healthy individuals.

Nutritional theories. While proper nutrition is essential for the well-being of a person with the illness, it is not likely that a lack of certain vitamins causes schizophrenia. Claims that promote megavitamin therapy have not been substantiated.

Some people do improve while taking vitamins. However, this can be due to concurrent use of antipsychotic medication, or to the overall therapeutic effect of a good diet, vitamin, and medication regime. Or, these individuals may be part of that group who will recover no matter what treatment is used.

Schizophrenia Is

- a brain disease, with concrete and specific symptoms due to physical and biochemical changes in the brain

- an illness that strikes young people in their prime—age of onset is usually between 16 and 25

- almost always treatable with medication

- more common than most people think. It affects 1 in 100 people worldwide.

Schizophrenia Is Not

- a "split personality"

- caused by childhood trauma, bad parenting, or poverty

- the result of any action or personal failure by the individual

Symptoms

Just as other diseases have signs or symptoms, so does schizophrenia. Symptoms are not identical for everyone. Some people may have only one episode of schizophrenia in their lifetime. Others may have recurring episodes, but lead relatively normal lives in between. Others may have severe symptoms for a lifetime.

Schizophrenia always involves a change in ability and personality. Family members and friends notice that the person is "not the same." Because they are experiencing perceptual difficulties—trouble knowing what is real from what is not real—the person who is ill often begins to withdraw as their symptoms become more pronounced. Deterioration is usually observed in:

- work or academic activities
- relationships with others
- personal care and hygiene

Characteristic Changes

Personality change is often a key to recognizing schizophrenia. At first, changes may be subtle, minor, and go unnoticed. Eventually, such changes become obvious to family, friends, classmates, or co-workers. There is a loss or lack of emotion, interest and motivation. A normally outgoing person may become withdrawn, quiet, or moody. Emotions may be inappropriate—the person may laugh in a sad situation, or cry over a joke—or may be unable to show any emotion at all.

Thought disorder is the most profound change, since it prevents clear thinking and rational response. Thoughts may be slow to form, or come extra fast, or not at all. The person may jump from topic to topic, seem confused, or have difficulty making simple decisions. Thinking may be colored by delusions—false beliefs that have no logical basis. Some people also feel they are being persecuted—convinced they are being spied on or plotted against. They may have grandiose delusions or think they are all-powerful, capable of anything, and invulnerable to danger. They may also have a strong religious drive, or believe they have a personal mission to right the wrongs of the world.

Perceptual changes turn the world of the ill person topsy-turvy. Sensory messages to the brain from the eyes, ears, nose, skin, and taste buds become confused—and the person may actually hear, see, smell, or feel sensations that are not real. These are called hallucinations.

People with schizophrenia will often hear voices. Sometimes the voices are threatening or condemning; they may also give direct orders such as, "kill yourself." There is always a danger that such commands will be obeyed.

People who are ill may also have visual hallucinations—a door in a wall where no door exists; a lion, a tiger, or a long-dead relative may suddenly appear. Colors, shapes, and faces may change before the person's eyes.

There may also be hypersensitivity to sounds, tastes, and smells. A ringing telephone might seem as loud as a fire alarm bell, or a loved one's voice as threatening as a barking dog. Sense of touch may also be distorted. Someone may literally "feel" their skin is crawling—or conversely, they may feel nothing, not even pain from a real injury.

Sense of self. When one or all five senses are affected, the person may feel out of time, out of space—free floating and bodiless—and non-existent as a person.

Someone who is experiencing such profound and frightening changes will often try to keep them a secret. There is often a strong need to deny what is happening, and to avoid other people and situations where the fact that one is "different" might be discovered. Intense misperceptions of reality trigger feelings of dread, panic, fear, and anxiety—natural reactions to such terrifying experiences.

Psychological distress is intense, but most of it remains hidden—so there may be strong denial, born out of fear. The pain of schizophrenia is further accentuated by the person's awareness of the worry and suffering they may be causing their family and friends.

People with schizophrenia need understanding, patience, and reassurance that they will not be abandoned.

Early Warning Signs

The following list of warning signs was developed by people whose family members have schizophrenia. Many behaviors described are within the range of normal responses to situations. Yet families sense—even when symptoms are mild—that behavior is "unusual;" that the person is "not the same." The number and severity of these symptoms differ from person to person—although almost everyone mentions "noticeable social withdrawal."

- deterioration of personal hygiene
- depression
- bizarre behavior

- irrational statements
- sleeping excessively or inability to sleep
- social withdrawal, isolation, and reclusiveness
- shift in basic personality
- unexpected hostility
- deterioration of social relationships
- hyperactivity or inactivity—or alternating between the two
- inability to concentrate or to cope with minor problems
- extreme preoccupation with religion or with the occult
- excessive writing without meaning
- indifference
- dropping out of activities—or out of life in general
- decline in academic or athletic interests
- forgetting things
- losing possessions
- extreme reactions to criticism
- inability to express joy
- inability to cry, or excessive crying
- inappropriate laughter
- unusual sensitivity to stimuli (noise, light, colors, textures)
- attempts to escape through frequent moves or hitchhiking trips
- drug or alcohol abuse
- fainting
- strange posturing
- refusal to touch persons or objects; wearing gloves, etc.
- shaving head or body hair
- cutting oneself; threats of self-mutilation
- staring without blinking—or blinking incessantly
- flat, reptile-like gaze
- rigid stubbornness
- peculiar use of words or odd language structures
- sensitivity and irritability when touched by others

What Is It Like to Have Schizophrenia?

Despite her illness, Janice Jordan has successfully accomplished work as a technical editor for over 20 years and has completed a book of poetry based on her experiences.

> The schizophrenic experience can be a terrifying journey through a world of madness no one can understand, particularly the person traveling through it. It is a journey through a world that is deranged, empty, and devoid of anchors to reality. You feel very much alone. You find it easier to withdraw than cope with a reality that is incongruent with your fantasy world. You feel tormented by distorted perceptions. You cannot distinguish what is real from what is unreal. Schizophrenia affects all aspects of your life. Your thoughts race and you feel fragmented and so very alone with your "craziness..."

> I have suffered from schizophrenia for over 25 years. In fact, I can't think of a time when I wasn't plagued with hallucinations, delusions, and paranoia. At times, I feel like the operator in my brain just doesn't get the message to the right people. It can be very confusing to have to deal with different people in my head. When I become fragmented in my thinking, I start to have my worst problems. I have been hospitalized because of this illness many times, sometimes for as long as 2 to 4 months.

> I do know that I could not have made it as far as I have today without the love and support of my family, my therapists, and my friends. It was their faith in my ability to overcome this potentially devastating illness that carried me through this journey.

> ...So many wonderful medications are now available to help alleviate the symptoms of mental illness. It is up to us, people with schizophrenia, to be patient and to be trusting. We must believe that tomorrow is another day, perhaps one day closer to fully understanding schizophrenia, to knowing its cause, and to finding a cure...

—by Janice C. Jordan.
From "Adrift in an Anchorless Reality."

How Families Can Help

Get Proper Medical Help

- Take the initiative. If symptoms of schizophrenia are occurring, ask your doctor for an assessment or referral. Family members are usually the first to notice symptoms and suggest medical help. Remember, if the ill person accepts hallucinations and delusions as reality, they may resist treatment.

- Be persistent. Find a doctor who is familiar with schizophrenia. The assessment and treatment of schizophrenia should be done by people who are well-qualified. Choose a physician who has an interest in the illness, who is competent and has empathy with patients and their families. Remember—if you lack confidence in a physician or psychiatrist, you always have the right to seek a second opinion.

- Assist the doctor/psychiatrist. Patients with schizophrenia may not be able to volunteer much information during an assessment. Talk to the doctor yourself, or write a letter describing your concerns. Be specific. Be persistent. The information you supply can help the physician towards more accurate assessment and treatment.

Making the Most of Treatment

There may be exchanges between doctor and patient that the patient feels are of a highly personal nature and wants to keep confidential. However, family members need information related to care and treatment. You should be able to discuss the following with the doctor:

- signs and symptoms of the illness
- expected course of the illness
- treatment strategies
- signs of possible relapse
- other related information

Provide plenty of support and loving care. Help the person accept their illness. Try to show by your attitude and behavior that there is hope, that the disease can be managed, and that life can be satisfying and productive.

Help the person with schizophrenia maintain a record of information on:

- symptoms that have appeared

- all medications, including dosages

- effects of various types of treatment

Learn to Recognize Signs of Relapse

Family and friends should be familiar with signs of "relapse"— where the person may suffer a period of deterioration due to a flare up of symptoms. It helps to know that relapse signs often recur for an individual. These vary from person to person, but the most common signs are:

- increased withdrawal from activities

- deterioration of basic personal care

You should also know that:

- stress and tension make symptoms worse

- symptoms often diminish as the person gets older

Managing from Day to Day

- Ensure that medical treatment continues after hospitalization. This means taking medication and going for follow-up treatment.

- Provide a structured and predictable environment. The recovering patient will have problems with sensory overload. To reduce stress, keep routines simple, and allow the person time alone each day. Try to plan non-stressful, low-key regular daily activities, and keep "big events" to a minimum.

- Be consistent. Caregivers should agree on a plan of action and follow it. If you are predictable in the way you handle recurring concerns, you can help reduce confusion and stress for the person who is ill.

- Maintain peace and calm at home. Thought disorder is a great problem for most people with schizophrenia. It generally helps to keep voice levels down. When the person is participating in discussions, try to speak one at a time, and at a reasonably moderated pace. Shorter sentences can also help. Above all, avoid arguing about delusions (false beliefs).

- Be positive and supportive. Being positive instead of critical will help the person more in the long run. People with schizophrenia need frequent encouragement, since self-esteem is often very fragile. Encourage all positive efforts. Be sure to express appreciation for a job even half-done, because the illness undermines a person's confidence, initiative, patience, and memory.

- Help the ill person set realistic goals. People with schizophrenia need lots of encouragement to regain some of their former skills and interests. They may also want to try new things, but should work up to them gradually. If goals are unreasonable, or someone is nagging, the resulting stress can worsen symptoms.

- Gradually increase independence. As participation in a variety oasks and activities increases, so should independence. Set limits on how much abnormal behavior is acceptable, and consistently apply thensequences. Some relearning is usually necessary for skills such as handling money, cooking, and housekeeping. If outside employment is too difficult, try to help the person plan to use their time constructively.

Getting Treatment

How Can We Find Appropriate Medical Help?

Specifically, you need to find a doctor who:

- believes schizophrenia is a brain disease
- takes a detailed history
- screens for problems that may be related to other possible illnesses
- is knowledgeable about antipsychotic medications
- follows up thoroughly
- adjusts the course of treatment when necessary
- reviews medications regularly

- is interested in the patient's entire welfare, and makes appropriate referrals for aftercare, housing, social support, and financial aid

- explains clearly what is going on

- involves the family in the treatment process

How Is Schizophrenia Treated?

Although schizophrenia is not yet a "curable" disease, it is treatable. The proper treatment of schizophrenia includes the following:

- *Medication.* Most patients with schizophrenia have to take medication regularly to keep their illness under control.

- *Education.* Patients and their families must learn all they can about schizophrenia. They should also be directly included in planning the treatment program.

- *Family counseling.* Since the patient and the family are often under enormous emotional strain, it may be advantageous to obtain counseling from professionals who understand the illness.

- *Hospitalization and regular follow-up.* If someone becomes acutely ill with schizophrenia, they will probably require hospitalization.

- *Residential and rehabilitation programs.* Social skills training, along with residential, recreational, and vocational opportunities tailored to people with mental illness are very important. Used as part of the treatment plan, they can result in improved outcomes for even the most severely disabled people.

- *Self-help groups.* Families can be very effective in supporting each other and in advocating for much-needed research, public education, and community and hospital-based programs. People with mental illness can also provide consultation and advocacy in these areas, as well as offering peer support to other individuals with schizophrenia.

- *Nutrition, rest and exercise.* Recovery from schizophrenia, as with any illness, requires patience. It is aided by a well-balanced diet, adequate sleep, and regular exercise. However, the illness and the side effects of medication can interfere with proper eating, sleeping, and exercise habits. There may be appetite loss, lack of motivation, and withdrawal from normal daily activity. Someone who is ill may simply forget to eat, or become very suspicious about food, so supervision of daily routines may be required. If you are a family member or friend who is trying to help—be patient. Above all, don't take seeming carelessness or disinterest personally.

- *Electroconvulsive therapy (ECT)*. ECT is not normally used for patients with schizophrenia unless they are also suffering from extreme depression, are suicidal for long periods, and do not respond to medication or other treatments.

Medication Update

Trying to understand a bewildering array of medication terminology can be frustrating. It's always a good idea to learn at least some of the technical "lingo" that mental health professionals use. Generally, medications for treating psychotic symptoms of schizophrenia are referred to as antipsychotics, or sometimes neuroleptics.

"Standard" Antipsychotics

Until recently, doctors referred to antipsychotic medications neuroleptics because of their tendency to cause neurological side effects. Medications that have been around for a number of years are now called "standard" antipsychotics. Examples of standard antipsychotics include Thorazine, Mellaril, Modecate, Prolixin, Navane, Stelazine, and Haldol.

"Atypical" Antipsychotics

Four common atypical antipsychotics are risperidone (Risperdal), clozapine (Clozaril), olanzapine (Zyprexa) and the newest medication, quetiapine (Seroquel).

Recovery

Some of the most recent and hopeful news in schizophrenia research is emerging from studies in the field of psychosocial "rehab." New studies challenge several long-held myths in psychiatry about the inability of people with schizophrenia to recover from their illness. It now appears that such myths, by maintaining an overall pessimism about outcomes, may significantly reduce patients' opportunities for improvement and/or recovery.

In fact, the long-term perspective on schizophrenia should give everyone a renewed sense of hope and optimism. According to Dr. G. Gross, author of a 22-year study of 508 patients with schizophrenia:

> "...schizophrenia does not seem to be a disease of slow, progressive deterioration. Even in the second and third decades of illness, there is still potential for full or partial recovery."

After three decades of empirical study, it is now clear that good rehabilitation programs are an important part of treatment strategy. In addition, where family input is solicited and families are included as part of the treatment "team," patient outcomes are greatly improved.

Families need and want education, information, coping and communication skills, emotional support, and to be treated as collaborators. For this reason, knowledgeable clinicians will make a special effort to involve family members. Once a relationship is established, clinician, patient and family can work together to identify needs and appropriate interventions. Everyone should be able to have realistic yet optimistic expectations about improvement and possible recovery.

Studies show that families who are supportive, non-judgmental, and, most especially, non-critical, can do much to help patients recover. On the other hand, patients who are around chaotic or volatile family members usually have a more difficult time, and have to return to hospital more often.

Since we now know this, it is important for family members to assess their own coping skills and try to anticipate and adapt to the ups and downs of the illness. Calm assurance, assistance, and support from family members can make a difference to the person with schizophrenia.

FAQs—Frequently Asked Questions

What Are My Chances of Developing Schizophrenia?

There is no way of knowing exactly who will get schizophrenia. However, about 1 in 100 people worldwide will develop the illness. Since schizophrenia tends to run in families, your chances may be higher if someone in your family has the disease.

Can Children Develop Schizophrenia?

Yes. In rare instances, children as young as five have been diagnosed with the illness. They are often described as being different from other children from an early age. Most people with schizophrenia, however, do not show recognizable symptoms until adolescence or young adulthood.

Myths and Misconceptions

Society's knowledge of major mental illness lags way behind the facts. People with schizophrenia are victims of this general ignorance. In truth, they are victims twice over. First, they have an incurable, chronic brain disease that they must learn to live with as best they can. Next, because of their illness, they are discriminated against.

What is the biggest problem for people with mental illness? Most say it's that others do not accept them. Once they have learned to manage their symptoms, they still have to face overwhelming difficulties with friends, housing, and work. They feel the sting of discrimination in almost everything they do. Old friends and even some family members are uncomfortable in their presence. So they become isolated, cut off from society.

No wonder so many people with schizophrenia feel they don't belong; that they are "different;" that they are not respected or valued. Widespread, hurtful ignorance leads to the terrible social isolation and loneliness that can become the most disabling feature of the illness.

Chapter 11

Managing Attention Deficit/ Hyperactivity Disorder (ADHD) in Teenagers

Attention Deficit Hyperactivity Disorder (ADHD), once called hyper kinesis or minimal brain dysfunction, is one of the most common mental disorders among children. It affects 3 to 5 percent of all children, perhaps as many as 2 million American children. Two to three times more boys than girls are affected. On the average, at least one child in every classroom in the United States needs help for the disorder. ADHD often continues into adolescence and adulthood, and can cause a lifetime of frustrated dreams and emotional pain.

But there is help...and hope. In the last decade, scientists have learned much about the course of the disorder and are now able to identify and treat children, adolescents, and adults who have it. A variety of medications, behavior-changing therapies, and educational options are already available to help people with ADHD focus their attention, build self-esteem, and function in new ways.

Understanding the Problem

What Are the Symptoms of ADHD?

At present, ADHD is a diagnosis applied to children and adults who consistently display certain characteristic behaviors over a period of

Excerpted from "Attention Deficit Hyperactivity Disorder," National Institute of Mental Health, National Institutes of Health (NIH), U.S. Department of Health and Human Services,NIH Publication No. 96-3572, http://www.nimh. nih.gov/publicat/adhd.cfm, printed 1994, reprinted 1996, last updated March 10, 2000.

87

time. The most common behaviors fall into three categories: inattention, hyperactivity, and impulsivity.

Inattention. People who are inattentive have a hard time keeping their mind on any one thing and may get bored with a task after only a few minutes. They may give effortless, automatic attention to activities and things they enjoy. But focusing deliberate, conscious attention to organizing and completing a task or learning something new is difficult.

Hyperactivity. People who are hyperactive always seem to be in motion. They can't sit still. They may dash around or talk incessantly. Sitting still through a lesson can be an impossible task. Hyperactive children squirm in their seat or roam around the room. They might wiggle their feet, touch everything, or noisily tap their pencil. Hyperactive teens and adults may feel intensely restless. They may be fidgety or they may try to do several things at once, bouncing around from one activity to the next.

Impulsivity. People who are overly impulsive seem unable to curb their immediate reactions or think before they act. As a result they may blurt out inappropriate comments. They may run into the street without looking. Their impulsivity may make it hard for them to wait for things they want or to take their turn in games. They may grab a toy from another child or hit when they're upset.

To assess whether a person has ADHD, specialists consider several critical questions: Are these behaviors excessive, long-term, and pervasive? That is, do they occur more often than in other people the same age? Are they a continuous problem, not just a response to a temporary situation? Do the behaviors occur in several settings or only in one specific place like the playground or the office? The person's pattern of behavior is compared against a set of criteria and characteristics of the disorder. These criteria appear in a diagnostic reference book called the *DSM* (short for the *Diagnostic and Statistical Manual of Mental Disorders*).

According to the diagnostic manual, there are three patterns of behavior that indicate ADHD. People with ADHD may show several signs of being consistently inattentive. They may have a pattern of being hyperactive and impulsive. Or they may show all three types of behavior.

According to the *DSM*, signs of inattention include:

- becoming easily distracted by irrelevant sights and sounds
- failing to pay attention to details and making careless mistakes
- rarely following instructions carefully and completely
- losing or forgetting things like toys, or pencils, books, and tools needed for a task

Some signs of hyperactivity and impulsivity are:

- feeling restless, often fidgeting with hands or feet, or squirming
- running, climbing, or leaving a seat, in situations where sitting or quiet behavior is expected
- blurting out answers before hearing the whole question
- having difficulty waiting in line or for a turn

Because everyone shows some of these behaviors at times, the DSM contains very specific guidelines for determining when they indicate ADHD. The behaviors must appear early in life, before age 7, and continue for at least 6 months. In children, they must be more frequent or severe than in others the same age. Above all, the behaviors must create a real handicap in at least two areas of a person's life, such as school, home, work, or social settings. So someone whose work or friendships are not impaired by these behaviors would not be diagnosed with ADHD. Nor would a child who seems overly active at school but functions well elsewhere.

ADHD is a serious diagnosis that may require long-term treatment with counseling and medication. So it's important that a doctor first look for and treat any other causes for these behaviors.

What Causes ADHD?

Understandably, one of the first questions parents ask when they learn their child has an attention disorder is "Why? What went wrong?"

Health professionals stress that since no one knows what causes ADHD, it doesn't help parents to look backward to search for possible reasons. There are too many possibilities to pin down the cause with certainty. It is far more important for the family to move forward in finding ways to get the right help.

Scientists, however, do need to study causes in an effort to identify better ways to treat, and perhaps some day, prevent ADHD. They are finding more and more evidence that ADHD does not stem from home environment, but from biological causes. When you think about it, there is no clear relationship between home life and ADHD. Not all children from unstable or dysfunctional homes have ADHD. And not all children with ADHD come from dysfunctional families. Knowing this can remove a huge burden of guilt from parents who might blame themselves for their child's behavior.

ADHD is not usually caused by:

- too much TV
- food allergies
- excess sugar
- poor home life
- poor schools

Getting Help

How Is ADHD Identified and Diagnosed?

Many parents see signs of an attention deficit in toddlers long before the child enters school. But in many cases the teacher is the first to recognize that a child is hyperactive or inattentive and may consult with the school psychologist. Because teachers work with many children, they come to know how "average" children behave in learning situations that require attention and self control. However, teachers sometimes fail to notice the needs of children who are quiet and cooperative.

Types of Professionals Who Make the Diagnosis

School-age and preschool children are often evaluated by a school psychologist or a team made up of the school psychologist and other specialists. But if the school doesn't believe the student has a problem, or if the family wants another opinion, a family may need to see a specialist in private practice. In such cases, who can the family turn to? What kinds of specialists do they need?

What Are the Educational Options?

Children with ADHD have a variety of needs. Some children are too hyperactive or inattentive to function in a regular classroom, even with medication and a behavior management plan. Such children may be placed in a special education class for all or part of the day. In some schools, the special education teacher teams with the classroom teacher to meet each child's unique needs. However, most children are able to stay in the regular classroom. Whenever possible, educators prefer to not to segregate children, but to let them learn along with their peers.

Children with ADHD often need some special accommodations to help them learn. For example, the teacher may seat the child in an area with few distractions, provide an area where the child can move around and release excess energy, or establish a clearly posted system of rules and reward appropriate behavior. Sometimes just keeping a card or a picture on the desk can serve as a visual reminder to use the right school behavior, like raising a hand instead of shouting out, or staying in a seat instead of wandering around the room. Giving a child extra time on tests can make the difference between passing and failing, and gives her a fairer chance to show what she's learned. Reviewing instructions or writing assignments on the board, and even listing the books and materials they will need for the task, may make it possible for disorganized, inattentive children to complete the work.

Table 11.1. Types of professionals.

Speciality	Can diagnose ADHD	Can prescribe medications, if needed	Provides counseling or training
Psychiatrists	yes	yes	yes
Psychologists	yes	no	yes
Pediatricians or family physicians	yes	yes	no
Neurologists	yes	yes	no

The family can start by talking with the child's pediatrician or their family doctor. Some pediatricians may do the assessment themselves, but more often they refer the family to an appropriate specialist they know and trust. In addition, state and local agencies that serve families and children, as well as some of the volunteer organizations listed in the back of this *Sourcebook*, can help identify an appropriate specialist.

Many of the strategies of special education are simply good teaching methods. Telling students in advance what they will learn, providing visual aids, and giving written as well as oral instructions are all ways to help students focus and remember the key parts of the lesson.

Students with ADHD often need to learn techniques for monitoring and controlling their own attention and behavior. The process of finding alternatives to interrupting the teacher makes them more self-sufficient and cooperative.

Because schools demand that children sit still, wait for a turn, pay attention, and stick with a task, it's no surprise that many children with ADHD have problems in class. Their minds are fully capable of learning, but their hyperactivity and inattention make learning difficult. As a result, many students with ADHD repeat a grade or drop out of school early. Fortunately, with the right combination of appropriate educational practices, medication, and counseling, these outcomes can be avoided.

Some Coping Strategies for Teens and Adults with ADHD

- When necessary, ask the teacher or boss to repeat instructions rather than guess.

- Break large assignments or job tasks into small, simple tasks. Set a deadline for each task and reward yourself as you complete each one.

- Each day, make a list of what you need to do. Plan the best order for doing each task. Then make a schedule for doing them. Use a calendar or daily planner to keep yourself on track.

- Work in a quiet area. Do one thing at a time. Give yourself short breaks.

- Write things you need to remember in a notebook with dividers. Write different kinds of information like assignments, appointments, and phone numbers in different sections. Keep the book with you all of the time.

- Post notes to yourself to help remind yourself of things you need to do. Tape notes on the bathroom mirror, on the refrigerator, in your school locker, or dashboard of your car— wherever you're likely to need the remainder.

- Store similar things together. For example, keep all your Nintendo disks in one place, and tape cassettes in another. Keep canceled checks in one place, and bills in another.

- Create a routine. Get yourself ready for school or work at the same time, in the same way, every day.

- Exercise, eat a balanced diet, and get enough sleep.

What Treatments Are Available?

For decades, medications have been used to treat the symptoms of ADHD. Three medications in the class of drugs known as stimulants seem to be the most effective in both children and adults. These are methylphenidate (Ritalin), dextroamphetamine (Dexedrine or Dextrostat), and pemoline (Cylert). For many people, these medicines dramatically reduce their hyperactivity and improve their ability to focus, work, and learn.

Unfortunately, when people see such immediate improvement, they often think medication is all that's needed. But these medicines don't cure the disorder, they only temporarily control the symptoms. Although the drugs help people pay better attention and complete their work, they can't increase knowledge or improve academic skills. The drugs alone can't help people feel better about themselves or cope with problems. These require other kinds of treatment and support.

For lasting improvement, numerous clinicians recommend that medications should be used along with treatments that aid in these other areas. There are no quick cures. Many experts believe that the most significant, long-lasting gains appear when medication is combined with behavioral therapy, emotional counseling, and practical support. Some studies suggest that the combination of medicine and therapy may be more effective than drugs alone. NIMH is conducting a large study to check this.

Use of Stimulant Drugs

Stimulant drugs, such as Ritalin, Cylert, and Dexedrine, when used with medical supervision, are usually considered quite safe. Although they can be addictive to teenagers and adults if misused, these medications are not addictive in children.

Other types of medication may be used if stimulants don't work or if the ADHD occurs with another disorder. Antidepressants and other medications may be used to help control accompanying depression or anxiety. In some cases, antihistamines may be tried. Clonidine, a drug normally used to treat hypertension, may be helpful in people with both ADHD and Tourette's syndrome. Although stimulants tend to be more effective, clonidine may be tried when stimulants don't work or can't be used. Clonidine can be administered either by pill or by skin patch and has different side effects than stimulants. The doctor works closely with each patient to find the most appropriate medication.

The Medication Debate

As useful as these drugs are, Ritalin and the other stimulants have sparked a great deal of controversy. Most doctors feel the potential side effects should be carefully weighed against the benefits before prescribing the drugs. While on these medications, some children may lose weight, have less appetite, and temporarily grow more slowly. Others may have problems falling asleep. Some doctors believe that stimulants may also make the symptoms of Tourette's syndrome worse, although recent research suggests this may not be true. Other doctors say if they carefully watch the child's height, weight, and overall development, the benefits of medication far outweigh the potential side effects. Side effects that do occur can often be handled by reducing the dosage.

Treatments to Help People with ADHD and Their Families Learn to Cope

Medication can help to control some of the behavior problems that may have lead to family turmoil. But more often, there are other aspects of the problem that medication can't touch. Even though ADHD primarily affects a person's behavior, having the disorder has broad emotional repercussions. For some children, being scolded is the only attention they ever get. They have few experiences that build their sense of worth and competence. If they're hyperactive, they're often told they're bad and punished for being disruptive. If they are too disorganized and unfocused to complete tasks, others may call them lazy. If they impulsively grab toys, butt in, or shove classmates, they may lose friends. And if they have a related conduct disorder, they may get in trouble at school or with the law. Facing the daily frustrations that can come with having ADHD can make people fear that they are strange, abnormal, or stupid.

Often, the cycle of frustration, blame, and anger has gone on so long that it will take some time to undo. Both parents and their children may need special help to develop techniques for managing the patterns of behavior. In such cases, mental health professionals can counsel the child and the family, helping them to develop new skills, attitudes, and ways of relating to each other. In individual counseling, the therapist helps children or adults with ADHD learn to feel better about themselves. They learn to recognize that having a disability does not reflect who they are as a person. The therapist can also help people with ADHD identify and build on their strengths, cope with daily problems, and control their attention and aggression. In group counseling, people learn that they are not alone in their frustration and that others want to help. Sometimes only the individual with ADHD needs counseling support. But in many cases, because the problem affects the family as well as the person with ADHD, the entire family may need help. The therapist assists the family in finding better ways to handle the disruptive behaviors and promote change. If the child is young, most of the therapist's work is with the parents, teaching them techniques for coping with and improving their child's behavior.

Controversial Treatments

Understandably, parents who are eager to help their children want to explore every possible option. Many newly touted treatments sound reasonable. Many even come with glowing reports. A few are pure quackery. Some are even developed by reputable doctors or specialists—but when tested scientifically, cannot be proven to help.

Here are a few types of treatment that have not been scientifically shown to be effective in treating the majority of children or adults with ADHD:

- biofeedback
- restricted diets
- allergy treatments
- medicines to correct problems in the inner ear
- megavitamins
- chiropractic adjustment and bone re-alignment
- treatment for yeast infection
- eye training
- special colored glasses

A few success stories can't substitute for scientific evidence. Until sound, scientific testing shows a treatment to be effective, families risk spending time, money, and hope on fads and false promises.

Sustaining Hope

Can ADHD Be Outgrown or Cured?

Even though most people don't outgrow ADHD, people do learn to adapt and live fulfilling lives. With effective combinations of medicine, new skills, and emotional support, people with ADHD can develop ways to control their attention and minimize their disruptive behaviors. They may find that by structuring tasks and controlling their environment, they can achieve personal goals. They may learn to channel their excess energy into sports and other high energy activities. They can identify career options that build on their strengths and abilities.

As they grow up, with appropriate help from parents and clinicians, children with ADHD become better able to suppress their hyperactivity and to channel it into more socially acceptable behaviors, like physical exercise or fidgeting. And although we know that half of all children with ADHD will still show signs of the problem into adulthood, we also know that the medications and therapy that help children also work for adults.

All people with ADHD have natural talents and abilities that they can draw on to create fine lives and careers for themselves. In fact, many people with ADHD even feel that their patterns of behavior give them unique, often unrecognized, advantages. People with ADHD tend to be outgoing and ready for action. Because of their drive for excitement and stimulation, many become successful in business, sports, construction, and public speaking. Because of their ability to think about many things at once, many have won acclaim as artists and inventors. Many choose work that gives them freedom to move around and release excess energy. But some find ways to be effective in quieter, more sedentary careers. Sally, a computer programmer, found that she thinks best when she wears headphones to reduce distracting noises. Some people strive to increase their organizational skills. Others who own their own business find it useful to hire support staff to provide day-to-day management.

What Are Sources of Information and Support?

Several publications, organizations, and support groups exist to help individuals, teachers, and families to understand and cope with attention disorders. Other resources are outpatient clinics of children s hospitals, university medical centers, and community mental health centers. Please see the Additional Help and Information section of this *Sourcebook* for contact information and further resources.

Chapter 12

Oppositional Defiant Disorder (ODD) and Conduct Disorder (CD) in Children and Adolescents

Oppositional Defiant Disorder (ODD)

What Is It?

ODD is a psychiatric disorder that is characterized by two different sets of problems. These are aggressiveness and a tendency to purposefully bother and irritate others. It is often the reason that people seek treatment. When ODD is present with ADHD (Attention Deficit Hyperactivity Disorder), depression, Tourette's, anxiety disorders, or other neuropsychiatric disorders, it makes life with that child far more difficult. For example, ADHD plus ODD is much worse than ADHD alone, often enough to make people seek treatment. The criteria for ODD are:

A pattern of negativistic, hostile, and defiant behavior lasting at least six months during which four or more of the following are present:

- often loses temper

- often argues with adults

- often actively defies or refuses to comply with adults' requests or rules

Jim Chandler, MD, FRCPC, "Oppositional Defiant Disorder (ODD) and Conduct Disorder (CD) in Children and Adolescents: Diagnosis and Treatment," http://www.klis.com/chandler/pamphlet/oddcd/oddcdpamphlet.htm, last updated February 14, 2001, downloaded July 10, 2001. Reprinted with permission.

97

- often deliberately annoys people
- often blames others for his or her mistakes or misbehavior
- is often touchy or easily annoyed by others
- is often angry and resentful
- is often spiteful and vindictive

The disturbance in behavior causes clinically significant impairment in social, academic, or occupational functioning.

How Often Is "Often"?

All of the criteria above include the word "often." But what exactly does that mean? Recent studies have shown that these behaviors occur to a varying degree in all children. These researchers have found that the "often" is best solved by the following criteria.

Has occurred at all during the last three months

- is spiteful and vindictive
- blames others for his or her mistakes or misbehavior

Occurs at least twice a week

- is touchy or easily annoyed by others
- loses temper
- argues with adults
- actively defies or refuses to comply with adults' requests or rules

Occurs at least four times per week

- is angry and resentful
- deliberately annoys people

What Causes It?

No one knows for certain. The usual pattern is for problems to begin between ages 1–3. If you think about it, a lot of these behaviors are normal at age 2, but in this disorder they never go away. It does run in families. If a parent is alcoholic and has been in trouble with the law, their children are almost three times as likely to have ODD. That is, 18% of children will have ODD if the parents are alcoholic and the father has been in trouble with the law.

How Can You Tell If a Child Has It?

ODD is diagnosed in the same way as many other psychiatric disorders in children. You need to examine the child, talk with the child, talk to the parents, and review the medical history. Sometimes other medical tests are necessary to make sure it is not something else. You always need to check children out for other psychiatric disorders, as it is common the children with ODD will have other problems, too.

Who Gets It?

A lot of children! This is the most common psychiatric problem in children. Over 5% of children have this. In younger children it is more common in boys than girls, but as they grow older, the rate is the same in males and females.

ODD Rarely Travels Alone

It is exceptionally rare for a physician to see a child with only ODD. Usually the child has some other neuropsychiatric disorder along with ODD. The tendency for disorders in medicine to occur together is called comorbidity. Understanding comorbidity in pediatric psychiatry is one of the most important areas of research at this moment.

What Happens to Children Who Have This When They Grow Up?

There are three main paths that a child will take. First, there will be some lucky children who outgrow this. The exact number is not clear, but probably not the majority. The aggressiveness is very stable. That is, aggressive 2 year olds are likely to be aggressive 20 year olds. Only IQ is more stable over years than aggression.

Second, ODD may turn into conduct disorder (CD). This usually happens fairly early. That is, after a 3–4 years of ODD, if it hasn't turned into CD, it won't ever. What predicts a child with ODD getting CD? A history of a biologic parent who was a career criminal, and very severe ODD.

Third, the child may continue to have ODD. Recent work suggests that this is probably the most common path. If you look at a group of preschool boys who have ODD and check them out two years later, about 75% still have something wrong. Sometimes ODD at that age changes into something else, but that is rare. More often ADHD and ODD just continue on. The more common thing that happens is that children with ODD develop signs of mood disorders or anxiety as they get older. By the time these children are in the end of elementary school, about 25% will have mood or anxiety problems which are disabling. That means that it is very important to watch for signs of mood disorder and anxiety as children with ODD grow older.

Will Children with ODD End up as Criminals?

Probably not unless they develop conduct disorder. Even then many will grow out of it. Life may not be easy. People with ODD who are grown up often do best if they can work for themselves and stay away from alcohol. However their tendency to irritate others often leads to a lonely life.

My Father in Law Says the Whole Problem Is My Husband and I. My Daughter Convinced Him That She Is a Victim of Uncaring Parents. How Often Does This Happen?

Too often! Children and adolescents with ODD produce strong feelings in people. They are trying to get a reaction out of people, and they are often successful. Common ones are: inciting spouses to fight with each other and not focus on the child, making outsiders believe that all the fault lies with the parents, making certain susceptible people believe that they can "save" the child by doing everything the child wants, setting parents against grandparents, setting teachers against parents, and inciting the parents to abuse the child. I frequently see children with ODD in which teachers and parents and sometimes others are all fighting amongst each other rather than with the child who is causing all the turmoil in the first place.

Conduct Disorder (CD)

In some ways, conduct disorder (CD) is just a worse version of ODD. However recent research suggests that there are some differences. Children with ODD seem to have worse social skills than those with CD. Children with ODD seem to do better in school. Conduct disorder is the most serious childhood psychiatric disorder. Approximately 6–10% of boys and 2–9% of girls have this disorder. Here is the definition:

A repetitive and persistent pattern of behavior in which the basic rights of others or major society rules are violated. At least three of the following criteria must be present in the last 12 months, and at least one criterion must have been present in the last 6 months. The problem causes significant impairment in social, academic, and occupational functioning.

Aggression to People and Animals

- often bullies, threatens, or intimidates others
- often initiates physical fights
- has used a weapon that can cause serious physical harm to others (a bat, brick, broken bottle, knife, gun)
- physically cruel to animals
- physically cruel to people
- has stolen while confronting a victim (mugging, purse snatching, extortion, armed robbery)

Destruction of Property

- has deliberately engaged in fire setting with the intention of causing serious damage
- has deliberately destroyed other's property other than by fire setting

Deceitfulness or Theft

- has broken into someone else's house, building or car
- often lies to obtain goods or favors or to avoid work
- has stolen items of nontrivial value without confronting a victim (shoplifting, forgery)

Serious Violations of Rules

- often stays out at night despite parental prohibitions, beginning before 13 years of age
- has run away from home overnight at least twice without returning home for a lengthy period
- often skips school before age 13

Diagnosis

Conduct disorder is diagnosed like all things in pediatric psychiatry. The child and the caregivers will be interviewed together and separately to go over the history and check out all other possible comorbid conditions. Usually there are school reports, too. The child is examined to look for signs of many disorders. This usually includes some school work, some parts of the physical exam, and getting the child's perspective on things. Occasionally, there are lab tests and x-rays to do.

Prognosis and Course of Conduct Disorder

Perhaps about 30% of conduct disorder children continue with similar problems in adulthood. It is more common for males with CD to continue on into adulthood with these types of problems than females. Females with CD more often end up having mood and anxiety disorders as adults. Substance abuse is very high. About 50–70% of ten year olds with conduct disorder will be abusing substances four years later. Cigarette smoking is also very high. A recent study of girls with conduct disorder showed that they have much worse physical health. Girls with conduct disorder were almost 6 times more likely to abuse drugs or alcohol, eight times more likely to smoke cigarettes daily, where almost twice as likely to have sexually transmitted diseases, had twice the number of sexual partners, and were three times as likely to become pregnant when compared to girls without conduct disorder.

Looked at from the other direction, by the time they are adults, 70% of children no longer show signs of conduct disorder. Are they well? Some are, but what often happens is that the comorbid problems remain or get worse. A girl with CD and depression may end up as an adult with depression, but no conduct disorder. The same pattern can be true of CD plus bipolar disorder and other disorders.

Families and CD

It is not unusual to see signs of stress in the parents and other siblings when a child has CD. One of the hardest questions is figuring out whether or not difficulties in the family are causing CD or whether the stress of CD is causing family problems. Often it is impossible to determine this, or there are reasons to suggest both the CD is causing the family problems and the family is causing the CD to be worse. CD is a very difficult problem to live with. It would be very unusual to see a family where it was not causing grave distress. This obviously needs to be addressed in any treatment plan.

What Can Be Done?

Treat Comorbid Disorders

CD plus ADHD. Recent studies have shown that treating CD plus ADHD with stimulants helps the conduct disorder and the ADHD symptoms. This effect appears independent of how bad the ADHD is. Since 60–70% of children who go to a clinic for help with CD also have ADHD, this is extremely important. Serious consideration should be given to medically treating all children with CD plus ADHD. Although this type of medical intervention does not make the children "normal," it can make a big difference. It often means that the non-medical interventions will work much better.

CD plus depression. Recent work also suggests that treating depression in the context of CD is effective. While Prozac was used in this study, most likely other drugs in that same family would be effective.

CD plus substance abuse, movement disorders, bipolar disorder, psychosis, pervasive developmental disorders. Although there is not as much data on these areas, it is a good idea to always vigorously treat any disorder which is comorbid with CD. The importance of treating comorbid conditions cannot be overstated.

Non-Medical Strategies for ODD and CD

Containment. The essence of this group of interventions is to make it impossible for ODD or CD to "work." That is, it is a way of making sure all these attempts to irritate and annoy others and to cause fighting between others are not successful. There are three elements to this.

1. Come together. The most common thing I see in children with ODD (except for aggressiveness) is that a lot of the suffering that the child inflicts on others is blamed on others. Children and adolescents with ODD convince mothers that fathers have mistreated them. They convince parents that the teachers are treating their child unfairly. They convince teachers that the parents are bad, etc. You have to come together and

never believe anything the child with ODD tells you about how others treat them. Instead, all parties need to talk directly with each other without the child as an intermediary. Sometimes parole officers, parents, teachers and others have to all sit down together for the purpose of making it impossible for the child to play one person or group off against another.

2. Have a plan. That is, a plan to deal with all of this oppositional and defiant behavior. If you react on the spur of the moment, your emotions will guide you wrongly in dealing with children and adolescents with ODD. They will work to provoke intense feelings in everyone. Everyone needs to agree on what happens when the child with ODD does certain things. What do we do if she disrupts class, annoys others incessantly, fights, has a major temper tantrum, states she is going to kill herself or run away? You need a behavior modification or management plan. For behavior modification to work, the program must target a few important clear cut behaviors, and it must be consistent. There is no bending of rules in this sort of thing: no difference between the baby-sitter, mom, or dad.

3. Decide what you are going to ignore. Most children and adolescents with ODD are doing too many things you dislike to include every one of them in a behavior management plan. The main caregivers have to decide ahead of time what sort of thing will just be ignored.

4. Try very hard not to show any emotion when reacting to the behaviors of children and adolescents with ODD. The worst thing to do with a kid with ODD is to react strongly and emotionally. This will just make the child push you that same way again. You do not want the child to figure out what really bugs you. You want to try to remain as cool as possible while the child is trying to drive you over the edge. This is not easy. Once you know what you are going to ignore and what will be addressed through behavior modification, it should be far easier not to let your feelings get the best of you.

Make sure that you are as healthy and strong as you can be. Children and adolescents with ODD will find the weakness in the family system and exploit it. Is there tension between father and mother? They will aim to worsen this. Trouble with the in-laws? These children and adolescents will try to exploit this. Are you out of shape and exhausted after work? That's when they will be most trying. Are you worried or depressed about something? They will try to figure it out and torment you. Dealing with a child with ODD is very exhausting and trying. It will take about 1/3 to 1/4 of all your emotional, mental, and physical resources. If you knew that you would be chopping wood for four hours every day, you would make sure you got enough rest, a good diet, and had plenty of time to relax. The same is true for dealing with ODD in the long term. You have to take care of yourself in ways you would not have to if your child did not have ODD.

Limit television. Television is a major force in our lives. Study after study have shown that television is filled with violence, drug and alcohol use, and sexuality. The average child spends at least 2–3 hours a day watching this stuff. Many children spend 4–6 hours a day watching this. It should not be any wonder then that children who watch a lot of TV are more violent, are more likely to do drugs, and are preoccupied with sex. In a child with a problem like ADHD or ODD, this is clearly something that needs to be done.

Eliminate or reduce video and computer games. Anyone who has ever seen a child play Nintendo can see that there is a very potent force at work here. Unfortunately, the vast majority of computer and video games are violent and are becoming more graphic, not less, in their depiction of violence. As mentioned above, large amounts of television viewing can cause increased psychiatric problems for children. Although there is a less research on games, the same trend is there.

Enlist others to help you. Caring for a child with ODD can take a lot out of anyone, especially if you are one of the main people the child is trying to aggravate. Some children with ODD and more children with ODD plus other psychiatric problems can require an incredible amount of patience, energy, and determination. Often this is more than any one or two human beings can provide. There is no natural law that states that all children can be managed by one or two reasonable parents. Many children are born who require three to five full-time parents. You may have one!

First think who in your family can take care of this child reasonably well for an hour? a day? a weekend? a week? Try what is available publicly. Daycare for little kids? After school programs for older children and adolescents? Big brother and big sisters?

Hospitalize the child. Some children with ODD plus a few other psychiatric diagnoses or CD are just totally out of control. They have everyone fighting with each other, are controlling the family, and are causing so much chaos that caregivers can only concentrate on surviving each minute. Sometimes putting the child in the child psychiatric ward can do wonders. You get some rest, and most importantly have some time to figure out what to do next with the assistance of the child psychiatric ward staff.

Full time parenting. If you are the full time parent with a child like this, it is a full time job. That means that either both parents/caregivers work part time or one works and the other doesn't. Don't expect to both work full time outside the home. It won't work. You won't spend every minute with the child, but by the time you address all the needs of the child and yourself and your family, there will be no time for work, too.

Someone to talk to. Whether it is your spouse, relative, friend, pastor, or a counselor, you need to be able to talk to someone with total frankness, especially if things go wrong. You cannot do it yourself.

Medical Interventions

When do you consider medications? There are three reasons to consider this

1. if medically treatable co-morbid conditions are present (ADHD, depression, tic disorders, seizure disorders, psychosis)

2. if non-medical interventions are not successful

3. when the symptoms are very severe

In choosing drugs for ODD, I look for drugs that have been proven safe in children, have no long term side effects, and have been found in research studies to be effective in extremely aggressive children and adolescents or in co-morbid conditions which children with CD often have. Each drug has certain problems that need to be watched for.

Clonidine

This drug was originally developed for treating blood pressure and it is very safe. It turns out to be useful for a lot of things. Tics, severe ADHD, detoxifying heroin addicts, menopausal flushing, and sometimes autism with hyperactivity or severe aggression are the usual indications. The good thing about this is that it never aggravates tics, works when autism is present, and works in very aggressive children and adolescents who never sleep. It is safe for pre-schoolers and comes in a pill called dixarit that is sweet tasting and looks exactly like smarties. As a result, children and adolescents will easily take it. It also comes in a larger size. It is my first choice when tics are present. It is also used in autism, preschoolers, and very aggressive children and adolescents with ADHD and insomnia.

And the bad side? About one out of every 10 to 20 people who take this will become depressed. It comes on within about 3–4 days and after the drug is stopped, it can take 3–4 days to clear.

This drug also has an effect on the heart. It can lower the pulse and blood pressure. To be cautious, I check an EKG before I start the drug and once the child is on it. I also check their blood pressure and pulse at every visit.

It will make some children sedated, but usually by cutting back the dose you can avoid this.

Risperidone

This drug was initially developed to be a safer drug for adult schizophrenia. It was then found to be effective in children with schizophrenia and other psychoses. Then it was found to be helpful in some children with tic disorders. Based on those findings it has been used in conduct disorder. There are some promising studies that show that this drug can help some of the core conduct disorder symptoms. When a group of hospitalized aggressive children with conduct disorder and borderline mental retardation were given an average of 2 mg of Risperidal a day about half of the children were a lot better and another quarter were somewhat better. Violence against others, verbal abuse, and property damage all significantly decreased. Another recent study found that risperidone was very helpful to children with conduct disorder when compared to placebo. These drugs were very well tolerated. These studies are probably the most exciting news for the medical treatment of CD in 20 years.

Weight gain is the biggest problem with this drug. Most studies show that some children gain from 10–35 lbs taking these drugs. Stiffness, restlessness, and tremor—these occasionally happen with these drugs, too, but to a much less extent than with the others. Tardive Dyskinesia (a movement disorder) can still occur, but only in 3–4 per 100,000.

This drug can also cause something called Neuroleptic Malignant Syndrome. This is a rare reaction to antipsychotic medication where people are very ill and have a fever, stiffness, and they are not thinking clearly. It can be very serious and has even caused deaths.

Other Medications in the Same Family as Risperidone

There are two other drugs in the same family as Risperidone which are new. One is Zyprexa (olanzepine). It has some of the same side effects as Risperidone but has only been used in a small number of children. The other is Seroquel, (quetiapine). This has also been tried on only a few children with conduct disorder. However, it is quite likely that these drugs will also be found to be helpful in CD.

Anti-Convulsants

It has been known for sometime that children and adults with brain damage can have severe temper problems. The drugs Tegretol (carbamazepine) and Epival (divalproex [trade name in the U.S. is Depakote]) have successfully been used to treat the temper problems in people with brain damage. These drugs are usually used for seizures and bipolar disorder. Recently, there have been some studies of these drugs in children and adults with severe problems with aggression and temper who do not have any brain damage. Most of these are in adults and show some of the same difficult personality characteristics that children with ODD show. Although there is not a lot of data, so far it does look promising.

While both Epival and Tegretol are safe to use in children, they are not without side effects.

Conclusion

ODD and CD are bad problems. There is no one thing that will probably fix them. Make sure you are not prematurely ruling out any of the possible interventions above. If you are not careful, it can destroy you long before it ruins the kid. If nothing is done, the outcome can be dismal. It is absolutely key to keep working to do everything you can to keep this problem from devastating your life and your child's.

Chapter 13

Mental Health Professionals for Adolescents

Being Prepared: Know When to Seek Help for Your Child

Parents are usually the first to recognize that their child has a problem with emotions or behavior. Still, the decision to seek professional help can be difficult and painful for a parent. The first step is to gently try to talk to the child. An honest open talk about feelings can often help. Parents may choose to consult with the child's physicians, teachers, members of the clergy, or other adults who know the child well. These steps may resolve the problems for the child and family.

This chapter contains text from "Being Prepared: Know When to Seek Help for Your Child" Facts for Families No. 24, September 1999, http://www.aacap.org/publications/factsfam/whenhelp.htm, "Being Prepared: Knowing Where to Find Help for Your Child" Facts for Families No. 25, updated August 1999, http://www.aacap.org/publications/factsfam/wherehlp.htm, "Being Prepared: Understanding Your Mental Health Insurance" Facts for Families No. 26, updated November 1999, http://www.aacap.org/publications/factsfam/insuranc.htm, "What Is Psychotherapy for Children and Adolescents?" Facts for Families No. 53, November 1995, http://www.aacap.org/publications/factsfam/therapy.htm, "Comprehensive Psychiatric Evaluation," Facts for Families No. 52, November 1995, http://www.aacap.org/publications/factsfam/eval.htm, and "Psychiatric Medications for Children and Adolescents Part III: Questions to Ask," Facts for Families No. 51, November 1995, http://www.aacap.org/publications/factsfam/medquest.htm. All documents copyright 1997 by the American Academy of Child and Adolescent Psychiatry (AACAP). Reprinted with permission AACAP. Despite their age, documents published in 1995 contain useful information about mental health professionals for adolescents.

Following are a few signs which may indicate that a child and adolescent psychiatric evaluation will be useful for pre-adolescents and adolescents.

- marked change in school performance

- inability to cope with problems and daily activities

- marked changes in sleeping and/or eating habits

- many physical complaints

- sexual acting out

- depression shown by sustained, prolonged, negative mood and attitude, often accompanied by poor appetite, difficulty sleeping, or thoughts of death

- abuse of alcohol and/or drugs

- intense fear of becoming obese with no relationship to actual body weight, purging food or restricting eating

- persistent nightmares

- threats of self-harm or harm to others

- self-injury or self destructive behavior

- frequent outbursts of anger, aggression

- threats to run away

- aggressive or non-aggressive consistent violation of rights of others; opposition to authority, truancy, thefts, or vandalism

- strange thoughts and feelings; unusual behaviors

If problems persist over an extended period of time and especially if others involved in the child's life are concerned, consultation with a child and adolescent psychiatrist or other clinician specifically trained to work with children may be helpful.

Being Prepared: Know Where to Find Help for Your Child

Parents are often concerned about their child's emotional health or behavior but they don't know where to start to get help. The mental health system can sometimes be complicated and difficult for parents to understand. A child's emotional distress often causes disruption to both the parent's and the child's world. Parents may have difficulty being objective. They may blame themselves or worry that others such as teachers or family members will blame them.

If you are worried about your child's emotions or behavior, you can start by talking to friends, family members, your spiritual counselor, your child's school counselor, or your child's pediatrician or family physician about your concerns. If you think your child needs help, you should get as much information as possible about where to find help for your child. Parents should be cautious about using Yellow Pages phone directories as their only source of information and referral. Other sources of information include:

- employee assistance program through your employer

- local medical society, local psychiatric society

- local mental health association

- county mental health department

- local hospitals or medical centers with psychiatric services

- department of psychiatry in nearby medical school

- national advocacy organizations (for example, Federation of Families for Children's Mental Health, National Mental Health Organization)

- national professional organizations (American Academy of Child and Adolescent Psychiatry, American Psychiatric Association)

The variety of mental health practitioners can be confusing. There are psychiatrists, psychologists, psychiatric social workers, psychiatric nurses, counselors, pastoral counselors, and people who call themselves therapists. Few states regulate the practice of psychotherapy, so almost anyone can call herself or himself a psychotherapist.

Child and adolescent psychiatrist. A child and adolescent psychiatrist is a licensed (M.D. or D.O.) physician who is a fully trained psychiatrist and who has two additional years of advanced training beyond general psychiatry with children, adolescents, and families. Child and adolescent psychiatrists who pass the national examination administered by the American Board of Psychiatry and Neurology are board certified in child and adolescent psychiatry. Child and adolescent psychiatrists provide medical/psychiatric evaluation and a full range of treatment interventions for emotional and behavioral problems and psychiatric disorders. As physicians, child and adolescent psychiatrists can prescribe and monitor medications.

Psychiatrist. A psychiatrist is a physician (a medical doctor) whose education includes a medical degree (M.D. or D.O.) and at least four additional years of study and training. Psychiatrists are licensed by the states as physicians. Psychiatrists who pass the national examination administered by the American Board of Psychiatry and Neurology are board certified in psychiatry. Psychiatrists provide medical/psychiatric evaluation and treatment for emotional and behavioral problems and psychiatric disorders. As physicians, psychiatrists can prescribe and monitor medications.

Psychologist. Some psychologists possess a master's degree (M.S.) in psychology while others have a doctoral degree (Ph.D., Psy.D, or Ed.D) in clinical, educational, counseling or research psychology. Psychologists are licensed by most states. Psychologists can provide psychological evaluation and treatment for emotional and behavioral problems and disorders. Psychologists also provide psychological testing and assessments.

Social worker. Some social workers have a bachelor's degree (B.A., B.S.W., or B.S.), however most social workers have earned a master's degree (M.S. or M.S.W.). In most states social workers can take an examination to be licensed as clinical social workers. Social workers provide most forms of psychotherapy.

Parents should try to find a mental health professional who has advanced training and experience with children, adolescents, and families. Parents should always ask about the professionals training and experience. However, it is also very important to find a comfortable match between your child, your family, and the mental health professional.

Being Prepared: Understanding Your Mental Health Insurance

Insurance benefits for mental health services have changed a lot in recent years. These changes are consistent with the nationwide trend to control the expense of health care. It is important to understand your mental health care coverage so that you can be an active advocate for your child's needs within the guidelines of your particular plan. Here are some useful questions to ask when evaluating the mental health benefits of an insurance plan or HMO:

- Do I have to get a referral from my child's primary care physician or employee assistance program to receive mental health services?

- Is there a "preferred list of providers" or "network" that you must see? Are child psychiatrists included? What happens if I want my child to see someone outside the network?

- Is there an annual deductible that I pay before the plan pays? What will I actually pay for services? What services are paid for by the plan: office visits, medication, respite care, day hospital, inpatient?

- Are there limits on the number of visits? Will my provider have to send reports to the managed care company?

- What can I do if I am unhappy with either the provider of the care or the recommendations of the "utilization review" process?

- What hospitals can be used under the plan?

- Does the plan exclude certain diagnoses or pre-existing conditions?

- Is there a "lifetime dollar limit" or an "annual limit" for mental health coverage, and what is it?

- Does the plan have a track record in your area?

Some of the language used in describing your health care plan may be unfamiliar to you. Managed care refers to the process of someone reviewing and monitoring the need for and use of services. Your insurance company may do its own review and monitoring or may hire a "managed care company" to do the reviewing. The actual review of care is commonly known as "utilization review" and is done by professionals, mostly social workers and nurses, known as "utilization reviewers" or "case managers." The child psychiatrist treating your child may have to discuss the treatment with a reviewer in order for the care to be authorized and paid for by your insurance. The reviewers are trained to use the guidelines developed by your health care plan. A review by a child and adolescent psychiatrist reviewer usually must be specially requested.

The review process often takes place over the telephone. Written treatment plans may also be required. Some plans may require that the entire medical record be copied and sent for review. Reviewers usually authorize payment for a limited number of outpatient sessions or a few days of inpatient care. In order for additional treatment to be authorized, the psychiatrist must call the reviewer back to discuss the child's progress and existing problems. Managed care emphasizes short term treatment with a focus on changing specific behaviors.

Preferred providers are groups of doctors, social workers, or psychologists which your insurer has agreed to pay. If you choose to see doctors outside of this list, (out of network caregivers), your insurer may not pay for the services. You will still be responsible for the bill. Similarly, care given in hospitals designated as "in network" is paid for by your insurance, while care given in hospitals "out of network" is usually not paid by your insurance and becomes your responsibility. Even when using preferred providers and in network hospitals, utilization reviewers still closely monitor treatment.

Another change is the variety of services and diagnosis paid for by different plans. In the past, only inpatient care and outpatient care was covered by insurance. Now, depending upon your particular plan, other services such as day hospital, home-based care, and respite care may also be covered. These lower cost services may offer advantages to inpatient hospitalization.

A limiting feature of some mental health care plans is a low lifetime maximum or a low annual dollar amount that can be used for mental health care. (i.e. Once this amount is used, plan coverage ends.) You, as parent or guardian, are responsible for paying the non-covered bill. If your child/adolescent needs continued care, you may need to seek help from your state public mental health system. This usually means changing doctors, which may disrupt your child's care.

It is important to understand as much as possible about your particular insurance plan. Understanding your coverage will put you in a better position to help your child. Sometimes you may need to advocate for services that are not a part of your plan, but which you and your child's psychiatrist feel are necessary. Advocacy groups may provide you with important information about local services. The support of other parents is also useful and important when engaged in advocacy efforts.

What Is Psychotherapy for Children and Adolescents?

Psychotherapy refers to a variety of techniques and methods used to help children and adolescents who are experiencing difficulties with emotion and behavior. Although there are different types of psychotherapy, each relies on communications as the basic tool for bringing about change in a person's feelings and behaviors. Psychotherapy may involve an individual child, group or family. In children and adolescents, playing, drawing, building, and pretending, as well as talking, are important ways of sharing feelings and resolving problems.

As part of the initial assessment, the child and adolescent psychiatrist will determine the need for psychotherapy. This decision will be based upon such things as the child's current problems, history, level of development, ability to cooperate in treatment, and what interventions are most likely to help with the presenting concerns. Psychotherapy is often used in combination with other treatments (medication, behavior management, or work with the school). The relationship that develops between the therapist and the patient is very important. The child or adolescent must feel comfortable, safe, and understood. This type of trusting environment makes it much easier for the child to express his/her thoughts and feelings and to use the therapy in a useful way.

Psychotherapy helps children and adolescents in a variety of ways. They receive emotional support, resolve conflicts with people, understand feelings and problems, and try out new solutions to old problems. Goals for therapy may be specific (change in behavior, improved relations with friends), or more general (less anxiety, better self-esteem). The length of psychotherapy depends on the complexity and severity of problems. Child and adolescent psychiatrists are specifically trained and skilled to provide psychotherapy.

Parents should ask the following questions:

- Why is psychotherapy being recommended?

- What are some of the results I can expect to see?

- How long will my child be involved in therapy?

- How frequently will the doctor want to see my child?

- Will the doctor be meeting with just my child or the entire family?

- How will we (the parents) be informed about our child's progress and how can we help?

- How soon can we expect to see some changes?

A child and adolescent psychiatrist will be able to provide you with answers to your questions and concerns.

Comprehensive Psychiatric Evaluation

Evaluation by a child and adolescent psychiatrist is appropriate for any child or adolescent with emotional or behavioral problems. Most children and adolescents with serious emotional and behavioral problems need a comprehensive psychiatric evaluation.

Comprehensive psychiatric evaluations usually require several hours over one or more office visits for the child, parents, and family. With the parents' permission, other significant people (such as the family physician, school personnel, or other relatives) may be contacted for additional information.

The comprehensive evaluation frequently includes the following:

- description of present problems and symptoms
- information about health, illness and treatment (both physical and psychiatric)
- parent and family histories
- information about the child's development
- information about school and friends
- information about family relationships
- psychiatric interview of the child or adolescent
- if needed, laboratory studies such as blood tests, x-rays, or special assessments (for example, psychological, educational, speech, and language evaluation)

The child and adolescent psychiatrist then develops a formulation. The formulation describes the child's problems and explains them in terms that the parents and child can understand. Biological, psychological, and social parts of the problem are combined in the formulation with the developmental needs, history, and strengths of the child or adolescent.

Time is made available to answer the parents' and child's questions. Parents often come to such evaluations with many concerns, including:

- Is my child normal? Am I normal? Am I to blame?
- Am I silly to worry?
- Can you help us? Can you help my child?
- Does my child need treatment? Do I need treatment?

- What is wrong? What is the diagnosis?

- What are your recommendations? How can the family help?

- What will treatment cost, and how long will it take?

Parents are often worried about how they will be viewed during the evaluation. The child and adolescent psychiatrist is there to support the family and to be a partner, not to judge or blame. They listen to concerns, and help the child or adolescent and his/her family define the short and long-term goals of the evaluation. Parents should always ask for explanations of words or terms they do not understand.

When a treatable problem is identified, recommendations are provided and a specific treatment plan is developed. Child and adolescent psychiatrists are specifically trained and skilled in conducting comprehensive psychiatric evaluations with children, adolescents, and families.

Psychiatric Medications for Children and Adolescents: Questions to Ask

Medication may be an important part of treatment for some psychiatric disorders in children and adolescents. Psychiatric medication should only be used as one part of a comprehensive treatment plan. Ongoing evaluation and monitoring by a physician is essential. Parents should be provided with complete information when psychiatric medication is recommended as part of their child's treatment plan. Children and adolescents should be included in the discussion about medications, using words they understand. By asking the following questions, children, adolescents, and their parents will gain a better understanding of psychiatric medications:

- What is the name of the medication? Is it known by other names?

- What is known about its helpfulness with other children who have a similar condition to my child?

- How will the medication help my child? How long before I see improvement? When will it work?

- What are the side effects which commonly occur with this medication?

- What are the rare or serious side effects, if any, which can occur?

- Is this medication addictive? Can it be abused?

- What is the recommended dosage? How often will the medication be taken?

- Are there any laboratory tests (e.g. heart tests, blood test, etc.) which need to be done before my child begins taking the medication? Will any tests need to be done while my child is taking the medication?

- Will a child and adolescent psychiatrist be monitoring my child's response to medication and make dosage changes if necessary? How often will progress be checked and by whom?

- Are there any other medications or foods which my child should avoid while taking the medication?

- Are there any activities that my child should avoid while taking the medication? Are any precautions recommended for other activities?

- How long will my child need to take this medication? How will the decision be made to stop this medication?

- What do I do if a problem develops (e.g. if my child becomes ill, doses are missed, or side effects develop)?

- What is the cost of the medication (generic vs. brand name)?

- Does my child's school nurse need to be informed about this medication?

Treatment with psychiatric medications is a serious matter for parents, children, and adolescents. Parents should ask these questions before their child or adolescent starts taking psychiatric medications. Parents and children/adolescents need to be fully informed about medications. If, after asking these questions, parents still have serious questions or doubts about medication treatment, they should feel free to ask for a second opinion by a child and adolescent psychiatrist. Parents seeking a referral for any reason to a local child and adolescent psychiatrist may contact the AACAP, 3615 Wisconsin Avenue, NW, Washington, D.C. 20016.

Part Two

Physical Health Issues
Affecting Adolescents

Chapter 14

Acne

No one knows for sure exactly what causes acne vulgaris, the technical name for the zit attack. But researchers do know that it usually starts in adolescence and that heredity plays a big role. If one of your parents had acne, there's a good chance you'll develop it. If both of them had serious pimple problems, then your chances are even higher.

About 85 percent of the U.S. population between ages 12 and 25 develops some form of the skin condition. Most teens who get acne have the milder form, called noninflammatory acne, and get just a few blackheads or whiteheads every now and then. But some people suffer from the more severe form, called inflammatory acne, and have a constant outbreak covering the face, and sometimes also the neck, back, chest, and groin. These pus-filled pimples and cysts can cause deep pitting and scarring.

Acne develops when glands that produce an oily substance called sebum begin to work overtime, possibly due to hormone changes that are at their peak in the teen years. One of the jobs of the sebum is to carry cells shed by the glands to the surface of the skin. But because the excess sebum is blocking the openings of the glands, called ducts, both cells and sebum accumulate, forming a plug called a comedo. If the plug stays below the surface of the skin, it is light in color and called a whitehead. If the plug enlarges and pops out, the tip looks

---

Judith Levine Willis, "On the Teen Scene: Acne Agony," *FDA Consumer*, July-August 1999, http://www.fda.gov/opacom/catalog/ots_acne.html, Food and Drug Administration (FDA) Pub. No. 00-1197. This reprint contains revisions made in November 1999.

dark and it's called a blackhead. This isn't dirt and it won't wash away. The darkness is due to a buildup of melanin, the dark pigment in the skin. If the process continues, a pimple forms.

What Causes Acne?

Acne most often starts at around age 11 for girls and 13 for boys. Scientists think a hormone called androgen plays a role in acne. Among other things, androgen stimulates the sebum-producing glands. After puberty, boys produce 10 times as much androgen as girls, and so it's not surprising that more boys than girls develop severe cases of acne. Also, bacteria called *Corynebacterium acnes*, which cause skin fats to break down into irritating chemicals, can directly contribute to an outbreak.

Other things that can cause acne, or make it worse, are certain drugs, such as those used to treat epilepsy or tuberculosis; exposure to industrial oils, grease, and chemicals; and stress and strong emotions (which may account for the big date breakout). Some oily cosmetics and shampoos can, on rare occasions, trigger acne in people who are prone to get it.

The American Academy of Dermatology says it's a good idea for acne sufferers to check with a dermatologist to ensure the skin condition really is acne. Rashes from other sources, such as make-up and oral medicine, can create acne-like symptoms.

Many young women notice that they get more pimples around the time of their menstrual periods. In fact, some studies have shown that up to 70 percent of women notice their acne worsening the week before their periods.

You may have heard that certain foods, such as chocolate, nuts, cola drinks, potato chips, french fries, and other "junk food" cause acne or make it worse. But there's no scientific evidence to back up these claims. Still, if you notice that outbreaks increase after you eat certain foods, it makes sense to eat as little of them as possible.

Oily skin and hair don't actually cause acne, experts say. Although there is an association between the severity of acne and the amount of oil a person's skin produces, not all people with oily skin have acne. And some people with dry skin do!

Does Anything Help?

In one Swedish study, most people's acne improved after exposure to the sun. But not all doctors agree that sunlight is helpful. Some say it may just be relaxing in the sun that makes the pimples vanish.

At any rate, the idea that the sun improves acne by drying out greasy skin doesn't hold water; sun and heat increase oil production.

Mild acne can often be cleared up simply by washing your face once or twice daily and avoiding any food or drink you think triggers an outbreak. If these measures alone don't work, you may want to try one of the acne medicines that you apply directly to the skin and that are sold without a prescription. They may contain benzoyl peroxide, sulfur, resorcinol, or salicylic acid, all of which the Food and Drug Administration (FDA) has found effective for treating mild acne.

All of these drugs are "peeling agents," which cause irritation and drying that help the body loosen plugs and shed dead cells. The drugs also can keep bacteria from forming, which reduces the fatty acids that contribute to acne.

(FDA officials are concerned about what happens when skin treated with benzoyl peroxide is exposed to sun. Research done so far hasn't shown the combination to be harmful. But the agency is reviewing other studies to ensure the safety of benzoyl peroxide products.)

What won't work is picking at pimples. This can injure skin and underlying tissues. If you have acne that won't clear up with home treatment, see a dermatologist, a doctor who specializes in treating skin problems.

Sometimes dermatologists use instruments called comedo extractors to remove blackheads. They may also surgically drain large pustules or abscesses.

There are also drugs that can be prescribed for more severe cases. These include both topical and oral antibiotics such as tetracycline and erythromycin, and Retin-A (tretinoin), a derivative of vitamin A that comes in cream, gel or liquid. Another acne drug, Accutane (isotretinoin), is also derived from vitamin A. But this medication, taken by mouth, has serious side effects and isn't for everybody.

In very rare instances, where these measures don't work or haven't been used before the acne causes permanent skin damage, plastic surgery can be used to smooth over deeply pitted and scarred skin.

Acne may be an inevitable companion of the teen years. But today, with proper measures, it can usually be controlled before it becomes totally unsightly. And if pimples pop up for that big evening, don't let it get you down—your date will probably have a few, too.

One Acne Drug Causes Birth Defects

There is one medication for acne that teenage girls should be particularly cautious of. The name of the drug is Accutane (isotretinoin).

It's a capsule taken by mouth that is derived from vitamin A, and for some time it has been known to cause birth defects.

Accutane is approved by FDA for treating severe cystic acne for people whose skin condition does not sufficiently improve with other treatments, including antibiotics taken by mouth. Accutane completely clears acne in many people, but there continues to be concern about its use in young women who may become pregnant.

The instructions that doctors receive for prescribing the drug warn:

- There is an extremely high risk that a deformed infant will result if pregnancy occurs while taking Accutane, even for short periods.

- Accutane is not to be given to a woman of childbearing age (any menstruating female) unless she has "severe disfiguring cystic acne" that does not improve with standard therapies and unless certain precautions are taken.

- Before prescribing Accutane to women of childbearing age, the doctor should give the patient an information sheet that includes statements about the drug's ability to cause birth defects. The patient is asked to initial these statements and to sign an authorization for treatment. If the patient is a minor, a parent or guardian's initials and signature are required.

Another acne medication, Retin-A (tretinoin), is also derived from vitamin A, but it is applied to the skin, not taken by mouth, and there have been no reports of birth defects related to its use.

—by Judith Levine Willis

Judith Levine Willis is a member of FDA's public affairs staff. Sharon Snider, an FDA press officer, also contributed to this article.

Chapter 15

Using Cosmetics Safely

A sea of cosmetics crowds the drugstore shelves, luring you with claims of romance, popularity and beauty. To be happy, you must use these products! Or so the advertisers would have you believe.

Do they work? Will you be the most beautiful, the most successful, and the most radiant person if you use these products? Where does the hype end and the help begin?

Cosmetics are defined in the Federal Food, Drug, and Cosmetic Act as "articles (other than soap) intended to be applied to the human body for cleansing, beautifying, promoting attractiveness, or altering the appearance without affecting the body's structure or functions."

The following are all considered cosmetics:

- skin care creams, lotions, powders
- perfume, cologne, toilet water
- makeup (lipstick, foundation, blush)
- nail polish, polish remover, cuticle softener
- hair coloring preparations
- deodorants

Laura Bradbard, "On the Teen Scene: Cosmetics and Reality," *FDA Consumer*, November 1993, revised May 1994, Food and Drug Administration (FDA) Pub. No. 94-5015, http://vm.cfsan.fda.gov/~dms/cos-teen.html. Reviewed in February 2001 by Dr. David A. Cooke, MD, Diplomate, American Board of Internal Medicine.

- shaving cream, aftershave, skin conditioner
- shampoos (except dandruff shampoos)
- bath oils and bubble bath
- mouthwash and toothpaste (with whiteners it is considered a drug)

Skin Care

Cosmetics can't work miracles, but they can help keep your skin clean and looking moist and soft. They also can temporarily close pores, plump up skin to make it appear smoother, and give you a rosy glow or blush.

Many cosmetic products are designed to protect the skin of people over 30 against dryness and the accompanying wrinkles. But these aren't the concerns of most teens. The biggest skin problem for most teenagers is acne. Some studies show that all adolescents have acne to some degree because when puberty hits, your skin starts secreting more oil. This contributes to blackheads and pimples, which cause your pores to stretch a little bit. Although acne cannot be avoided simply by washing your face, the oils on the surface of your skin can be diminished by frequent washing with cleansers made for that purpose. And there are many treatments available for acne both in over-the-counter and prescription strengths.

If, while trying to decrease the oily shine on your face, you make your skin overly dry, or if you're spending a lot of time outdoors in very cold weather, you may want to use a moisturizer. "Teens really should only use a water-based moisture lotion labeled 'non-comedogenic,' which means it doesn't clog pores," says Dr. Barry Leshin, MD, associate professor of dermatology at the Wake Forest School of Medicine. "Heavier oil-based moisturizers can cause acne cosmetica—an [acne-like] skin condition directly attributed to the use of cosmetics."

Ingredients

What cosmetics can or cannot do for your complexion is determined by the ingredients of the cosmetics and your own complexion. Cosmetics contain ingredients from nature and from the laboratory. Some work well for cleaning, others are good for lubricating—and some don't do very much at all.

It's a good idea to read the labeling on cosmetics to find out what the product contains. Some ingredients, such as alcohol and mineral oil, are fairly common. Others seem more unusual and may require some explanation. Here are some examples.

- *Liposomes:* Microscopic sacs manufactured from natural or synthetic fatty substances which include phospholipids (components of cell membranes). When properly mixed with water, phospholipids can "trap" any substance that will dissolve in water or oil. Manufacturers say that liposomes act like a delivery system, depositing product ingredients into the skin. When the liposomes "melt," the ingredients, such as moisturizers, are released.

- *Aloe vera:* A plant from the lily family, aloe vera in large amounts has anti-irritant properties. Although it's an ingredient in many skin lotions, it would take much more aloe vera than most products contain for the anti-irritant properties to work.

- *Vitamins:* Foods containing vitamins A, D, E, K, and some of the B complex group are necessary in diets to maintain healthy skin and hair but, according to Dr. Leshin, "There is no evidence that vitamins or other additives are advantageous when applied to the skin."

Allergies

Overuse of some cosmetics can cause allergies and other skin problems. Ingredients such as fragrance and preservatives can cause allergic reactions in some people. Skin reactions, which doctors call contact dermatitis, should be taken seriously. Even if you've used a cosmetic for years with no problems, you can develop an allergic reaction as you become sensitized to one or more of the ingredients.

Some cosmetics are labeled "allergy-tested" or "hypoallergenic," but products with these claims don't always offer a solution to cosmetic allergies. "Hypoallergenic" means only that the manufacturer feels that the product is less likely to cause an allergic reaction. Before placing this claim on the label, some companies conduct tests, and others simply don't include perfumes or other common problem-causing ingredients in their products. The claim "dermatologist-tested" on some cosmetic products only means that a skin doctor has tested the product to see if it will generally cause allergenic problems. Other label claims that carry no guarantee that they won't cause reactions include "sensitivity-tested" and "non-irritating."

"Natural" ingredients are extracted directly from plants or animal products as opposed to being produced synthetically. Natural ingredients can cause allergic reactions. If you have an allergy to certain plants or animals, you could have an allergic reaction to cosmetics containing those ingredients. For instance, "lanolin," extracted from sheep wool, is an ingredient in many moisturizers and is a common cause of allergies.

Marcia Sheets, a substitute teacher in Sykesville, Md., has tried to use cosmetics for years, but even those claiming to be allergy-free have created problems for her.

"I've had hives and swollen eyes, I've sneezed because of perfumes, and I've had blotchy skin—even from some products that are supposed to be gentle. If you have allergies, you just don't use the stuff. Over the years, I've figured out what I can use and what I can't."

If you have an allergic reaction to a cosmetic, you should stop using all cosmetics until you call your doctor, who will then try to determine which ingredient, or combination of ingredients, caused the reaction.

Cosmetic Safety

Serious problems from cosmetic use are rare, but sometimes problems arise with specific products. The Food and Drug Administration (FDA) warned consumers last February about the danger of using aerosol hairspray near heat, fire, or while smoking. Until hairspray is fully dry, it can ignite and cause serious burns. Injuries and deaths have occurred from fires related to aerosol hairsprays.

Another problem can occur with aerosol sprays or powders: If they are inhaled, they can cause lung damage.

The most common injury from cosmetics is from scratching the eye with a mascara wand. Eye infections can result if eye scratches go untreated. Such infections can lead to ulcers on the cornea, loss of lashes, or even blindness. To play it safe, never try to apply mascara while riding in a car, bus, train, or plane. Sharing makeup can also lead to serious problems. Cosmetics become contaminated with bacteria the brush or applicator sponge picks up from the skin—and if you moisten brushes with saliva, the problem is much more severe. Washing your hands before using makeup will help prevent exposing the makeup to bacteria.

Artificial nails can be a source of problems, especially when not applied correctly. Artificial nails must be completely sealed because any space between the natural nail and the artificial nail gives fungal infection an opportunity to begin. Such infections can lead to permanent nail loss.

Sleeping while wearing eye makeup can cause problems, too. If mascara flakes into your eyes while you sleep, you might awaken with itching, bloodshot eyes, and possibly infections or eye scratches. To avoid eye infections or injury, remove all makeup before going to bed.

Other safety tips are:

- Keep makeup containers closed tight when not in use.

- Keep makeup out of the sunlight to avoid destroying the preservatives.

- Don't use eye cosmetics if you have an eye infection such as conjunctivitis (pink eye), and throw away any makeup you were using when you first discovered the infection.

- Never add any liquid to a product unless the instructions tell you to.

- Throw away any makeup if the color changes or an odor develops. Preservatives can degrade over time and may not be able to fight bacteria.

by Laura Bradbard

Laura Bradbard is a member of FDA's public affairs staff.

Chapter 16

A Hole in the Head?
A Parents' Guide to Tattoos,
Piercings, and Worse

"Doesn't that hurt?" asks Jessica Brown, age 10, as she rivets her gaze on the ivory spike through graduate student Shawn Arthur's nose. She stares at the needles skewering the skin on either side of his chest. "That's got to be painful."

Her parents, Mark and JoEllen Brown from Nanticoke, Pa., listen approvingly. After an afternoon of gaping at living canvases at the "Inkin' the Valley" body-art convention in Wilkes-Barre, Pa., Jessica no longer craves a tattoo. She says they "make people uglier." She'll settle for just a navel ring.

Jessica's parents might consider that a victory, given that teenagers today seem to comb the *National Geographic* for fashion tips. (Don't laugh. Branding, scarification, and stretched earlobe holes are showing up among kids in California and New York.) Tattoos and piercing are far more mainstream than most parents realize. In a forthcoming study of more than 2,100 adolescents from schools in eight states, Texas Tech University School of Nursing Prof. Myrna Armstrong found that 1 in 10 had a tattoo and that over half were interested in getting one. The young "body-art" enthusiasts came from all income levels and ethnic groups. A majority earned A's and B's.

What's a parent to do? Many child-raising experts would have you believe that resistance is futile. It isn't. But the social and commercial currents are powerful. Tattoos and piercings have become widely acceptable, if not respectable. They turn up on celebrities, in toy stores (the Tattoodles doll), and as games on the Internet (Piercing Mildred). Young Jessica can tick off every pierced part on her favorite pop singers, the Spice Girls. "I've got people bringing in pictures from *Glamour* magazine and wanting me to reproduce some star's tattoo," says Scranton, Pa., tattooer Marc Fairchild, who—like most professionals—refuses to work on minors. "Pamela Anderson has made me thousands with that barbed wire around her arm." One Miss America contestant even bared a bellybutton ring in this year's pageant.

That's why tattooing emerged as the country's sixth-fastest-growing retail business last year—after Internet and paging services and bagel, computer, and cellular phone shops. Since then, the industry has been expanding by more than one studio a day, to 2,926—a 13.9 percent jump in nine months. These brightly lighted establishments are springing up near suburban malls and colleges.

What the heck. While it may alarm parents, the body-art fad is "nothing pathological," says University of Missouri psychiatrist Armando Favazza, an authority on self-mutilation and author of Bodies Under Siege. Indeed, studies show that young people indulge in body art for many of the same reasons adults do: to differentiate themselves, commemorate an event in their lives, or simply for the heck of it. "I like expressing myself that way—it expresses me," explains senior Tiffanie Gillis, a former varsity volleyball and soccer player at Piedmont Hills High School in San Jose, Calif. She sports a dozen perforations in her ears, a pierced bellybutton, tongue, and nipple, and five discreet tattoos, including a cartoon character she now regrets inking on her ankle two years ago, at age 15. Though her father has begged her to stop, Gillis intends to get more markings when she turns 18 and no longer needs to fake parental consent. "To tell you the truth, it's addictive," she says.

"Frankly, I like being shocking," says alternative music fan Amy Elizabeth Eisenberg, 20, a former scholarship student in marine biology at the University of Maryland who got the first of her eight facial piercings at age 16. "Why not?"

How about the pain? Though tattoo and piercing initiates often ask about it, most experience only a modicum of discomfort. Biting your tongue hurts more than getting it pierced. Tattooing feels like hair electrolysis.

Parents would do better to emphasize the potential medical complications. Navel piercings can take 12 months to heal, for instance, and can hurt for much of that time, since they are prone to infection and easily irritated by waistbands. Tongues, though quick to mend, swell tremendously when first pierced and can remain tender. "I had to live on Slurpees for a week," recalls Bridget McNicholas, a 14-year-old sophomore from Bowie High School in Maryland who had her tongue pierced this summer. The health risks include hepatitis B and tetanus, as well as skin reactions that can occur with red and yellow dyes. An improperly placed piercing can damage nerves. Dentists have seen tongue studs cause problems from chipped teeth to speech impairment.

If a kid shows any concern about the pain, that could be an opening for parents to suggest faux piercings with magnetic studs or temporary tattoos such as mehndi skin paintings (below). Though many states ban the tattooing or piercing of minors, parents can't count on that to protect their kids. Wily teens will find ways to thwart ID checks and permission forms. Tiffanie Gillis got a friend's father to accompany her to the tattoo parlor at 15; she then returned alone, using that first tattoo as "proof" she was of age. When Philip Wheeles, an 18-year-old senior from Gaithersburg, Md., and his girlfriend drove three hours to Ocean City, Md., for her to get her tongue pierced two years ago, they grabbed a stranger off the boardwalk to sign the parental consent form. And those were legitimate establishments. Amateurs known as "scratchers," operating out of flea markets and fruit stands, rarely demand ID—or pay attention to hygiene. Kits that include needles and ink sell for a few hundred dollars through skin-art magazines.

Many teens resort to do-it-yourself jobs. Elizabeth Fisher, 15, an honors student in Manchester, Md., and her friend inked ladybugs on their ankles last summer. Her mother let her cover the mess with a professionally done blue bear rather than remove it.

Axl's Advice

For the parent of the persistent teen, there is the risky strategy of a field trip. "Luckily, we ran into people who said what we wanted to hear," says JoEllen Brown, mother of preteen Jessica.

Parents who feel they have exhausted all other avenues can still stress to their children the wise words of heavily tattooed rock star W. Axl Rose: Think before you ink.

"Start out small, and put it in an inconspicuous place," recommends Steven Snyder, an Owings Mills, Md., dermatologist and laser surgeon who has removed over 10,000 tattoos. The bulk of his business is older people who have spent years regretting their youthful exuberance and keeping the evidence covered in long sleeves or folks who broke up with the partners whose names are emblazoned on their bodies. Depending on the size and color—black ink is easier to remove than green—most tattoos take several painful laser sessions and cost between $800 and $1,600 to remove. Homemade jobs often prove more difficult than a professional piece because the ink may get etched deeper into the epidermis, or leave scars.

If all else fails, parents can still try to protect their kids from major damage. Visit several tattoo and piercing parlors. First impressions count for a lot: If a place isn't clean, walk away. "Ask to see the autoclave," recommends Las Vegas tattooer Mari DeVine, who says no one has ever asked to see hers in the three years since she opened Tattoos-R-Us. These sterilizers work like pressure cookers and can kill hepatitis B. Needles should come in sealed packages and be opened in front of you. Each pot of ink or petroleum jelly should be fresh for you. Tattooers and piercers should wear latex gloves. Guns used for punching holes in earlobes are inappropriate for other body parts. "Most piercing shops are dangerous and have no concept of what they're doing. You have to be really careful," says Jhan Dean Egg, a San Francisco piercer.

It may come as sweet consolation to learn that even the experts—tattooers, piercers, body-art enthusiasts—also grapple with dissuading their kids. "Ear piercing, that's where I draw the line," declares Jim McNulty, a heavily tattooed database administrator from Dickson City, Pa., whose 14-year-old, Ashley, wants to get a tongue stud and thinks navel rings are "the coolest-looking things in the world." For a tattoo, it's age 18 or no go. Reasons McNulty, "The larger tattoo is a decision on a lifestyle, not just what you want to wear on your body." Unless, of course, the whole point is to needle your parents.

—*With Rachel Lehmann-Haupt in San Francisco*

Clip and Paint: How to Save Your Skin

Think of magnetic jewelry as clip-on-earrings for the body-piercing set, and you've got the answer to many parents' nightmares. Introduced to cash in on the piercing craze about two years ago, the $6 jewelry attaches with a strong magnet at hard-to-get-to places like the upper ear, nose, or even the lip. New York manufacturer Gravity Free Factory estimates that it has single-handedly saved the world from getting more than 1 million new holes. A plus for parents: The small, faux lip stud and its magnet must be removed before meals.

Mehndi, the intricate Indian art of henna painting on skin, is the way to avoid the tiny holes of the tattooer's needles. Some beauty parlors, particularly those that employ Indian immigrants, now offer the designs. The harmless dyes last up to two months. Urban Outfitters, a teen clothing and accessories shop, sells an $18 henna tattoo kit that includes dye, two stencils, and instructions.

But it's not just teenagers who are experimenting with the safe alternatives. Rosemary Reed, manager of Toast & Strawberries in Washington, D.C., swears that her magnetic jewelry clientele is mainly "lawyers and Pentagon types."

The fake jewelry has some disadvantages, though. The likelihood of swallowing makes the magnets an unwise choice for tongues, though doctors say that a swallowed magnet should simply pass through the system. Wearing a stud on each side of the nose is also a bad idea; the magnets will probably attract each other. The fakes don't work on most navels. It's only the rare, deep "innie" bellybutton that can accommodate both stud and backing. And experienced piercers insist that magnetic studs look as unconvincing as a clip-on necktie.

—Linda Kulman

Exposing Skin Art

Unable to attend a body-arts convention? These sources of medical and legal information may help.

A videotape for schools that follows two teens through the tattooing process, from assessing the risks to exploring removal, can be ordered for $55 from Texas Tech University Health Sciences Center School of Nursing, 3601 4th Street, Room 2B164, Lubbock, TX 79430, or by calling (806) 743-2730.

The National Environmental Health Association is writing a "body-art model code" for state and local officials. The group can be reached at 720 S. Colorado Boulevard, South Tower, Suite 970, Denver, CO 80246, or at (303) 756-9090.

Along with providing a well-stocked list of frequently asked questions, the rec.arts.bodyarts home page offers links to the newsgroup, where people can seek guidance on procedures and care, or just swap experiences.

The Association of Professional Piercers posts its "Piercee's Bill of Rights" in member shops, alerting customers they should expect a "brand-new, completely sterilized needle, which is immediately disposed of in a medical sharps container."

Two safety guides from Health Edco, a health education company in Waco, Texas, cover topics from how to choose a piercer to after-care advice.

The Internet magazine Tattoos.Com has convention schedules as well as medical literature on health risks and preventive meaure.

Chapter 17

The Darker Side of Tanning

Public health experts and medical professionals are continuing to warn people about the dangers of ultraviolet (UV) radiation from the sun, tanning beds, and sun lamps. Two types of ultraviolet radiation are Ultra violet A (UVA) and Ultraviolet B (UVB). UVB has long been associated with sunburn while UVA has been recognized as a deeper penetrating radiation.

Although it's been known for some time that too much UV radiation can be harmful, new information may now make these warnings even more important. Some scientists have suggested recently that there may be an association between UVA radiation and malignant melanoma, the most serious type of skin cancer.

What Are the Dangers of Tanning?

UV radiation from the sun, tanning beds, or from sun lamps may cause skin cancer. While skin cancer has been associated with sunburn, moderate tanning may also produce the same effect. UV radiation can also have a damaging effect on the immune system and cause premature aging of the skin, giving it a wrinkled, leathery appearance.

"The Darker Side of Tanning," http://www.fda.gov/cdrh/tanning.html, copyright 1996 American Academy of Dermatology, updated February 1997. Reprinted with permission from the American Academy of Dermatology. All rights reserved.

But Isn't Getting Some Sun Good for Your Health?

People sometimes associate a suntan with good health and vitality. In fact, just a small amount of sunlight is needed for the body to manufacture vitamin D. It doesn't take much sunlight to make all the vitamin D you can use—certainly far less than it takes to get a suntan!

Are People Actually Being Harmed by Sunlight?

Yes. The number of skin cancer cases has been rising over the years, and experts say that this is due to increasing exposure to UV radiation from the sun, tanning beds, and sun lamps. More than 1 million new skin cancer cases are likely to be diagnosed in the U.S. this year.

But Aren't the Types of Skin Cancer Caused by the Sun, Tanning Beds, and Sun Lamps Easily Curable?

Not necessarily. Malignant melanoma, now with a suspected link to UVA exposure, is often fatal if not detected early. The number of cases of melanoma is rising in the U.S., with an estimated 38,300 cases and 7,300 deaths anticipated this year.

Why Doesn't the Skin of Young People Show These Harmful Effects?

Skin aging and cancer are delayed effects that don't usually show up for many years after the exposure. Unfortunately, since the damage is not immediately visible, young people are often unaware of the dangers of tanning. Physicians and scientists are especially concerned that cases of skin cancer will continue to increase as people who are now in their teens and twenties reach middle age.

But Why Is It That Some People Can Tan for Many Years and Still Not Show Damage?

People who choose to tan are greatly increasing their risk of developing skin cancer. This is especially true if tanning occurs over a period of years, because damage to the skin accumulates. Unlike skin cancer, premature aging of the skin will occur in everyone who is repeatedly exposed to the sun over a long time, although the damage may be less apparent and take longer to show up in people with darker skin.

Who Is at Greatest Risk in the Sun?

People with skin types I and II are at greatest risk. Which skin type are you?

Table 17.1. Skin Sunburn and Tanning History

Type	According to Skin Type
I	Always burns; never tans; sensitive ("Celtic")
II	Burns easily; tans minimally
III	Burns moderately; tans gradually to light brown (Average Caucasian)
IV	Burns minimally; always tans well to moderately brown (Olive Skin)
V	Rarely burns; tans profusely to dark (Brown Skin)
VI	Never burns; deeply pigmented, not sensitive (Black Skin)

Since Most Sun Lamps and Tanning Beds Emit UVA Radiation, Doesn't That Make Them Safer Than Natural Sunlight?

No. It's true that most sun lamps emit mainly UVA radiation, and that these so called "tanning rays" are less likely to cause a sunburn than UVB radiation from sunlight. But, contrary to the claims of some tanning parlors, that doesn't make them safe. UVA rays have a suspected link to malignant melanoma, and, like UVB rays, they also may be linked to immune system damage.

What's the Government's Position on Using Sun Lamp Products Found in Tanning Parlors and in Homes?

The Food and Drug Administration (FDA) and the Centers for Disease Control and Prevention (CDC) encourage people to avoid use of tanning beds and sun lamps.

What Do Medical Professionals Say about Tanning?

The American Medical Association (AMA) and the American Academy of Dermatology (AAD) have warned people for many years about the dangers of tanning. In fact, AMA and AAD have urged action that would ban the sale and use of tanning equipment for non-medical purposes. Doctors and public health officials have recommended the following steps to minimize the sun's damage to the skin and eyes:

- Plan your outdoor activities to avoid the sun's strongest rays. As a general rule, avoid the sun between 10 a.m. and 4 p.m.

- Wear protective covering such as broad brimmed hats, long pants and long sleeved shirts to reduce exposure.

- Wear sunglasses that provide 100% UV ray protection.

- Always wear a broad spectrum sunscreen with Sun Protection Factor (SPF) 15 or more, which will block both UVA and UVB when outdoors. Reapply it according to manufacturer's directions.

For more information on the levels of ultraviolet radiation reaching your area at noon, you can get the Ultraviolet Index (UVI) from local newspapers, radio, or TV in many cities. The UVI is a number from 0–10. The higher the number, the more intense the exposure.
If you believe that some damage has already been done:

- Seek immediate medical attention if you receive skin or eye damage from the sun or if you experience an allergic reaction to the sun.

- See your dermatologist or personal physician if you develop an unusual mole, a scaly patch or a sore that doesn't heal.

- Always wear a broad spectrum sunscreen with Sun Protection Factor (SPF) 15 or more.

Chapter 18

Cancer in Adolescents

An Introduction, The Disease, and Tips for Clinic Visits and Medical Procedures

Introduction

This text was written for you—a parent of a young person with cancer. It addresses some of the most common questions about cancer in the young, combining medical information with practical suggestions. Special consideration is given to the emotional impact of cancer on patients and family members. This chapter is designed to help you cope with the stress of a chronic disease that entails rigorous treatment, frequent visits to the doctor and hospital, interruptions in schooling and social activities, physical change, and perhaps most frightening of all, uncertainty about the future.

Because cancer in adults and children actually involves over 100 distinct diseases, and no two patients or families are alike, this chapter

This chapter contains text from "Young People with Cancer, A Handbook for Parents—Introduction, The Disease, Tips for Clinic Visits and Medical Procedures, and Coping with Cancer" Chapters 1–4, National Cancer Institute (NCI), National Institutes of Health (NIH), http://rex.nci.nih.gov/NCI_Pub_Interface/Young_People/yngconts.html, January 1993. Updated in January, 2001 by Dr. David A. Cooke, MD, Diplomate, American Board of Internal Medicine, and "Talking with Your Child about Cancer," NCI, NIH, http://rex.nci.nih.gov/NCI_Pub_Interface/Talking_to_kids/talking.html, January 1993. Reviewed in January, 2001 by Dr. David A. Cooke, MD, Diplomate, American Board of Internal Medicine.

cannot address every issue or situation that will arise. Instead, it provides a general view of childhood cancer: what to expect from it and how to deal with it.

Direct specific questions to your family physician and/or other members of the treatment team. If you want more information in special interest areas, you may want to refer to the section in this *Sourcebook* entitled "Additional Help and Information."

The terms used in this guide are those used by treatment team members when talking about your child's disease or treatment. Some of these at first may be unfamiliar to you. The glossary at the end of this *Sourcebook* defines terms used in this chapter and others that might be used by your doctor or others involved in your child's care.

The Disease

Cancer is actually a group of diseases, each with its own name, its own treatment, and its own chances of control or cure. It occurs when a particular cell or group of cells begins to multiply and grow uncontrollably, crowding out the normal cells. Cancer may take the form of leukemia, which develops from the white blood cells, or solid tumors, found in any part of the body.

Despite considerable and continuing research, no one knows why children get cancer. Some common misconceptions about cancer are addressed below:

1. So far as scientists have been able to determine, nothing you or your child did or didn't do caused the disease. Cancer in children is still a largely unexplained disease, and there is no evidence that you could have prevented it.

2. Few cases of childhood cancer are due to genetic (inherited) factors.

3. In almost all cases of childhood cancer, its appearance in one child does not mean that a brother or sister is more likely to develop it.

4. Cancer is not contagious. It cannot be spread from person to person like a cold, or from an animal to a person.

5. No food or food additive has been implicated as a cause of any childhood cancer.

Leukemia

Leukemia is a cancer of the blood and develops in the bone marrow, the body tissue that produces blood cells. The bone marrow is a jelly-like substance that fills the inside of the bones.

The bone marrow makes three kinds of cells:

1. Red blood cells (erythrocytes): They give the blood its red color. These cells pick up oxygen and carry it to the tissues. They are also known as RBCs.

2. Platelets (thrombocytes): They help stop bleeding if there is injury.

3. White blood cells (leukocytes): They fight infections. They are also known as WBCs. Leukemia develops in these blood cells. In leukemia, certain white blood cells escape the normal control mechanisms that direct their maturing. Instead of aging so they are able to assume certain functions, they remain young and continue to multiply. This can happen to any of three main kinds of white blood cells:

    *   neutrophils, which eat bacteria

    *   lymphocytes, which make substances to fight bacteria

    *   monocytes, which destroy foreign materials

Solid Tumors

The word tumor does not always imply cancer. Some tumors (collections of abnormally growing cells) are benign (not cancerous). In discussing tumors that are malignant (cancerous), however, the term solid tumor is used to distinguish between a localized mass of tissue and leukemia. (Leukemia is actually a type of tumor that takes on the fluid properties of the organ it affects—the blood.)

Treatment

When a diagnosis of cancer is confirmed, it is best for your child to begin treatment at a center that has an experienced staff and the resources to apply the most effective form(s) of treatment right from the beginning. Your family physician or pediatrician can help you find such a center where specialists in childhood cancer will be in charge of your child's care.

Your child's treatment will be based on medical advances learned from treating many other young people. For some types of cancer, treatment programs may be well established. However, research for effective treatments is constantly under way, and your child may be treated under a research protocol (or regimen), which is a general treatment plan that several hospitals use for treatment of one type of cancer. The protocol is carefully designed to establish the ideal type, frequency, and duration of treatment.

Still, because children's reactions to therapy vary, the treatments may need to be modified to allow for individual differences. If a child is unable to tolerate a treatment plan or protocol, and minor adjustments do not correct this, another treatment plan may be begun or a specially designed program created. Before any therapy begins, the doctor should discuss the treatment program with you, including benefits and risks, and obtain your consent. Depending on the hospital's policy on the age at which a patient's agreement is necessary to undertake therapy, your child may also be required to approve it.

The treatment plan may look complicated at first, but each of the steps will be carefully explained, and you will soon become familiar with the routine.

At the treatment center, your child may be seen by different physicians from time to time, all of whom will follow the basic treatment plan. Your child may also be examined by resident physicians, fellows, and medical students who are working in the center as part of the educational program in cancer medicine and pediatrics. All residents and fellows are experienced physicians who are near the end of their training period, and their work is supervised by a senior physician.

In addition to these physicians at the treatment center, your family physician or pediatrician may continue to play an active role in the care of your child. With current information on the therapy prescribed for your child, your doctor can remain a source of advice and treatment for routine medical care and problems. Especially if distance between your home and the treatment center is a factor, your local physician may be called on to do blood tests or administer chemotherapy prescribed by the center physicians; thus, the number of visits to the center may be reduced. If that is the case, your child's initial hospitalization or outpatient treatment will usually take place at the center, and you will return there for periodic checkups.

The exact type of treatment your child will receive depends on the type of cancer. Most patients receive surgery, radiation therapy, chemotherapy, or a combination of these. These treatments aim at bringing about a remission, the decrease or disappearance of symptoms of the cancer. There are two major phases of treatment: remission induction and remission maintenance. Remission induction attempts to establish a "clinical" remission, in which detectable cancer has been eliminated. If this phase is successful, maintenance therapy aims at reaching undetectable cancer cells, which experience has shown may remain in the body. Remission induction may be accomplished through surgery, radiation, or chemotherapy. Maintenance therapy involves the use of chemotherapy and may last only a few months or go on for several years.

Hospitalization

Hospitalization threatens the growing sense of independence in older children. The young person is taken to the doctor, taken to the hospital, given treatment. This role is passive rather than active. The lack of independence resulting from hospitalization and cancer treatment is particularly displeasing to the adolescent, who may frequently and loudly protest the forced dependence. It is not uncommon for adolescents to refuse treatment, break hospital rules, miss outpatient appointments, or undertake activities against the doctor's orders. Besides rebelling against the feelings of dependence, teenagers may be acting on the normal adolescent resistance to authority figures and reluctance to appear different from peers outside the hospital. Some hospitals have responded by relaxing certain rules so teenagers can dress in street clothes whenever possible and have visits from their friends. Hospitals may also fill the oncology ward's refrigerator with their patients' favorite foods. Parents can help by allowing the adolescent a share of the responsibility for his or her own care and by respecting the need for independence and privacy, hard as that may be under the circumstances. But more than anything else, your teenager needs to know that you are there if you are needed and that you can be relied on for honest, dependable answers.

Surgery

For many solid tumors, surgery is the primary and most effective treatment. For very large tumors, radiation or chemotherapy is often used before surgery to reduce the size of the tumor, make surgery safer for the patient, and lessen any physical or functional defects.

The young person facing surgery is likely to be afraid. To counter some of that fear, many hospitals prepare patients for surgery by letting them visit the operating and recovery rooms, where they can meet and talk with the people who will be present during the operation. These people explain what they will be doing and how they will look. This advance preparation can at least ease the shock and accompanying fear of the sterile operating room, strange equipment, and uniformed, masked personnel.

In addition, the patients should be encouraged to discuss their feelings and fears concerning surgery. Young people commonly worry about the anesthesia, whether there will be a lot of pain, how their bodies will be changed, and whether their parents will be there when they wake up. If an internal organ has been removed, some children feel a lack of wholeness afterward. Amputations for bone cancer, primarily osteosarcoma, may produce similar feelings. Amputation also means the young person must accept and learn to use an artificial limb.

Your child will have questions about the surgery, and these must be answered as honestly as possible, because the child may feel betrayed if what you said does not match up with what actually happened. You will want to learn as much about the operation as possible. The surgeon and other members of the treatment team can help you. If you wish, they may be able to arrange for your child to see and talk with another young person who has had the same type of surgery and is doing well. If a limb must be removed, the center's staff might show the child a prosthesis. If appropriate, your child may begin to practice walking with crutches even before amputation of the leg makes crutches temporarily necessary.

Chemotherapy

Chemotherapy is treatment with anticancer drugs. These drugs can be given orally (pills or liquids) or by injection. There are several types of injections: into a muscle (intramuscular, or IM), into a vein (intravenous, or IV), into an artery (intra-arterial), or into a cavity (intracavitary). Doctors also inject anticancer drugs into the spinal fluid (intrathecal, or IT) to treat brain tumors and to prevent central nervous system disease in leukemia. Often, special devices, such as catheters and pumps, are used to help deliver the drugs.

Insertion of the IV needle may be painful and, once in the vein, the drugs may cause an uncomfortable burning sensation. If the drug leaks from the vein, it may severely burn the skin, so care must be taken to make sure the IV line is securely in place, and the nurse or doctor must act immediately if the needle comes out of the vein.

Injections are generally given by physicians or nurses, but pills may be given at home. Older children, particularly adolescents, may wish to be responsible for taking and keeping track of their oral medication(s). However, it is still important for parents to be familiar with the medications and check to be sure they are being taken correctly.

Whether you or your child is responsible, you may want to develop a system for keeping track of when medications are taken. Marking a special calendar is one way of doing this.

Chemotherapy and its side effects. Once in the bloodstream, chemotherapeutic drugs are taken up by cells such as breast cancer that divide rapidly. In the cancer cell, the drugs act by interfering with the duplication and growth of the cell, primarily by preventing it from dividing or depriving it of a substance it requires to function, and the cell is eventually destroyed. Anticancer drugs can affect not only cancer cells but also other rapidly dividing normal cells such as those in the gastrointestinal tract, bone marrow, hair follicles, and reproductive system. Because of this, unwanted side effects of the treatment can and often do occur. Most side effects, however, are temporary.

One common side effect of chemotherapy is the reduction of the bone marrow's ability to produce the normal amount of blood cells. This may put your child at greater risk for anemia (if significantly fewer red blood cells are being produced), bleeding (if production of platelets is down), or infection (if the white cell count, particularly that of the neutrophils, is low). Doctors use colony stimulating factors (CSFs), hormone-like substances that regulate the production and function of blood cells, to promote the growth of infection-fighting white blood cells. Using CSFs lessens the risk of infection in patients with a low white blood cell count as a result of chemotherapy. In general, you or your child should be particularly alert to any signs of infection, bruising, or bleeding and notify your physician if they occur.

Common acute side effects:

- nausea and vomiting
- pain and burning at injection site

Less common acute side effects:

- allergic reactions (hives; rash; swelling of eyelids, hands, and feet; shortness of breath)
- drug extravasation (leaking of drug out of vein into skin)

147

Common delayed side effects:

- hair loss
- mouth soreness and ulcers
- constipation (especially with the drug vincristine)
- bone marrow depression (low blood counts)

Uncommon delayed side effects:

- jaundice (yellow tint to skin and eyes due to liver problems)
- hemorrhagic cystitis (bloody urine due to bladder irritation especially with the drug cyclophosphamide)
- mental or nervous system changes (lethargy, tiredness, lack of coordination)

Chemotherapy may cause some long-term side effects in several body organs. The physician can tell you more about these in relation to your child's specific care and treatment.

Radiation Therapy

Radiation therapy is treatment with high-energy x-rays. High levels of radiation can kill cells or keep them from growing and dividing. Radiation therapy is used to treat cancer because cancer cells are growing and dividing more rapidly than many of the normal cells around them. In addition, most normal cells appear to recover more fully from radiation effects than cancer cells.

Radiation may be used alone, in combination with surgery or chemotherapy, or both. There is no pain or discomfort during the treatment. It is much like having an ordinary x-ray taken, except that the child needs to hold still for a few minutes longer. In some cases, young children need to be sedated in order to hold still for the radiation treatment. You will not be allowed in the room during treatment, because this would expose you to needless x-rays. Younger children may find it frightening to be left alone in the room during radiation therapy. If you accompany your child to treatment, it may be reassuring to explain that you are just outside the room. In some hospitals, closed-circuit television or viewing windows allow you to watch your child receive treatment, and in these cases, the child may feel easier knowing that you can see him or her all during the treatment. Most radiation departments are willing to give you and your child a tour of the treatment area before the first treatment. During this time, the technologist will explain the machines. A trip to the radiation therapy room ahead of time may also help quiet fears about the equipment, especially its large size.

Side effects of radiation therapy and controlling them. Your child will not be radioactive during or after radiation therapy. Neither you nor anyone else need fear contact with the child. Among the real side effects of treatment, which vary according to the site receiving the radiation, are:

1. *Skin damage.* The skin in the treated area may be somewhat sensitive and therefore should be protected against exposure to sunlight and irritation. During treatment, it should not be exposed to sunlight. Your physician may also prescribe baby powder or cornstarch, an antibiotic ointment, or steroid cream to relieve itching and pain and to speed healing. Nothing, however, should be applied to the treatment area without the recommendation of the person in charge of the treatment.

2. *Sore mouth* (if the head and neck are within the irradiated area). Your physician may prescribe a mouth rinse, and the hints on mouth care provided in "Common Health Issues" will also help.

3. *Hair loss.* Hair is frequently lost from the area receiving the radiation therapy. This loss is usually temporary, with hair growth beginning about 3 months after the completion of treatment. Initial adjustment to even temporary hair loss can be difficult, but after a time, children are able to play, work, and go to school without undue embarrassment. Some will want to wear a wig, cap, or scarf.

4. *Nausea, vomiting, and headaches.* A few children have these symptoms following radiation therapy to specific sites, such as the head or abdomen. These problems may last for about 4 or 5 hours and can be relieved by medicines prescribed by your doctor. In terms of diet, small, frequent meals are recommended. You may want to see that your child eats 3 to 4 hours before treatment.

5. *Diarrhea after radiation to the abdomen* (or pelvic area). This condition usually responds to simple measures such as nonprescription drugs or medications prescribed by your doctor. A

low-residue diet avoiding fresh fruits, vegetables, and fried foods may also help. Occasionally, treatment will have to be suspended until the symptoms subside.

6. Late effects. Following irradiation to the brain and/or central nervous system, some children seem to be drowsy and need more sleep. This symptom may begin at various times, even as late as 5 to 7 weeks after therapy has been completed. It usually lasts about 5 to 10 days. Several days before the drowsiness occurs, the child may lose his appetite, have fever or headache, have nausea and vomiting, and be irritable in general. This is a temporary condition; nevertheless, it is important to report such symptoms to your physician. Other post therapy symptoms your doctor will want to evaluate are dizziness, sight disturbances, increased appetite, and stiff neck. None of these may occur, but if they do, you should contact the physician.

7. Long-term effects. Research suggests that radiation therapy to the head may affect intelligence and/or coordination, depending on several factors, including the age of the child at the time of exposure. In some cases, growth may be affected. Research also points to the increased possibility of developing a second tumor in an area treated with radiation. Your child's physician or radiation therapist can tell you more about these long-term effects in relation to your child and the treatment.

Unconventional Methods of Cancer Treatment

Unusual remedies and approaches to cancer treatment often achieve public notoriety. As the parent of a child with cancer, inevitably you will hear of these yourself or have them brought to your attention by others. Patients, particularly older ones, may also hear of such treatments.

These treatments may involve unusual forms of therapy or strict dietary regimens that are reported to cure cancer. Despite many claims, no dietary or vitamin therapy has ever been shown to cure or improve cancer, and many patients suffer more from these regimens than from conventional treatment. As a group, these treatment techniques have not been tested in the same strict method as have treatments employed by your physician. Reports of unconventional cures seldom provide enough information to compare their effectiveness with that of more conventional therapies. Be very suspicious of therapies that rely heavily on testimonials to prove themselves; they frequently are frauds. Also keep in mind that some of these therapies are not necessarily safe, and can even cause injuries or death.

The guarantee of cure these treatments offer may seem attractive when judged against the difficult treatment course of conventional therapies and the fact that your physician cannot absolutely predict the results of that treatment. If you develop an interest in an unconventional treatment or have any questions, discuss it with your physician, who should be able to provide or direct you to relevant information. The treatment team's primary concern is that your child receive the most effective treatment possible. If some magical, easy cure for cancer existed, caregivers would be the first to make it available.

Because many people have heard of these alternative methods of cancer treatment, you, or occasionally the older patient, may find yourself in the position of defending your decision to follow conventional treatment methods. This can be a frustrating situation and place a burden on you during an already stressful time. It is important to remember that suggestions are usually well intentioned and that they come from those who are not well informed about treatment advances. The best way to deal with this may be to provide these people with more information and make it clear that you appreciate their interest but that you feel your child is already receiving the best treatment available.

Common Health Issues

A number of routine health-related matters are common to all young people with cancer. Some of these are discussed below and should provide you with general information on issues of concern to you. You may want to check with your physician or others in the treatment center to see how these general statements apply to your child's specific situation.

Infections

Because of lowered white blood cell counts from chemotherapy, infections can be particularly serious. There is the potential for the development of serious and unusual infections, and any sign of infection, such as fever, should be reported to your child's physician as soon as possible.

To determine the cause of the infection, the physician may ask that cultures be taken of any sores as well as of the blood, urine, throat, and stool. If it is a bacterial infection, antibiotics will be given to control it. These may be given either orally or intravenously. Depending on the severity of the infection and your physician's policy, your child may be hospitalized. The cultures taken earlier will usually be repeated to check the course of the infection and the effectiveness of the antibiotic treatment.

Antibiotics will not be used if the infection is caused by a virus, because antibiotics are ineffective in treating viral infections. In these cases, chemotherapy may be stopped for a time and medication given to ease the symptoms while your child's blood counts and general condition are closely monitored.

Some viral infections, such as chickenpox, can be particularly dangerous to a child receiving chemotherapy, because complications from the infection may arise. Notify your child's physician immediately if your child has been exposed, because certain measures can be taken such as decreasing drug doses or using a special gamma globulin. If your child attends school, teachers should know to inform you at once if a schoolmate develops chickenpox.

Most children who have had chickenpox are immune for life and will not contract it, even if exposed while in relapse or on chemotherapy. However, some children on chemotherapy who have already had chickenpox may, when exposed to it again, develop shingles. This is a blistery-like skin rash that resembles chickenpox but, instead of appearing all over the body, is confined to one area. Although complications from shingles are less likely than from chickenpox, notify your physician if you suspect your child has shingles.

Regular or red measles (also known as rubeola or hard 9-day measles) may also be more serious for a child on chemotherapy. If the child is exposed to this type of measles, your physician should be notified. Regular gamma globulin may be given in an attempt to prevent or control the infection.

There is no evidence that infections play any role in activating the cancer or causing a relapse. As stated earlier, your child will tolerate most infections as well as if he or she did not have cancer. Chemotherapy may be stopped during the period of infection, depending on the severity of the infection and the child's white cell count. Your physician will be the best judge of whether this should be done.

Your child may miss some oral medications because of a gastrointestinal infection. Contact the physician or treatment center if this occurs. Brief interruptions of medicine for such reasons do not seem to jeopardize the welfare of the child.

Activities

Cancer and its management may seem to consume an overwhelming amount of your time. For the child, however, the best antidote to this unwelcome (and at times painful) attention is to encourage your child to live as normal and active a life as possible. Check with your physician to see if any special precautions should be taken.

If your child feels well, there is no need to insist on extra rest. However, there may be days, especially after chemotherapy or radiation therapy, when your child may seem lethargic or appear to need more rest. This is a normal result of the treatment. Other days normal levels of energy will return, and you should encourage your child to get regular rest and pursue normal activities.

In complete remission, there are usually no restrictions on activity.

Immunizations

Live virus vaccines (regular measles, German measles or rubella, mumps, polio) should not be given. They may be dangerous to a young person who is under medication that suppresses the normal response to these vaccines. Diphtheria, whooping cough, influenza, and tetanus immunizations (DPT or DT shots) are not "live" and are considered by some to be safe for those being treated for cancer. Ask your physician before allowing any immunizations to be given. If your child has never received the regular measles vaccine, report this to the physician.

Other Medications

A young person under treatment should not take any other medications without the physician's approval. It is important to note that some medications ordinarily used to treat common conditions should be avoided. For instance, when the child's platelet count is low, avoid aspirin and glyceryl guaiacolate (present in certain cough syrups). If your child is on prednisone or dexamethasone, avoid aspirin, because it may stimulate bleeding. If fever, pain, or aches are present, acetaminophen (aspirin-free pain reliever) may be used, but the presence of the condition (fever, pain, etc.) should be reported to the physician.

Dental Care

Ideally, your child should have a thorough oral examination and any necessary dental work before cancer treatment begins. This is not always possible. Although dental work may have to be delayed because of the cancer and side effects of treatment, it should not be neglected.

When blood counts are normal, dental work is an important part of overall health care, but you should cheek with the physician before scheduling dental work. Even checkups should be avoided when the blood count is low.

Bleeding

A low platelet count may predispose your child to bleeding. In that case, special precautions should be taken to curtail "contact" activities. For the older child, it is wise to limit activities such as football, soccer, skateboarding, or roller skating. To control episodes of sustained bleeding, remember the following:

- Apply pressure until the bleeding stops—a clean towel, handkerchief, or cloth firmly applied to the wound will slow or stop the bleeding.

- For nosebleeds, have the child sit up. Don't let your child lie down. Pinch the bridge of the nose over the bone for 10 minutes. The pressure must be tight on both sides to be effective.

- Notify the doctor promptly if bleeding continues.

Transfusions

If necessary, transfusions of whole blood or specific components of blood can be given to cancer patients. Blood transfusions may be given to control the anemia that may result from a low red blood cell count. The blood may be given as whole blood, which includes the plasma or liquid portion of the blood, or as "packed cells," a transfusion of blood from which the plasma has been removed.

Platelet transfusions may be given if your child has a low platelet count because of the disease or its treatment and is at increased risk for bleeding. Platelet transfusions are most commonly given if the patient is bleeding or is in a situation that will predispose to bleeding, such as preparing for surgery.

Because each individual has a characteristic blood type, tests are run to be sure the donor's blood is compatible with the recipient's. This process is called blood typing and cross-matching. In transfusions of white blood cells, the need for compatible tissue type between donor and recipient is greater, and siblings and parents of the patient often serve as donors. White cell transfusions may be given to a patient with a low white count and a serious infection that is not responding to treatment.

When to Call the Doctor

Ask when your child's physician should be called. Call when you have questions or if you are unsure whether something should be reported.

In general, you should let a physician or other team member know if your child has any of the following:

- a fever or other sign of infection

- exposure to a contagious infection, especially chickenpox or measles, unless your child is known to be immune from prior exposure or develops a contagious infection

- persistent headaches, pain, or discomfort anywhere in the body

- difficulty in walking or bending

- pain during urination or bowel movements

- reddened or swollen areas

- vomiting, unless you have been told that your child might vomit after chemotherapy or radiation

- problems with eyesight such as blurred or double vision

- bleeding. In addition to obvious bleeding such as nosebleeds, signs of bleeding can be seen in the stools (red or black), in the urine (pink, red, or brown), in vomit (red or brown, like coffee grounds), or the presence of multiple bruises

- other troublesome side effects of treatment such as mouth sores, constipation (beyond 2 days), diarrhea, and easy bruising

- marked depression or a sudden change in behavior

You should also check with your child's physician when your child is due to receive any kind of vaccination or any form of dental care.

Talking with Your Child about Cancer

Introduction

Learning that your child has cancer is perhaps the hardest news you ever have had to face. As a parent, you must now decide how to tell your child.

The questions that many parents ask are: "What should my child be told?" "Who should tell my child?" and "When should my child be told?" This text was written to help you answer these questions.

You probably already are asking, "Should I tell my child about the cancer at all?" In the past, children were often shielded from the diagnosis. But, studies show that most children know they have a serious illness despite attempts of parents and health care workers to protect them.

Most likely, your child already suspects that something is wrong. He or she may not feel well, is seeing the doctor more often, and has had some uncomfortable and frightening tests. Your child also may sense the anxiety and fears of family members and close friends.

Children who are not told about their illness often depend on their imagination and fears to explain their symptoms. Many children with cancer believe their illness is punishment for something they have done; as a result, they may feel unnecessary anxiety and guilt. Health professionals generally agree that telling children the truth about their illness decreases stress and guilt. Knowing the truth also increases a child's cooperation with treatment. In addition, talking about cancer often helps bring the family closer together and makes dealing with illness a little easier for everyone.

Who Should Tell My Child?

The answer to this question is personal. It depends on the relationship you have with your child and on your own feelings and attitudes. You may want to tell your child yourself, or you may want your child's doctor to help explain the illness. Either way, you or someone close to your child should offer support, encouragement, and love.

If you choose to tell your child yourself, talking to others might help you decide what to say. Health professionals such as your child's doctor, nurse, or social worker can offer ideas. Talk with parents of other children with cancer. Contact members of support groups such as the Candlelighters Childhood Cancer Foundation for advice (to find the Candlelighters chapter nearest you, contact the Candlelighters Childhood Cancer Foundation, 7910 Woodmont Avenue, Suite 460, Bethesda,

MD 20814, or call (800) 366-2223 or (301) 657-8401). Thinking about what you want to say, talking it over with other concerned adults, and rehearsing it with someone close to you will help you feel more at ease.

When Should My Child Be Told?

Because you are the best judge of your child's personality and moods, you are probably the best person to decide when your child should be told about the illness. There is no "right" moment to tell a child he or she has cancer. Try to choose a quiet time and place where you and your child can be alone. This will create a calm and support-ive atmosphere. It is probably best to talk with your child soon after diagnosis. Waiting days or weeks gives children more time to use their imagination and develop fears that may be hard to get rid of later.

What Should My Child Be Told?

Before you speak with your child, you need to understand the type of cancer he or she has and the treatment that will be given. This way, you will be prepared for questions. Your child will feel more secure if you can provide the correct information.

The amount of information and the way it should be told depend on the child's age and intellectual maturity. As a rule, a gentle, open, and honest approach is best. The following describes general stages in child development and what children are likely to understand about a serious illness at different ages. Please keep in mind that these are only general guidelines. Your child may fit into more than one or none of these categories.

7- to 12-Year-Olds

Children ages 7 to 12 years are still limited by their own experi-ences but are starting to understand relationships among several events. Thus, they see their illness as a set of symptoms. They are less likely to believe that their illness resulted from something they did. They understand that getting better comes from taking medicines and doing what the doctor says. Children at this age are able to co-operate with treatment.

An explanation of cancer to this child can be more detailed but should still include familiar situations. Comparisons also are use-ful in explaining cancer to children in this age group. You might say that there are different kinds of cells in the body, and these cells have different jobs to perform. Like people, these cells must work together to get their jobs done. Cancer cells can be described as "troublemakers," that disrupt the work of the good cells. Treatment helps to get rid of the "troublemakers" so the other cells can work together once again.

Although the understanding of death varies among 7- to 12-year olds, many children in this age group think or worry about dying. However, they often are afraid to say anything to you. Be open and honest with your child. Tell your child that you, the doctors, nurses, and others are doing everything they can to make the cancer cells go away. Reassure your child that a lot of children with cancer get better, but no matter what happens, you'll be there. If you are not sure what to say, ask the doctor, nurse, social worker, or chaplain for help.

12 Years and Older

Many children older than 12 years are able to understand complex relationships between events. They are able to think about things they have not experienced themselves. Teenagers still define illness by specific symptoms such as tiredness, and by limits on everyday activities, but they also understand the reasons for their symptoms. Thus, you can explain cancer as a disease in which a few cells in the body go "haywire." These "haywire" cells grow more quickly than normal cells, invade other parts of the body, and disrupt normal body functions. The goal of treatment is to kill the "haywire" cells. Then the body can function normally again, and the symptoms will go away.

Teenagers understand that cancer can lead to death. They need to be reassured that much progress has been made in treating childhood cancer. They also need to know that many children who have cancer survive their disease and live normal, healthy lives. In fact, the number of survivors is increasing all the time.

Keeping Lines of Communication Open

Throughout treatment and followup care, you should continue to talk openly with your child. Like many other children, your child may, with time, ask more complex questions. Setting up patterns of open communication early will support your child now and strengthen your relationship for years to come.

At times, you may feel strong emotions when you are with your child. You do not want to burden your child with your fear, anger, or sadness. But children often are aware of how you feel. In fact, children may hide their own feelings to protect their parents. You may want to discuss your feelings with your child if you think they interfere with your relationship. You can tell your child why you are sad. This reassures your child that you are not angry with him or her and also lets your child express feelings. Let your child know that it is okay to cry and be sad. This gives him or her permission to show feelings.

During treatment, it is important to remember that you, your child, and the health care team are partners. Children who truly feel like a member of this team are more likely to cooperate and to accept treatment. You can help your child by explaining what will happen and allowing him or her to make simple, safe decisions about care.

Questions Your Child May Ask

Children often are curious and may have many questions about their illness and treatment. Your child knows and trusts you and will expect you to respond to questions. Some children will ask questions right away, while others will ask them later. Here are some ideas to help you answer some of the questions your child is likely to ask.

"Why Me?"

Children, like adults, wonder why they have cancer. They may feel strongly that their cancer was caused by something they did. A child with cancer should be told honestly that no one—not even the experts—knows why a person develops cancer. Children need to be reassured that nothing they did, or didn't do, caused their disease. Children also need to know that their illness is not contagious—they did not "catch" cancer from someone else.

"Will I Get Well?"

Often, children know about family members or friends who have died from cancer. As a result, many children are afraid to ask if they will get well; they fear the answer will be "no." You should tell your child that cancer is a serious disease but that the medicine, x-rays, and/or an operation will help to get rid of the cancer. You should also tell your child that the doctors, nurses, and family are trying their best to cure the cancer. By using this approach, you are giving your child an honest, hopeful answer. Knowing there are caring people such as doctors, nurses, counselors, and others also may help your child feel more secure.

"What Will Happen to Me?"

When children are first diagnosed with cancer, many new and frightening things happen to them. While at the doctor's office, clinic, or hospital, they may see other children with cancer who are not feeling well, are bald, or have had amputations. A child may be too afraid to ask questions and may develop unrealistic fears about what will happen. For this reason, children should be told in advance about their treatment and possible side effects. They should know what will be done to help if side effects occur. Children also should know that there are many types of cancer and that what happens to another child will not necessarily happen to them, even if they have the same type of cancer or the same type of treatment.

Children should know about their treatment schedule. They also should be told about any changes in their schedule or in the type of treatment they receive. Having your child keep a calendar that shows the days for doctor's visits, treatments, or special tests will help prepare for these visits.

"Why Must I Take Medicines When I Feel Okay?"

Most of us link taking medicine to feeling sick. It's confusing to children to take medicines when they feel well. Answers to this question may relate back to the original explanation of the cancer. For example, children could be told that even though they are feeling well and have no signs of disease, the "bad-guy cells" are hiding. They must take the medicine for a while longer to help find the bad guys and stop them from coming back.

"What Should I Tell the Kids at School?"

Children with cancer are concerned about how their friends and schoolmates will react. This is especially true when they have missed a lot of school or return with obvious physical changes such as weight loss, weight gain, or hair loss. Encourage your child to keep in touch with close friends and classmates. Friends often want to know what happens when a child is away from school. Encourage your child to talk honestly about the disease and the kind of treatment being given. Suggest that your child reassure friends that they cannot "catch" cancer from anyone. You or one of the teachers at school also may be able to talk to other students.

Try to help your child understand that not all people, including some adults, know about cancer. People who don't understand cancer often act differently or may give your child incorrect information.

Such talks with others may cause your child to have doubts and fears despite all your reassurance. Ask your child about conversations with others so that you can correct any misunderstandings.

You may want to ask your child's doctor, nurse, or social worker about a school conference, classroom presentations, or a school assembly that includes a question and answer session to help other students better understand cancer and what is happening to your child. Your child's teachers or the school counselor can help.

Your child will learn two important lessons about how people react to illness. First, some people, no matter what they are told, may act different because they do not know much about cancer. Second, good friends will remain friends. They know your child is still the same friend as before.

"Will I Be Able to Do the Things I Did before I Got Cancer?"

The answer to this question is individual and depends on the child's type of cancer and treatment. Most likely, your child will need some restrictions at different times during treatment. Tell your child why the doctors or nurses think it's best to restrict certain activities and how long this will last. Help your child substitute one kind of activity for another. For example, you could suggest that friends come over to paint, have a snack, or play video games if the doctor feels that your child should not ride a bike because the chance of injury is high.

Coping with Cancer

Dealing with the Diagnosis

Even though many parents suspect what the outcome of their child's diagnostic tests will be, the diagnosis confirming these fears comes as a shock. Initial explanations of the disease and treatment may be lost as parents try to come to grips with the reality that their child has cancer. This initial confusion is common, and repeated explanations of the diagnosis, treatment, and possible outcome of the disease may be necessary. Because this is a time when many important decisions must be made, as a parent, you should not be hesitant or embarrassed about asking and re-asking questions about your child's disease and its treatment. Treatment centers often provide printed materials that give further explanations about cancer and its treatment and allow parents to absorb details at their own pace. Many materials are available from the National Cancer Institute (see the "Resources" section of this *Sourcebook* for contact information).

Parents' Initial Reactions

Parents may experience many feelings upon hearing that their child has cancer. Common reactions are denial, anger, guilt, grief, fear, and confusion. These reactions are natural and may be a way of helping you cope with the necessity of accepting a situation that you want to change but cannot. It is important to remember, however, that this is a time when your child needs your support and is particularly sensitive to your moods and feelings. Expressing these feelings too strongly may create problems for the child. A child, particularly an older child, who senses that parents do not want to acknowledge the disease, may try to protect them by not discussing his or her own feelings and fears. This feeling isolates the child from an important source of support and may only increase concerns, because the child may imagine the situation to be far worse than it actually is.

Although the diagnosis is usually definite once the test results have been examined, parents often ask for a second opinion from another physician. Your physician or treatment center can recommend someone to you, or you may wish to get a recommendation from another source. Second opinions are useful for confirming the diagnosis and reassuring parents about its accuracy and for confirming recommended treatment or exploration of another approach to treatment. However, once the diagnosis and treatment have been agreed upon by two physicians, seeking a third opinion may in fact reflect a parent's need to find another, more acceptable diagnosis. This puts an unfair burden on the sick child and delays treatment.

Accepting the Diagnosis

Gradually, parents realize that their child has cancer and nothing can change it. At this point they begin to cope with the diagnosis and their feelings about it. Some parents become angry. Targets for this anger may vary and can include God, themselves, the physician, or even the sick child for becoming ill. Because it is difficult to express anger toward the sick child, spouses and healthy children can become the scapegoats for unresolved feelings. Parents sometimes lose their tempers. Letting the anger out may occasionally be helpful. It is important to remember, however, that other members of the family experience similar feelings. Realizing that some reactions stem from this anger and talking things through with family members, treatment staff, or others who can give support may help in dealing with these feelings.

Feelings of guilt may stem from thinking that the child's illness is retribution for the parents' past mistakes. Parents may worry about how they treated the child or whether the child should or should not have received a certain vaccine. It may be difficult to accept that, despite all their efforts to understand the cause of their child's cancer, it will largely remain unexplained. One thing parents should remember is that, as far as scientists can determine, nothing they did or didn't do caused their child s illness.

Parents frequently blame themselves and their physicians for delays in diagnosis. All parents want to know when the cancer began, but there is no definite answer. The onset can be rapid or gradual. Because the early symptoms of cancer are often the same as those for common childhood illnesses, early diagnosis is sometimes very difficult even for physicians. Furthermore, medical evidence suggests that in most cases of childhood cancer, the success of therapy depends more on the type of tumor and appropriate treatment than the time of diagnosis.

Reassuring Your Child

Whatever you tell your child about the illness, he or she may bring up the issue of death and the fears it creates. Be prepared to cope with questions about death, even if they are painful. Refusing to discuss death may deny your child an outlet for some strong and possibly frightening feelings, and it will deny you the opportunity to offer comfort or reassurance. In addition to discussing the child's feelings and fears, it is important to stress to all young people with cancer the fact that cancer can be treated, that research for better methods is ongoing, and that treatments are improving all the time.

Finally, young people of all ages tend to feel guilt and anger at the time of a severe illness. Guilt feelings may stem from the often subconscious feeling that disease is a punishment for being bad. Your child, therefore, needs frequent reassurances that he or she has done nothing wrong and is loved. The child may direct anger inward or at you for letting the illness happen. It is important for you to remember that even when your child is angry with you, your child loves you.

Many parents fear they will say something wrong that will upset their child or cause undue distress. In honest discussions this rarely happens. Even if initially upset or angry, the child will eventually benefit from the sharing of concerns with loved ones.

By handling the situation as openly as possible, the parent and child are free to resume as normal a life as possible. Shared awareness among the young person, parents, and medical personnel frequently has a soothing effect. The child seems happier knowing about the disease than fearing the unknown. Medical care is more successful because the child can actively participate. Parents do not carry the extra burden of concealing the truth. Despite the uncertainties and the heartaches, everyone becomes more comfortable with the disease and with the future.

In addition to talking with their parents and caregivers, young people with cancer may want to read about cancer and hospitalization. Such materials may be obtained from the organizations listed in the "Resources" section of this *Sourcebook*.

Continuing Life

One of the challenges facing the family of a child with cancer is maintaining a normal life. This is not always an easy task, particularly during moments of high stress such as at the time of diagnosis and during the hospitalizations and relapses. Even when treatment is going successfully, the lives of the patient and family members are influenced by the disease and its treatment and side effects. Schedules are rearranged to accommodate hospitalization or clinic visits, family members may be separated, siblings may feel neglected. Everyone may be worried or tense.

Despite all this, the continued development of family members demands that life continue as normally as possible under the circumstances. To see that this happens, the sick child should be treated as normally as possible, the needs and feelings of the patient's siblings attended to, and prediagnosis sources of support kept open for both the parents and the child. In addition, new sources of support such as other parents of children with cancer and treatment team members, can help parents cope.

The Parents

To cope with the child's illness and the changes this brings in your own life, you may want to consider the following suggestions:

- Make a special effort to find private times to communicate with your spouse, or if you are a single parent, with others close to you. Don't allow all your discussions to revolve around the sick child. Make time to do things you enjoyed doing together before your child became sick.

- Find ways to reduce the frustration you may feel when clinic visits require waiting for procedures, test results, or consultations with physicians. When your child is hospitalized, try to make it as easy on yourself as possible. Bring something to read or do while the child is sleeping or doesn't need your individual attention.

- If work schedules permit and the distance between hospital and home is close enough, you and your spouse may alternate staying with the hospitalized child. Weekends may be a good time for a switch: the parent who has been at home or work can stay at the hospital, and the other parent can spend time at home with the other children and rest. This also allows both parents to become familiar with the child's life in the hospital and various aspects of treatment. It reduces the gap that may grow between parents when one becomes much more actively involved in the treatment than the other. If you are a single parent, other family members or friends who are close to the child may be able to stay at the hospital occasionally so you can rest.

- Don't hesitate to turn to treatment staff for support. Most treatment centers have psychologists, social workers, nurse clinicians, or chaplains available to talk about special concerns.

- You may want to look for other sources of support. Talk to other parents of children with cancer informally in the hospital or clinic. Your treatment center may have a parents' group supervised by a staff member for more formal discussions. In addition, organizations outside the center may also exist. Such groups may provide support and information on how others have dealt or are dealing with situations you are facing. One national group, the Candlelighters Childhood Cancer Foundation, has local chapters. Treatment center staff may be able to help you locate such a group.

When your child is in remission, it may be tempting to put all thoughts of the cancer out of your mind. And, indeed, this is a good time to get a rest from it and focus your attention on other segments of your life. However, this is also a good time to clear up any misconceptions about the cancer that the patient, siblings, or other family members and friends may have.

This is particularly true for the patient and siblings when treatment has been a lengthy process. You may need to initiate discussions to update information if you feel that this has not happened naturally during the course of treatment and that the child is concerned but reluctant to raise questions.

School. For the school-aged child, continuing with school is vital. School is the major activity of children the same age, and continuing to attend school will reinforce the child's sense of well-being. Furthermore, it prevents the child from falling behind others the same age in learning and in the emotional development that comes from participating in school and school activities. When your child is hospitalized, a special hospital school program may be available. If your child is receiving frequent treatments or is too ill to attend school while at home, a home tutor may be available through the school system (the treatment center may be able to help you arrange for this). But home tutoring should be undertaken with the understanding that it is directed toward easing the eventual return to school.

When the young person returns to school, the teachers, counselor, school nurse, and principal may need information about the cancer and its treatment, any absences necessary for treatment, and any restrictions on activity. Teachers should be encouraged to give normal, equal attention instead of granting special favors that the child's condition does not warrant.

Both you and your child may be anxious about the return to school. Your child may be uneasy about how classmates will react to any change in appearance such as hair or weight loss, weight gain, or loss of a limb through amputation. You may find yourself reluctant to allow the return because you are afraid your child will become ill or you find separation difficult. Both reactions are common, but your child should return to school. Accept the child's fear of rejection and try to help deal with it. Most young people and parents find that their fears are unwarranted. Usually, classmates accept the patient and condition, and the child gains a sense of self-confidence by resuming the former role as a student. Because classmates may have questions about the child's cancer and any changes in appearance, you may want to help your child anticipate these questions and answers to them.

Siblings. Siblings of cancer patients may have many different feelings about the patient, the illness, and the attention the patient receives. While sympathizing with their brother or sister who is ill, they may still feel some resentment and believe that they are being neglected. In many cases, this is true. During times of hospitalization or when the patient is not feeling well, attention may focus on the sick child. As parents, you may not be able to pay as much attention to the siblings as you did before. You may have to miss school functions or ball games in which the siblings are participating. You may have little emotional reserve left after dealing with your sick child to talk with siblings about their concerns, to play with them, or help with their homework.

When you do have the energy, try to make special time for the siblings. Encourage them to become involved in outside activities and make a point of recognizing their achievements. When you can, make plans to spend time alone with them and do things that interest them.

Others may focus special attention on the sick child. It is not unnatural, then, for siblings to resent the "privileged status" of the sick child in the family, neighborhood, and school and the lack of attention to their own needs. Talking with siblings about the special attention paid to the sick child, letting them know that feelings of resentment are natural, and enabling them to share in the family crisis will encourage healthy growth and maturity. Efforts should be made to give equal attention or explanations when this is not possible.

One way to help them to understand their brother's or sister's illness is by involving them in the treatment. Older children in particular welcome the opportunity to be taken into their parents' confidence and will often respond in helpful ways. Finding things for them to do for their sick brother or sister, or their worried parents, gives many young people a sense of belonging and usefulness that might otherwise be lacking in the family's focus on cancer.

Siblings may accompany you to the clinic when the patient gets treatment or, if possible, visit when the patient is hospitalized. This will allow them to see for themselves what the hospital, clinic, and treatment are like. If this is not possible because of distance, try to describe the setting and situation. Photographs may also be helpful. Siblings may need such concrete experiences or explanations to prevent the construction of fantasies about the hospital and the hospital experience. Fantasies may range from fearing that the patient is being tortured to believing that the patient is having a good time; siblings may be terrified or jealous.

Remember, the patient's brothers and sisters may be asked questions about the illness by schoolmates or others in the community. They should have enough information to answer these questions. In fact, you might want to help them anticipate questions or comments and discuss possible answers.

Chapter 19

Teens and Risk Factors for Heart Disease

Chapter Contents

Section 19.1

Smoking, Fatty Diet Affect Teens'
Heart Disease Risk

"Smoking, Fatty Diet Affect Teens' Heart Disease Risk,"1997 Lubbock Ava-
lanche, www.lubbockonline.com/news/012897/smoking.htm; Reprinted with
permission of The Associated Press; and Kathleen M. Sardegna, M.D. and Jennifer M. H. Loggie, M.D.,

Teenagers may increase their risk of heart disease later in life by
smoking or eating fatty foods, according to a study of autopsy results
that found artery blockage in young people who died accidentally. The
study found dramatic differences in the severity of fatty deposits on
the arteries of teen-agers and other young people, depending on
whether they smoked or ate diets rich in fat. Fatty deposits and lesions were found in the major arteries of young people with high levels of cholesterol in their blood, according to the autopsies performed
on 1,079 men and 364 women between the ages of 15 and 34.

The amount of fatty deposits increased with age, and the difference between subjects with high and low cholesterol showed up as
early as age 15, according to the study published in Arteriosclerosis,
Thrombosis and Vascular Biology.

Although studies based on autopsies of American soldiers killed
during the Korean and Vietnam wars found similar results, this is
first large sample of data from young women, said Dr. Basil Rifkind,
of the National Heart, Lung and Blood Institute, which sponsored the
research. The researchers said their study disproves the notion that
women, who generally have heart attacks 10 years later then men,
do not have to alter their diets as early in life as men.

"It pretty firmly adds another large piece to the jigsaw puzzle and
says the problems of diet and heart disease is something that starts
off early in life," Rifkind said.

A childhood diet rich in fatty foods can begin the progression toward heart disease later in life, the researchers concluded. Children
who eat a lot of cheeseburgers and milkshakes increase their risk of

heart attacks if they do not change their dietary habits by young adulthood. "The saturated fat intake and the calories a single meal of that sort provides is tremendous and make you use up your daily rations in one meal," Rifkind said.

The heart institute's National Cholesterol Education Program recommends that all children over the age of 2 keep fat consumption under 30 percent of daily calories and saturated fat under 10 percent. But there has been a debate among scientists about how early dietary changes are needed to reduce the risk of heart disease later in life.

Section 19.2

Hypertension in Teens

Only during the past two decades have we come to recognize that primary hypertension and atherosclerosis have their origins in childhood. These conditions, which often are associated with overweight and lipid abnormalities, affect millions of adults in the US and are responsible for many illnesses and deaths. Overweight individuals with hypertension often have elevated levels of triglycerides and low-density lipoprotein (LDL) cholesterol and low levels of high-density lipoprotein (HDL) cholesterol. And with obesity rising steadily, hypertension in the young is likely to become increasingly prevalent.

Population studies show that about 2% of children and adolescents have persistent hypertension, although one study in an inner city found 15% of teenagers with the condition. Most hypertensive young people have primary—that is, essential—hypertension, and their condition is mild. More severe hypertension in children and adolescents often is secondary to a renal parenchymal or renovascular problem.

Given the seriousness of the conditions with which hypertension is associated, clinicians need to know how to recognize it in patients of various ages and sizes, and how to determine its cause. Hypertension in adolescents can be particularly hard to manage because teens make their own lifestyle choices.

Defining Hypertension

Blood pressure rises steadily from infancy until about 18 years of age; therefore, in adolescents, no single cut-point denotes hypertension. Hypertension in the young has been defined as a systolic or diastolic blood pressure at or above the 95th percentile for age and sex on three or more separate occasions. In teenagers, the 95th percentiles for systolic and diastolic blood pressure are close to the 140/90-mm-Hg cut-point used for diagnosing hypertension in adults, making elevated blood pressure relatively easy to recognize. In younger children, however, hypertension is sometimes overlooked because practitioners find it difficult to memorize the 95th percentile levels for each age and do not have readily available standards to which to refer.

In 1993, researchers published new blood pressure standards—based on height as well as age and gender—for seated children from 1 through 17 years old, drawn from data collected by the National Heart, Lung & Blood Institute (NHLBI). Although weight and height have long been known to be correlates of blood pressure, these investigators determined that height is a better correlate for children and teenagers because of the prevalence of obesity in young people in this country.

Pediatrics published an update of NHLBI research, including the newest national blood pressure standards for children and adolescents including what the standards are for adolescents age 12 to 17. To apply height-related standards, you need to measure each patient, plot the height on a standard growth curve, and use the table to ascertain the 90th and 95th percentiles for blood pressure for height, age, and sex. Using this practice, fewer tall but more short youngsters are labeled as hypertensive than under earlier standards.

Chronic hypertension is defined neither by how long the patient has had the condition (which may never be ascertained) nor by the blood pressure level. Instead, clinical findings of a causative underlying condition make the diagnosis. Whereas acute hypertension usually accompanies an acute disease, persistent hypertension may present without other signs and symptoms.

Remedy 1: Diet and Exercise

Because few controlled clinical trials of dietary intervention or drug therapy have been undertaken in teenagers with hypertension, management is based largely on information extrapolated from studies of adults. Nonpharmacologic approaches, which include management of obesity, exercise, and intakes of sodium and potassium, generally are first-line therapy for patients with mild hypertension.

Controlling obesity. Some patients with secondary hypertension are overweight, but this is usually less of a problem than with primary hypertension. During the past two decades, the number of adolescents who are obese has increased by 39%. This means that about 21% of adolescents in the US are obese; a disproportionate number of youngsters in this group are black adolescent females, Hispanic, Native American, or of low socioeconomic status. About 70% of these obese young people will continue to be obese as adults.

Both genetic and environmental factors contribute to being overweight. Lifestyle factors associated with obesity in adolescence include inactivity, which is promoted by excessive television viewing, and a high percentage of calories from fat in the diet rather than just a high intake of total calories. In addition, teenagers may persistently overeat to cope with stress and traumatic events within the family or social environment.

Unfortunately, treatment for obesity is often frustrating for patient and clinician alike, particularly when the patient is not motivated to make the necessary lifestyle changes. When the adolescent is ready to pursue weight management, however, an individualized program for modifying food intake and increasing physical activity can be implemented. Fully inform the patient's family about the program and solicit its active support. For adolescents who have not finished growing, weight maintenance may be the most appropriate initial goal.

Some authorities recommend that fat intake represent 25% to 30% of total calories consumed per day, with no more than 10% of calories coming from saturated fat. Adolescents exceed these levels if they regularly eat foods with a natural high fat content, fried foods, processed snack foods with added fats, baked goods, high-fat dairy products, and foods made or served with mayonnaise, salad dressing, margarine, butter, or gravy. By learning to read the nutrition labels on packaged products, the adolescent and family members who do the grocery shopping can avoid foods high in total and saturated fats. In addition, since many high-fat foods are also high in sodium and salt, they will learn to identify some salty foods to avoid. They should be warned that foods labeled "lite" or "healthy" are not necessarily low in fat, sodium, and calories.

Promoting exercise. Encourage all teenagers with hypertension, obese or not, to engage in aerobic exercise. Recommend brisk walking, swimming, soccer, basketball, and low-impact aerobic dancing classes or exercise videos, but caution sedentary individuals to phase into these activities gradually. Encourage young people not accustomed to exercising to get together with a family member or friend. As a method of keeping track of exercise patterns, having patients keep a diary yields more accurate information than questioning during office visits.

Decreasing sodium intake. Most people with mild hypertension are advised to reduce intake of sodium chloride. Patients receiving antihypertensive drugs for more severe hypertension also should avoid excessive intake of sodium chloride, which can override the effect of diuretics and increase urinary potassium losses.

Dietary counseling must be directed at the adolescent and family and be repetitive and ongoing. Adolescents, who often eat many meals outside their homes, should be aware of the sodium, fat, and caloric content of foods at fast-food chains, information that is readily available. Although sodium sufficient to support normal growth and development during adolescence is 500 mg/day, dietary surveys estimate that Americans have a daily sodium intake of 1,800 to 5,000 mg, with some reporting levels as high as 8,000 mg.

Sodium apparently elevates blood pressure more in individuals who are "salt sensitive" than in those who are not. Unfortunately, no simple test can determine whether an individual is salt sensitive, so all hypertensive teens should reduce their sodium intake.

It is not known to what level sodium chloride must be reduced to lower blood pressure in teenagers. Consequently, we recommend an arbitrary and safe level of 1,500 to 2,500 mg of sodium per day, which many teenagers find difficult not to exceed. In one of the few controlled clinical trials of sodium reduction in US children, researchers found it impossible to get boys to comply with a low sodium diet for an extended period.

In our experience, few adolescents go farther than refraining from adding salt to cooked foods even though we give them detailed information, both orally and in writing, about the sodium content of a wide variety of foods, including junk and fast foods. We also teach them how to read food labels and what levels of sodium chloride to avoid. Some stop adding salt to their food but substitute ketchup or some other salty condiment, and enough adolescents drink pickle juice that we inquire about it routinely.

Reduction of dietary sodium should be accomplished gradually. Food frequency questionnaires are available to help assess adolescents' sodium and salt intake.

Increasing potassium intake. Primitive peoples who ingest a diet high in potassium tend not to develop the rise in blood pressure seen among aging individuals in westernized societies. It therefore has been suggested that in moderating hypertension the dietary sodium-potassium ratio may be more important than sodium intake alone.

No definitive data support the use of potassium supplementation in treating hypertensive adolescents, however. In one multiyear clinical trial with normotensive youths, potassium supplementation lowered blood pressure in girls but not in boys. This finding was confounded by the boys' failure to adhere to a reduction in sodium intake. In addition, the studied population was not representative of the ethnic mix in the US population. Nonetheless, it may be reasonable to encourage all adolescents to eat a diet rich in potassium since these foods—primarily fruits and vegetables—are an important part of any healthy diet. Daily servings of such foods will exceed the 2,000 mg/day of potassium that is the estimated minimum daily requirement for teenagers.

Dietary calcium. The role dietary calcium plays in the regulation of blood pressure remains controversial, and there is no scientific basis for advising hypertensive adolescents to increase their dietary calcium intake beyond the 1,200 mg/day needed for skeletal growth and increasing bone density.

Avoiding smoking and drinking. Since smoking, like hypertension, is a risk factor for coronary artery disease, it should be avoided. Chronic use of alcohol can increase hypertension, and teenagers should limit their consumption.

Remedy 2: Medication

When an adolescent's blood pressure is clearly and persistently abnormal (greater than 140/90) physicians generally are not reluctant to start antihypertensive drugs if the hypertension has an underlying cause. Because the outcome for teenagers with primary hypertension is unclear, however, physicians sometimes hesitate to begin drug therapy. Yet many teenagers with primary hypertension have several cardiovascular risk factors and remain hypertensive as adults, and a significant number eventually develop target organ damage. In addition, many hypertensive young people are overweight and have great difficulty making recommended lifestyle changes.

Therefore, it increasingly is our practice to begin antihypertensive drugs if 6 to 12 months of a dietary and exercise regimen has failed to improve the blood pressure, especially if there is a strong family history of hypertension or evidence of end organ damage.

We do not tell patients that treatment will be lifelong, and we continue to encourage them to reduce their sodium and fat intake and to exercise regularly. Some adolescents are more successful with these interventions as they get older.

The entire spectrum of drugs used to treat hypertension in adults also has been used to treat adolescents. Because clinical trials with these agents in the young population have been few, adverse effects on cognitive function are unknown. Other long-term adverse effects also have not been studied.

Angiotensin-converting enzyme (ACE) inhibitors and calcium channel-blocking agents are common first choices. Teenagers seem to accept these agents more easily than older drugs because they often can be taken just once a day. They also have fewer side effects, though they are relatively expensive. An additional advantage is that the newer classes of drugs do not affect lipid levels.

The choice of antihypertensive drugs can be tailored somewhat to the individual patient's gender, race, lifestyle, level of activity, and the presence of co-existing health problems. For example, a beta-blocker may alleviate the headaches of a migraine sufferer as well as lower blood pressure. In adults, the blood pressure response to calcium channel-blocking drugs and diuretics is better in blacks than in whites, whereas whites may respond better to ACE inhibitors. In obese adolescents, who are likely to be "salt sensitive," a diuretic might be the initial drug of choice; however, thiazides may alter lipids, cause hypokalemia and hyperuricemia, and interfere with glucose metabolism and/or utilization.

The beta-blocking drugs are not indicated for young athletes, in whom they may decrease exercise tolerance. However, they may be ideal agents for hypertension associated with a hyperdynamic cardiovascular state, since they lower heart rate and cardiac output.

Special Problems

Compliance, a problem when treating hypertension in adults, is an even bigger issue with adolescents. Hypertensive adolescents who are school athletes and those who become pregnant present special challenges.

Compliance. Except when it is persistently severe or acute in onset, hypertension is usually asymptomatic. Consequently, many adolescents with hypertension have difficulty acknowledging that they have a serious health problem. This works against making lifestyle changes and leads to noncompliance with drug regimens and missed appointments. The situation is even worse if the teen feels well, but the prescribed medication makes her feel unwell.

For a young person accustomed to a diet high in junk foods, dietary restrictions for improving blood pressure are an imposition. It's particularly difficult for adolescents, who do not want their peers to see them as "different," to resist the temptation to eat pizza with their friends.

In addition, overweight is often a family problem, and an adolescent's relatives may not be willing to change diet and exercise patterns even if they also are hypertensive. The problem is compounded when the family lives in an area in which it is unsafe or inconvenient to exercise, or cultural cooking habits are at odds with a low-fat, low-sodium diet. It's not easy for a teenager to eat a healthy diet and exercise regularly alone, especially if she is depressed and has low self-esteem. College students living in a dormitory may also find it difficult to reduce sodium intake.

Another problem is that few third-party payers will fund nutritional counseling, behavior modification, and organized exercise programs. Recommended changes and prescribed drugs may impose costs that a family can ill afford.

The teenage athlete. Athletic teenagers generally can continue to participate in most sports, although we recommend that those with moderate or severe hypertension wait until the drug regimen brings blood pressure under control. We also avoid sodium reduction during the summer months for those exercising heavily.

Weight lifting is sometimes a component of training for competitive athletics or a way to build body strength and improve appearance. When it is part of a balanced exercise program, including aerobic exercise, weight lifting is probably acceptable. Competitive weight training and power lifting should be discouraged, however.

Pregnancy and contraception. Young women with hypertension should be educated about contraception and know that blood pressure normally is lower than usual during the early and middle stages of pregnancy, gradually returning to nonpregnancy levels—or sometimes higher—during the third trimester. In some parts of the southern US preeclampsia and gestational hypertension are the most frequent causes of hypertension in teenage females, many of whom eventually develop essential hypertension.

Ideally, pregnancy should be carefully planned and supervised. Treatment for hypertension, which is most likely to develop during the last trimester, is limited to a small group of drugs known to be effective and safe for the fetus. This does not include the ACE inhibitors or calcium channel-blocking drugs. Both the hypertensive female teenager and her fetus are at more risk for illness and death than normotensive pregnant adolescents.

In young women with hypertension, the risk of pregnancy outweighs the risk of proper contraception. Hypertension associated with oral contraceptive use is generally mild and, under proper surveillance, hypertensive adolescents may take birth control pills. If hypertension worsens, it may be preferable to prescribe antihypertensive drugs than to discontinue the contraceptive.

The question of continuity. Unfortunately, it is not yet clear which individuals with primary hypertension in adolescence will continue to be hypertensive as adults. Although population studies of children and adolescents show that childhood hypertension is likely to continue into adulthood, some hypertensive teenagers become normotensive.

Prematurely labeling an adolescent as hypertensive can be damaging. It may make it problematic to obtain life and health insurance and to pursue certain career choices. These issues pose difficult management choices.

On Their Own

Much of the management of hypertension is the responsibility of the individual adolescent and family. Even when hypertensive adolescents do not adhere to recommended therapy, catastrophic events are rare, which buttresses patients' conviction that nothing is really wrong. Although the condition is hard for patients to understand and frustrating for physicians to treat, it's important to try, and the occasional success is rewarding for all concerned.

Chapter 20

Juvenile Rheumatoid Arthritis

What Is Arthritis?

Arthritis means joint inflammation, and refers to a group of diseases that cause pain, swelling, stiffness and loss of motion in the joints. "Arthritis" is often used as a more general term to refer to the more than 100 rheumatic diseases that may affect the joints but can also cause pain, swelling, and stiffness in other supporting structures of the body such as muscles, tendons, ligaments, and bones. Some rheumatic diseases can affect other parts of the body, including various internal organs. Children can develop almost all types of arthritis that affect adults, but the most common type of arthritis that affects children is juvenile rheumatoid arthritis.

What Is Juvenile Rheumatoid Arthritis?

Juvenile rheumatoid arthritis (JRA) is arthritis that causes joint inflammation and stiffness for more than 6 weeks in a child of 16 years of age or less. Inflammation causes redness, swelling, warmth, and soreness in the joints, although many children with JRA do not complain of joint pain. Any joint can be affected and inflammation may limit the mobility of affected joints.

Excerpted from "Questions and Answers about Juvenile Rheumatoid Arthritis," National Institute of Arthritis and Musculoskeletal and Skin Diseases (NIAMS), National Institutes of Health (NIH), Pub. No. AR-112QA, http://www.nih.gov/niams/healthinfo/juvarthr.htm, May, 1998, e-text posted October, 1998.

Doctors classify three kinds of JRA by the number of joints involved, the symptoms, and the presence or absence of certain antibodies in the blood (antibodies are special proteins made by the immune system). These classifications help the doctor determine how the disease will progress:

Pauciarticular. Pauciarticular (paw-see-are-tick-you-lar) means that four or fewer joints are affected. Pauciarticular is the most common form of JRA; about half of all children with JRA have this type. Pauciarticular disease typically affects large joints, such as the knees. Girls under age 8 are most likely to develop this type of JRA.

Some children have special proteins in the blood called antinuclear antibodies (ANAs). Eye disease affects about 20 to 30 percent of children with pauciarticular JRA. Up to 80 percent of those with eye disease also test positive for ANA and the disease tends to develop at a particularly early age in these children. Regular examinations by an ophthalmologist (a doctor who specializes in eye diseases) are necessary to prevent serious eye problems such as iritis (inflammation of the iris) or uveitis (inflammation of the inner eye, or uvea). Many children with pauciarticular disease outgrow arthritis by adulthood, although eye problems can continue and joint symptoms may recur in some people.

Polyarticular. About 30 percent of all children with JRA have polyarticular disease. In polyarticular disease, five or more joints are affected. The small joints, such as those in the hands and feet, are most commonly involved, but the disease may also affect large joints. Polyarticular JRA often is symmetrical, that is, it affects the same joint on both sides of the body. Some children with polyarticular disease have a special kind of antibody in their blood called IgM rheumatoid factor (RF). These children often have a more severe form of the disease, which doctors consider to be the same as adult rheumatoid arthritis.

Systemic. Besides joint swelling, the systemic form of JRA is characterized by fever and a light pink rash, and may also affect internal organs such as the heart, liver, spleen, and lymph nodes. Doctors sometimes call it Still's disease. Almost all children with this type of JRA test negative for both RF and ANA. The systemic form affects 20 percent of all children with JRA. A small percentage of these children develop arthritis in many joints and can have severe arthritis that continues into adulthood.

How Is Juvenile Rheumatoid Arthritis Different from Adult Rheumatoid Arthritis?

The main difference between juvenile and adult rheumatoid arthritis is that many people with JRA outgrow the illness, while adults usually have lifelong symptoms. Studies estimate that by adulthood, JRA symptoms disappear in more than half of all affected children. Additionally, unlike rheumatoid arthritis in an adult, JRA may affect bone development as well as the child's growth.

Another difference between JRA and adult rheumatoid arthritis is the percentage of people who are positive for RF. About 70 to 80 percent of all adults with rheumatoid arthritis are positive for RF, but fewer than half of all children with rheumatoid arthritis are RF positive. Presence of RF indicates an increased chance that JRA will continue into adulthood.

What Causes Juvenile Rheumatoid Arthritis?

JRA is an autoimmune disorder, which means that the body mistakenly identifies some of its own cells and tissues as foreign. The immune system, which normally helps to fight off harmful, foreign substances such as bacteria or viruses, begins to attack healthy cells and tissues. The result is inflammation—marked by redness, heat, pain, and swelling. Doctors do not know why the immune system goes awry in children who develop JRA. Scientists suspect that it is a two-step process. First something in a child's genetic makeup gives them a tendency to develop JRA; and then an environmental factor, such as a virus, triggers the development of JRA.

What Are the Symptoms and Signs of Juvenile Rheumatoid Arthritis?

The most common symptom of all types of JRA is persistent joint swelling, pain, and stiffness that typically is worse in the morning or after a nap. The pain may limit movement of the affected joint although many children, especially younger ones, will not complain of pain. JRA commonly affects the knees and joints in the hands and feet. One of the earliest signs of JRA may be limping in the morning because of an affected knee. Besides joint symptoms, children with systemic JRA have a high fever and a light pink rash. The rash and fever may appear and disappear very quickly. Systemic JRA also may cause the lymph nodes located in the neck and other parts of the body

181

to swell. In some cases (less than half), internal organs including the heart, and very rarely, the lungs may be involved.

Eye inflammation is a potentially severe complication that sometimes occurs in children with pauciarticular JRA. Eye diseases such as iritis and uveitis often are not present until some time after a child first develops JRA.

Typically, there are periods when the symptoms of JRA are better or disappear (remissions) and times when symptoms are worse (flares). JRA is different in each child—some may have just one or two flares and never have symptoms again, while others experience many flares or even have symptoms that never go away.

Does Juvenile Rheumatoid Arthritis Affect Physical Appearance?

Some children with JRA may look different because they have growth problems. Depending on the severity of the disease and the joints involved, growth in affected joints may be too fast or too slow, causing one leg or arm to be longer than the other. Overall growth may also be slowed. Doctors are exploring the use of growth hormones to treat this problem. JRA also may cause joints to grow unevenly or to one side.

Children with JRA also may look different because of medication. Corticosteroids, a type of medication sometimes used to treat JRA, can result in weight gain and a round face. When the doctor stops giving the medication, these side effects may disappear.

How Is Juvenile Rheumatoid Arthritis Diagnosed?

Doctors usually suspect JRA, along with several other possible conditions, when they see children with persistent joint pain or swelling, unexplained skin rashes and fever, or swelling of lymph nodes or inflammation of internal organs. A diagnosis of JRA also is considered in children with an unexplained limp or excessive clumsiness.

No one test can be used to diagnose JRA. A doctor diagnoses JRA by carefully examining the patient and considering the patient's medical history and the results of laboratory tests that help rule out other conditions.

- *Symptoms:* One important consideration in diagnosing JRA is the length of time that symptoms have been present. Joint swelling or pain must last for at least 6 weeks for the doctor to consider a diagnosis of JRA. Because this factor is so important, it may be useful to keep a record of the symptoms, when they first appeared, and when they are worse or better.

- *Laboratory Tests:* Laboratory tests, usually blood tests, cannot by themselves provide the doctor with a clear diagnosis. But these tests can be used to help rule out other conditions and to help classify the type of JRA that a patient has. Blood may be taken to test for RF or ANA, and to determine the erythrocyte sedimentation rate (ESR).

  - ANA is found in the blood more often than RF, and both are found in only a small portion of JRA patients. The RF test helps the doctor tell the difference among the three types of JRA.

  - ESR is a test that measures how quickly red blood cells fall to the bottom of a test tube. Some people with rheumatic disease have an elevated ESR or "sed rate" (cells fall quickly to the bottom of the test tube), showing that there is inflammation in the body. Not all children with active joint inflammation have an elevated ESR.

- *X-Rays:* X-rays are needed if the doctor suspects injury to the bone or unusual bone development. Early in the disease, some x-rays can show cartilage damage. In general, x-rays are more useful later in the disease, when bones may be affected.

- *Other diseases:* Because there are many causes of joint pain and swelling, the doctor must rule out other conditions before diagnosing JRA. These include physical injury, bacterial infection, Lyme disease, inflammatory bowel disease, lupus, dermatomyositis, and some forms of cancer. The doctor may use additional laboratory tests to help rule out these and other possible conditions.

Who Treats Juvenile Rheumatoid Arthritis? What Are the Treatments?

A pediatrician, family physician, or other primary care doctor frequently manages the treatment of a child with JRA, often with the help of other doctors. Depending on the patient's and parents' wishes and the severity of the disease, the team of doctors may include pediatric rheumatologists (doctors specializing in childhood arthritis), ophthalmologists (eye doctors), orthopaedic surgeons (bone specialists), and physiatrists (rehabilitation specialists), as well as physical and occupational therapists.

The main goals of treatment are to preserve a high level of physical and social functioning and maintain a good quality of life. To achieve these goals, doctors recommend treatments to reduce swelling; maintain full movement in the affected joints; relieve pain; and identify, treat, and prevent complications. Most children with JRA need medication and physical therapy to reach these goals.

Several types of medication are available to treat JRA: nonsteroidal anti-inflammatory drugs (NSAIDs) which includes aspirin, ibuprofen, and naproxen sodium; disease-modifying anti-rheumatic drugs (DMARDs); methotrexate; and corticosteroids.

In addition to medications, physical therapy is an important part of a child's treatment plan. Exercise can help to maintain muscle tone and preserve and recover the range of motion of the joints. A physical therapist can design an appropriate exercise program for a person with JRA. The physical therapist also may recommend using splints and other devices to keep joints growing evenly.

How Can the Family Help a Child Live Well with JRA?

JRA affects the entire family who must cope with the special challenges of this disease. JRA can strain a child's participation in social and after-school activities and make school work more difficult. There are several things that family members can do to help the child do well physically and emotionally.

- Treat the child as normally as possible.

- Ensure that the child receives appropriate medical care and follows the doctor's instructions. Many treatment options are available, and because JRA is different in each child, what works for one may not work for another. If the medications that the doctor prescribes do not relieve symptoms or if they cause unpleasant side effects, patients and parents should discuss other choices with their doctor. A person with JRA can be more active when symptoms are controlled.

- Encourage exercise and physical therapy for the child. For many young people, exercise and physical therapy play important roles in treating JRA. Parents can arrange for children to participate in activities that the doctor recommends. During symptom-free periods, many doctors suggest playing team sports or doing other activities to help keep the joints strong and flexible and to provide play time with other children and encourage appropriate social development.

- Work closely with the school to develop a suitable lesson plan for the child and to educate the teacher and the child's classmates about JRA. Some children with JRA may be absent from school for prolonged periods and need to have the teacher send assignments home. Some minor changes such as an extra set of books, or leaving class a few minutes early to get to the next class on time can be a great help. With proper attention, most children progress normally through school.

- Explain to the child that getting JRA is nobody's fault. Some children believe that JRA is a punishment for something they did.

- Consider joining a support group. The American Juvenile Arthritis Organization runs support groups for people with JRA and their families. Support group meetings provide the chance to talk to other young people and parents of children with JRA and may help a child and the family cope with the condition.

Do Children with Juvenile Rheumatoid Arthritis Have to Limit Activities?

Although pain sometimes limits physical activity, exercise is important to reduce the symptoms of JRA and maintain function and range of motion of the joints. Most children with JRA can take part fully in physical activities and sports when their symptoms are under control. During a disease flare, however, the doctor may advise limiting certain activities depending on the joints involved. Once the flare is over, a child can start regular activities again.

Swimming is particularly useful because it uses many joints and muscles without putting weight on the joints. A doctor or physical therapist can recommend exercises and activities.

What Are Researchers Trying to Learn about Juvenile Rheumatoid Arthritis?

Scientists are investigating the possible causes of JRA. Researchers suspect that both genetic and environmental factors are involved in development of the disease and they are studying these factors in detail. To help explore the role of genetics, the National Institute of Arthritis and Musculoskeletal and Skin Diseases (NIAMS) has established a research registry for families in which two or more siblings have JRA. NIAMS also funds a Multipurpose Arthritis and Musculoskeletal Diseases Center (MAMDC) that specializes in research on pediatric rheumatic diseases including JRA.

Research doctors are continuing to try to improve existing treatments and find new medicines that will work better with fewer side effects. For example, researchers are studying the long-term effects of the use of methotrexate in children.

Chapter 21

Scoliosis in Children and Adolescents

What Is Scoliosis?

Scoliosis is a sideways curvature of the spine, or backbone. The bones that make up the spine are called vertebrae. Some people who have scoliosis require treatment. Other people, who have milder curves, may only need to visit their doctor for periodic observation. The section "Does Scoliosis Have to Be Treated?" describes how doctors decide whether or not to treat scoliosis.

Who Gets Scoliosis?

People of all ages can have scoliosis, but this chapter focuses on children and adolescents. Of every 1,000 children, 3 to 5 develop spinal curves that are considered large enough to need treatment. Adolescent idiopathic scoliosis (scoliosis of unknown cause) is the most common type and occurs after the age of 10. Girls are more likely than boys to have this type of scoliosis.

Since scoliosis can run in families, a child who has a parent, brother, or sister with idiopathic scoliosis should be checked regularly for scoliosis by the family physician.

Idiopathic scoliosis can also occur in children younger than 10 years of age, but is very rare. Early onset or infantile idiopathic scoliosis

Excerpted from "Questions and Answers about Scoliosis in Children and Adolescents," National Institute of Arthritis and Musculoskeletal and Skin Diseases (NIAMS), National Institutes of Health (NIH), http://www.nih.gov/ niams/healthinfo/scochild.htm, e-text posted October, 1998.

187

occurs in children less than 3 years old. It is more common in Europe than in the United States. Juvenile idiopathic scoliosis occurs in children between the ages of 3 and 10.

What Causes Scoliosis?

In 80 to 85 percent of people, the cause of scoliosis is unknown; this is called idiopathic scoliosis. Before concluding that a person has idiopathic scoliosis, the doctor looks for other possible causes, such as injury or infection. Causes of curves are classified as either nonstructural or structural.

- *Nonstructural (functional) scoliosis:* A structurally normal spine that appears curved. This is a temporary, changing curve. It is caused by an underlying condition such as a difference in leg length, muscle spasms, or inflammatory conditions such as appendicitis. Doctors treat this type of scoliosis by correcting the underlying problem.

- *Structural scoliosis:* A fixed curve that doctors treat case by case. Sometimes structural scoliosis is one part of a syndrome or disease, such as Marfan's syndrome, an inherited connective tissue disorder. In other cases it occurs by itself. Structural scoliosis can be caused by neuromuscular diseases (such as cerebral palsy, poliomyelitis, or muscular dystrophy), birth defects (such as hemivertebra, in which one side of a vertebra fails to form normally before birth), injury, certain infections, tumors (such as those caused by neurofibromatosis, a birth defect sometimes associated with benign tumors on the spinal column), metabolic diseases, connective tissue disorders, rheumatic diseases, or unknown factors (idiopathic scoliosis).

How Does the Doctor Diagnose Scoliosis?

The doctor takes the following steps to evaluate a patient for scoliosis: 1) medical history, 2) physical examination, 3) x-ray evaluation, 4) curve measurement (the doctor measures the spinal curve on the x-ray image).

Does Scoliosis Have to Be Treated? What Are the Treatments?

Many children who are sent to the doctor by a school scoliosis screening program have very mild spinal curves that do not need treatment. When a child does need treatment, the doctor may send him or her to an orthopedic spine specialist.

The doctor will suggest the best treatment for each patient based on the patient's age, how much more he or she is likely to grow, the degree and pattern of the curve, and the type of scoliosis. The doctor may recommend observation, bracing, or surgery.

- *Observation:* Doctors follow patients without treatment and re-examine them every 4 to 6 months when the patient is still growing (is skeletally immature) and has an idiopathic curve of less than 25 degrees.

- *Bracing:* Doctors advise patients to wear a brace to stop a curve from getting any worse when the patient has any of the following qualities (as a child nears the end of growth, the indications for bracing will depend on how the curve affects the child's appearance, whether the curve is getting worse, and the size of the curve):

    - is still growing and has an idiopathic curve that is more than 25 to 30 degrees.

    - has at least 2 years of growth remaining, has an idiopathic curve that is between 20 and 29 degrees, and, if a girl, has not had her first menstrual period.

    - is still growing and has an idiopathic curve between 20 and 29 degrees that is getting worse.

- *Surgery:* Doctors advise patients to have surgery to correct a curve or stop it from worsening when the patient is still growing, has a curve that is more than 45 degrees, and has a curve that is getting worse.

Are There Other Ways to Treat Scoliosis?

Some people have tried other ways to treat scoliosis, including manipulation by a chiropractor, electrical stimulation, dietary supplements, and corrective exercises. So far, studies of the following treatments have not been shown to prevent curve progression, or worsening:

- chiropractic manipulation
- electrical stimulation
- nutritional supplementation

- exercise: (Studies have shown that exercise alone will not stop progressive curves. However, patients may wish to exercise for the effects on their general health and well being.)

Which Brace Is Best?

The decision about which brace to wear depends on the type of curve and whether the patient will follow the doctor's directions about how many hours a day to wear the brace.

Braces can be custom made or can be made from a pre-fabricated mold. All must be selected for the specific curve problem and fitted to each patient. To have their intended effect (to keep a curve from getting worse), braces must be worn every day for the full number of hours prescribed by the doctor until the child stops growing.

Surgery

Patients and parents who are anticipating surgery may want to ask their doctor following questions:

- What are the benefits from surgery for scoliosis?

- What are the risks from surgery for scoliosis?

- What techniques will be used for the surgery?

- What devices will be used to keep the spine stable after surgery?

- Where will the incisions be made?

- How straight will the patient's spine be after surgery?

- How long will the hospital stay be?

- How long will it take to recover from surgery?

- Is there chronic back pain after surgery for scoliosis?

- Will the patient's growth be limited?

- How flexible will the spine remain?

- Can the curve worsen or progress after surgery?

- Will additional surgery be likely?

- Will the patient be able to do all the things he or she wants to do following surgery?

Can People with Scoliosis Exercise?

Exercise does not make scoliosis worse. In fact, it is very important for all people, including those with scoliosis, to exercise and remain physically fit. Girls have a higher risk than boys of developing osteoporosis (a disorder that results in weak bones that can break easily) later in life. The risk of osteoporosis is reduced in women who exercise regularly all their lives; and weight-bearing exercise, such as walking, running, soccer, and gymnastics, increases bone density and helps prevent osteoporosis. For both boys and girls, exercising and participating in sports also improves their general sense of well being.

Chapter 22

Asthma and Physical Activity in School

Introduction

Lifelong physical fitness is an important goal for all students. Yet students with asthma frequently restrict their physical activities—and about 1 child in every 15 has asthma. Much of this restriction is unnecessary—children with asthma can and should be physically active. This presents a challenge to classroom teachers, physical education teachers, and coaches.

What Is Asthma?

Asthma is a chronic lung condition with ongoing airway inflammation that results in recurring acute episodes (attacks) of breathing problems such as coughing, wheezing, chest tightness, and shortness of breath. These symptoms occur because the inflammation makes the airways overreact to a variety of stimuli including physical activity, upper respiratory infections, allergens, and irritants. Exposure to these stimuli—often called triggers—creates more swelling and blocking of the airways. Asthma episodes can be mild, moderate, or even life-threatening. Vigorous exercise will cause symptoms

"Asthma and Physical Activity in the School: Making a Difference," National Heart, Lung, and Blood Institute (NHLBI), National Institutes of Health (NIH), http://www.nhlbi.nih.gov/health/public/lung/asthma/phy_astr.htm, September 1995. Updated in February 2001 by Dr. David A. Cooke, MD, Diplomate, American Board of Internal Medicine.

for most students with asthma if their asthma is not well-controlled. Some students experience symptoms only when they exercise. However, today's treatments can successfully control asthma so that students can participate fully in physical activities most of the time.

Asthma varies from student to student and often from season to season. This is why physical education teachers and coaches need to understand what asthma is and what the individual needs of their students are. At times, programs for students with asthma may need temporary modification, such as varying the type, length, and/or frequency of activity. At all times, students with asthma should be included in activities as much as possible. Remaining behind in the gym or library or frequently sitting on the bench can set the stage for teasing, loss of self-esteem, unnecessary restriction of activity, and low levels of physical fitness.

Helping Students Control Their Asthma

Getting control of asthma means recognizing asthma triggers (the factors that make asthma worse or cause an asthma episode), avoiding or controlling these triggers, following an asthma management plan, and having convenient access to asthma medications. It also means modifying physical activities to match the students' current asthma status.

Recognize Asthma Triggers

Asthma Triggers

- exercise—running or playing hard—especially in cold weather
- upper respiratory infections—colds or flu
- laughing or crying hard
- allergens
- pollens—from trees, plants and grasses, including freshly cut grass
- animal dander from pets with fur or feathers
- dust and dust mites—in carpeting, pillows and upholstery
- cockroach droppings
- molds
- irritants

- cold air
- strong smells and chemical sprays, including perfumes, paint and cleaning solutions, chalk dust, lawn and turf treatments
- weather changes
- cigarette and other tobacco smoke

Each student with asthma has a list of triggers that can make his or her condition worse—that is, that increase airway inflammation and/or make the airways constrict, which makes breathing difficult.

Avoid or Control Asthma Triggers

Some asthma triggers—like pets with fur or feathers—can be avoided. Others—like physical exercise—are important for good health and should be controlled rather than avoided.

Actions to Consider

Identify students' known asthma triggers and eliminate as many as possible. For example, keep animals with fur out of the classroom. Consult the students' asthma management plans for guidance (see the next section).

Follow the Asthma Management Plan

A student's asthma management plan is developed by the student, parent/guardian, and health care provider. Depending on the student's needs, the plan may be a brief information card or a more extensive individualized health plan (IHP). The following section lists what asthma plans typically contain. A copy of the plan should be on file in the school office or health services office, with additional copies for the student's teachers and coaches. The plan—as well as the student's asthma medications—should be easily available for all on- and off-site activities before, during and after school.

Supporting and encouraging each student's efforts to follow his or her asthma management plan is essential for the student's active participation in physical activities. Students with asthma need understanding from both teachers and students in dealing with their asthma. If students with asthma are teased about their condition, they may be embarrassed, avoid using their medication, or cut class. If students with asthma are encouraged to "tough it out," they may risk health problems or just give up.

Ensure That Students with Asthma Have Convenient Access to Their Medications

Many students with asthma require two different medications: one for daily control and prevention, the other to treat and relieve symptoms. These medications are usually taken by metered-dose inhaler. Preventive asthma medications are taken daily and usually can be scheduled for before and after school hours. However, some students may need to take preventive daily medication during school hours. All students with asthma need to have their medication that relieves symptoms available at school in case of unexpected exposure to asthma triggers, or an asthma episode. In addition, students with asthma often benefit from using their inhaled medication 5–10 minutes before exercise. If accessing the medication is difficult, inconvenient, or embarrassing, the student may be discouraged and fail to use the inhaler as needed. The student's asthma may become unnecessarily worse and his or her activities needlessly limited.

Modify Physical Activities to Match Current Asthma Status

Students who follow their asthma management plans and keep their asthma under control can usually participate vigorously in the full range of sports and physical activities. Activities that are more intense and sustained—such as long periods of running, basketball, and soccer—are more likely to provoke asthma symptoms or an asthma episode. However, Olympic medallists with serious asthma have demonstrated that these activities are possible with good asthma management.

When a student experiences asthma symptoms, or is recovering from a recent asthma episode, exercise should be temporarily modified in type, length, and/or frequency to help reduce the risk of further symptoms. The student also needs convenient access to his or her medications.

Actions to Consider

- Include adequate warm-up and cool-down periods. These help prevent or lessen episodes of exercise-induced asthma.

- Consult the student's asthma management plan, parent/guardian, or health care provider on the type and length of any limitations. Assess the student and school resources to determine how the student can participate most fully.

- Remember that a student who experiences symptoms or who has just recovered from an asthma episode is at even greater risk for additional asthma problems. Take extra care. Observe for asthma symptoms, and check the student's peak flow if he or she uses a peak flow meter. Review the student's asthma management plan if there are any questions.

- Monitor the environment for potential allergens and irritants, for example, a recently mowed field or refinished gym floor. If an allergen or irritant is present, consider a temporary change in location.

- Make exercise modifications as necessary to get appropriate levels of participation. For example, if running is scheduled, the student could walk the whole distance, run part of the distance, alternate running and walking.

- Keep the student involved when any temporary but major modification is required. Ask the student to act, for example, as a scorekeeper, timer, or equipment handler until he or she can return to full participation. Dressing for a physical education class and participating at any level is better than being left out or left behind.

Recognizing Symptoms and Taking Appropriate Action

Recognizing asthma symptoms and taking appropriate action in response to the symptoms is crucial to asthma treatment and control.

Symptoms That Require Prompt Action

Acute symptoms require prompt action to help students resume their activities as soon as possible. Prompt action is also required to prevent an episode from becoming more serious or even life-threatening. The following section lists the symptoms that indicate an acute asthma episode and the need for immediate action. The student's asthma plan and the school's emergency plan should be easily accessible so that all staff, substitutes, volunteers, and aides know what to do.

Acute Symptoms Requiring Prompt Action

- coughing or wheezing
- difficulty in breathing

197

- chest tightness or pressure—reported by the student

- other signs, such as low peak flow readings as indicated on the asthma management plan

Symptoms of exercise-induced asthma (coughing, wheezing, pain or chest tightness) may last several minutes to an hour or more. These symptoms are quite different from breathlessness (deep, rapid breathing) that quickly returns to normal after aerobic exercise.

Actions to Take

- Stop the student's current activity.

- Follow the student's asthma management/action plan.

- Help the student use his or her inhaled medication.

- Observe for effect.

Get Emergency Help

- if the student fails to improve

- if any of the symptoms listed on the student's asthma plan as emergency indicators are present

- if any of the following symptoms are present (consider calling 911):

  - the student is hunched over, with shoulders lifted, and straining to breathe

  - the student has difficulty completing a sentence without pausing for breath

  - the student's lips or fingernails turn blue

Signs That May Indicate Poorly Controlled Asthma

Students may have symptoms that do not indicate an acute episode needing immediate treatment, but instead indicate that their asthma is not under complete control. The following is a list of these signs.

- a persistent cough

- coughing, wheezing, chest tightness, or shortness of breath after vigorous physical activity, on a recurring basis

- low level of stamina during physical activity or reluctance to participate

The teachers and coaches who supervise students' physical activities are in a unique position to notice signs that a child who struggles with physical activity might in fact have asthma. Because exercise provokes symptoms in most children with poorly controlled asthma, the student may need to be evaluated by his or her health care provider. It may also be that the student simply needs to follow his or her asthma management plan more carefully.

Actions to Consider

- Share observations of the symptoms with the school nurse and the student's parents or guardians. Helping students get the medical attention they need is an important way to help children become active and take control of their condition.

- Provide students convenient access to their asthma medication.

Confusing Signs: Is It an Asthma Episode or a Need for More Support?

At some times teachers and coaches may wonder if a student's reported symptoms indicate a desire for attention or a desire not to participate in an activity. At other times it may seem that students are overreacting to minimal symptoms.

It is always essential to respect the student's report of his or her own condition. If a student regularly asks to be excused from recess or avoids physical activity, a real physical problem may be present. It also may be that the student needs more assistance and support from his or her teacher and coach in order to become an active participant.

Actions to Consider

- Talk with the student to:
  - learn his or her concerns about asthma and activity.
  - offer reassurance that you understand the importance of appropriate modifications or activity limits.
  - develop a shared understanding about the conditions that require activity modifications or medications.

- Consult with the school nurse, parent/guardian, or health care provider to find ways to ensure that the student is safe, feels safe, and is encouraged to participate actively.

- If the student uses a peak flow meter, remind him or her to use it. This may help the student appreciate his or her asthma status and appropriate levels of activity.

Peak Flow Monitoring

There are different types of peak flow meters available. A peak flow meter is a small device that measures how well air moves out of the airways. Monitoring peak flow helps a student determine changes in his or her asthma and identify appropriate actions to take.

Each student has his or her personal best peak flow reading. This number should be noted in the student's asthma plan or school health file. A peak flow reading of less than 80 percent of the student's personal best indicates the need for action. A student should avoid running and playing until the peak flow reading returns or exceeds 80 percent of the personal best.

A peak flow reading is only one indicator of asthma problems. Symptoms such as coughing, wheezing, and chest tightness are also indicators of worsening asthma. Follow the student's individual plan or the school plan if you observe any of the signs or symptoms listed in the asthma emergency section or in the student's own plan.

Chapter 23

Minimizing the Risk of Injury in High School Athletics

Sports Injury Prevention, Children and Adolescents

Each year, more than 775,000 children under age 15 are treated in hospital emergency rooms for sports injuries. In fact, sports injuries are the number one reason for emergency department visits among children. Many of these injuries can be prevented if parents get involved and make sure their children wear protective gear, follow the rules of play, and are physically and emotionally prepared to play the sport.

Tips for Preventing Sports Injuries

To help your child avoid sports injuries, follow these safety tips from the American Academy of Pediatrics, the American Academy of Orthopaedic Surgeons, the National SAFE KIDS Campaign, and other sports and health organizations.

- Before your child starts a training program or enters a competition, take him or her to the doctor for a physical exam. The doctor can help assess any special injury risks your child may have.

This chapter contains text from "Sports Injury Prevention, Children and Adolescents," Centers for Disease Control and Prevention (CDC), SafeUSA website, http://www.cdc.gov/safeusa/sports/child.htm, last updated July 12, 2001, and "Minimizing the Risk of Injury in High School Athletics," National Athletic Trainers' Association (NATA), http://www.nata.org/publications/brochures/minimizingtherisks.htm, May 5, 2000, copyright 2000 NATA, reprinted with permission.

- Make sure your child wears all the required safety gear every time he or she plays and practices. Know how the sports equipment should fit your child and how to use it. If you're not sure, ask the coach or a sporting goods expert for help. Set a good example—if you play a sport, wear your safety gear, too.

- Insist that your child warm up and stretch before playing, paying special attention to the muscles that will get the most use during play (for example, a pitcher should focus on warming up the shoulder and arm).

- Teach your child not to play through pain. If your child gets injured, see your doctor. Follow all the doctor's orders for recovery, and get the doctor's OK before your child returns to play.

- Make sure first aid is available at all games and practices.

- Talk to and watch your child's coach. Coaches should enforce all the rules of the game, encourage safe play, and understand the special injury risks that young players face.

- If you're not sure if it's safe for your child to perform a certain technique or move (such as heading a soccer ball or diving off the highest platform), ask your pediatrician and the coach about it.

- Above all, keep sports fun. Putting too much focus on winning can make your child push too hard and risk injury.

How do you know if your child is ready to play a sport? The American Academy of Pediatrics recommends that you wait until your child is six years old to play team sports. Most children younger than that don't understand the concept of team play. With older children, you should decide if it's OK for them to play based on their physical and emotional development and their eagerness to play. Your child's doctor can help you make this decision. Remember, pushing children to play a sport before they're ready, or when they don't want to, can increase their risk of getting hurt.

Who Is Affected?

Close to 6 million high school students play team sports, and another 20 million children take part in recreational or competitive sports out of school. Sports activities help children and adolescents stay fit, learn about teamwork, and develop self-confidence. But playing a sport also brings the risk of injury. Each year, over 775,000 children under age 15 are treated in hospital emergency departments for sports-related injuries. About 80 percent of these injuries are from playing football, basketball, baseball, or soccer.

Most sports-related injuries in children—about two-thirds of them—are sprains (involving ligaments, which connect one bone to another) and strains (involving muscles). Only 5 percent of sports injuries involve broken bones. The majority of injuries are mild, but they can cause great inconveniences for both children and their parents during the healing process. And if not allowed to heal properly, a minor injury can become a more serious one that interferes with proper growth and causes life-long problems.

Minimizing the Risk of Injury in High School Athletics

Athletics are an important part of the high school experience for many students. Sports can provide a positive learning environment that will help student-athletes in many aspects of their lives. And like pep rallies, Friday night football, and cross-town rivalries—injuries are an inevitable part of high school athletics regardless of the preventive measures taken. Students can, however, reduce their risk of injury by following several basic steps. One of the most important is proper overall conditioning, which can also enhance rehabilitation and shorten the "down time" of athletes.

The following guidelines have been developed based on interviews with a number of certified athletic trainers around the country. This listing is not all-inclusive, but is designed to provide guidance.

In addition to these general guidelines, the National Athletic Trainers' Association encourages all athletes to develop the specific skills involved in their sport and to be aware of the rules governing their athletic endeavors.

It is essential to remember that medical, legal, financial, and professional standards, limitations, and requirements change continually and vary from place to place, person to person and setting to setting. These guidelines must not, therefore, be taken to represent uniformly applicable national standards.

General Guidelines

Every student-athlete should receive a pre-participation physical exam, including a general exam and an orthopedic exam. The general exam should include checks on height, weight, blood pressure, pulse, respiration, eye, ear, nose, chest, and abdomen. The orthopedic exam should focus on joint flexibility, joint range of motion, and a re-examination of past bone and joint injuries.

Athletes should work with athletic trainers and coaches year-round to ensure they maintain their condition with appropriate exercises and nutrition. In addition, athletes should engage in appropriate conditioning programs for a minimum of six weeks before the start of daily practice.

Athletes should focus on developing muscular strength and endurance, cardiovascular fitness, and flexibility.

Good nutritional practices incorporate the basic food groups: grains, fruits and vegetables, dairy, and meat/poultry/fish. Athletes' diets should be high in complex carbohydrates while also including essential proteins and fats.

Athletes practicing or playing in warmer climates should become acclimatized to high levels of activity in hot weather. Practice should be held early in the morning or late in the afternoon.

Limit workouts and practices to no more than two hours.

The night before an event, athletes should hydrate with electrolyte fluids to reduce the risk of dehydration.

Fluid breaks should be offered at least every 45 minutes, and athletes should be entitled to unrestricted amounts of fluids to help prevent dehydration and other forms of heat-related illness.

All athletes should use appropriate equipment that fits properly. This equipment should be checked before and after each use to ensure that it is in proper working condition, and replaced or repaired immediately if any problems are noted.

Appropriate protective equipment should be worn in all practices as well as during competitions.

Shoes should fit appropriately and provide the necessary support for each individual sport.

Foot diseases, such as athlete's foot, should be treated immediately and fully to avoid more extensive problems.

Mouth guards should be used in all collision sports, including ice hockey, football and rugby; and recommended for all sports where contact could occur, including basketball, baseball, lacrosse, soccer, etc. Not only do they help to prevent dental injuries, but they can also absorb shocks from blows to the jaw or head and reduce the severity of these blows.

Players should stretch properly before and after workouts of any kind.

A minimum 15-minute warm-up period before any game or practice, and an appropriate cool-down period afterward, is recommended. Athletes should also warm up for five minutes during any prolonged breaks in activity (including half time, between periods, etc.).

Ice should be available on the sidelines of every game and practice to apply to appropriate injuries.

Injuries involving bones or joints should be examined by a licensed physician.

All injuries should be evaluated immediately.

Parents should be aware of who is responsible for injury care at their child's school. Parents should ask if this person is qualified to handle all injuries and provide proper instruction and rehabilitation, as well as whether he or she is available for both practice and games.

Every school with an athletic program should have a written emergency plan which is reviewed regularly and addresses every level of medical care for injured athletes.

Every school should be encouraged to develop an Injury Protection Manual, which answers any questions a parent may have about the way an injury is to be handled and who will be primarily responsible. The school should distribute this manual to all athletes' parents.

The athletic department should be encouraged to have an Emergency Medical Authorization Card on file for every athlete. This card gives parental permission for emergency medical care if it is required. The card should include name, address, parents' home and work phone numbers, etc.

The athletic department should be encouraged to have parents sign a waiver that indicates they are aware of the inherent risk of injury to their children.

Coaches should be certified in first aid and CPR and, where possible, earn a state- or nationally-approved certificate to coach specific sports.

All individuals involved in the athletes' health and safety—including athletic trainers, coaches, physicians, emergency medical personnel (paramedics and EMTs), school administrators and parents—should be encouraged to maintain cooperative liaisons.

Football-Specific Guidelines

- Intentional spearing of opponents should be discouraged.

- Blocking below the waist should be minimized during practice.

- Block and tackle with the head up to reduce the risk of neck injuries.

- In addition to total strengthening and conditioning, football-specific conditioning exercises should strengthen the neck to allow players to keep their heads firmly erect while making contact during blocks or tackles.

- Make sure the practice and playing areas are safe. Look for holes, broken glass, and other hazards on and around the practice field, game field and blocking sleds.

- Ample fluid replacement should be available at all times.

Basketball-Specific Guidelines

- Players should focus on conditioning exercises for the total body, including upper and lower extremities.

- Players should focus on good warm-up and stretching prior to any ballistic movements.

- Footwear should fit properly to minimize the risk of ankle- and foot-related injuries.

- Replace footwear when the shock absorption is no longer adequate.

Soccer-Specific Guidelines

- Players should be encouraged to wear appropriate shin guards during practice and play.

- Provide fluids on the sidelines throughout practice and games. Although soccer requires non-stop play with no time outs, athletes should be encouraged to come to the sidelines or touch line where they can replenish fluids without penalty.

- Warm up for approximately 15 minutes, beginning for half that time without a ball. Warm-up exercises should include light jogging and stretching. Without these warm-ups, the explosive action of shooting can result in strained muscles.

- Adhere to the rules of the game when tackling.

- Although soccer does not provide time outs, injuries should be evaluated immediately to ensure the athlete is not worsening the injury.

Baseball/Softball-Specific Guidelines

- Most injuries in baseball and softball involve the throwing arm and shoulder, but these injuries usually result through a gradual process. Athletes should not abuse the throwing arm by overusing it.

- Players should incorporate conditioning and stretching exercises for the shoulder into their overall program.

- It is to the player's advantage to warm up and cool down the throwing arm properly to minimize the risk of injuries.

- Condition all shoulder muscles, emphasizing muscles in the back of the shoulder that are required to stop the pitching motion. Muscles in the front of the arm are naturally stronger— shoulder injuries can result from weaker muscles in the back.

Track and Field-Specific Guidelines

- Stretching is key to minimizing the risk of injury in every event.

- Conditioning programs should concentrate on muscular strength, muscular endurance, and flexibility. Individual event training should be emphasized.

- All athletes involved in running events should work to maintain year-round cardiovascular endurance.

- Before and after each event, athletes should warm up and cool down, stretch, and hydrate with fluids.

- Special attention should be paid to the nutritional needs of the endurance athlete.

Wrestling-Specific Guidelines

- Depleting food and fluid to make a particular weight class may be detrimental to the health and safety of the athlete. Body composition and weight loss should be closely monitored.

- Wrestlers should be encouraged to wear protective headgear that provides ear protection.

- Wrestlers should be encouraged to wear protective knee pads.

- To reduce the risk of skin diseases, wrestlers should shower before and after workouts; wash their workout clothes daily; dry their skin adequately; clean mats daily; avoid wearing street shoes on wrestling mats or wrestling shoes off the mats; wipe headgear down with alcohol pads after each use; and conduct daily total body skin inspections.

- Wrestlers with open wounds, broken skin or diseases of the skin should be discouraged from participating until the skin is healed or the wrestler has been cleared to participate by a licensed physician. If allowed to wrestle, the athlete should have the affected skin covered to prevent cross-contamination.

- Proper strength and conditioning regimes should be encouraged.

Volleyball-Specific Guidelines

- An overall strength base with emphasis on leg, back, and posterior shoulder (rotator cuff) strengthening during pre-season is vital.

- Proper equipment should include volleyball-specific shoes and knee pads for shock absorption.

- A proper warm-up and stretching program should emphasize the shoulder, low back, and legs. Do not start spiking before warm-up stretching for the shoulder. After stretching, start throwing a volleyball easily, gradually increasing intensity until the muscles are warm.

- Advanced drills and conditioning, such as plyometrics or jump training, should not be conducted unless the athlete has been tested and can demonstrate balance, flexibility, and strength.

- Ample fluid replacement should be available at all times.

Chapter 24

Should Teens Go on Diets?

What do the hula hoop, "high-protein diets," and wearing your clothes backwards have in common? They are all fads. Fads come and go, but when it comes to fad diets, the health effects can be permanent—especially for teenagers.

Not all teens who go on diets need to lose weight. Pressure from friends—and sometimes parents—to be very slim may create a distorted body image. Having a distorted body image is like looking into a funhouse mirror: You see yourself as fatter than you are.

A national survey of 11,631 high school students conducted by the national Centers for Disease Control and Prevention found that more than a third of the girls considered themselves overweight, compared with fewer than 15 percent of the boys. More than 43 percent of the girls reported that they were on a diet—and a quarter of these dieters didn't think they were overweight. The survey found that the most common dieting methods used were skipping meals, taking diet pills, and inducing vomiting after eating.

"The teenage years are a period of rapid growth and development," points out Ronald Kleinman, M.D., chief of the Pediatric Gastrointestinal and Nutrition Unit of Massachusetts General Hospital in Boston. He explains that fad dieting can keep teenagers from getting the

Excerpted from Ruth Papazian, "On the Teen Scene: Should You Go on a Diet," *FDA Consumer*, September 1993, http://www.fda.gov/opacom/catalog/ots_diet.html, Food and Drug Administration (FDA) Pub. No. 97-1214. The version below is from a reprint of the original article and contains revisions made in May 1994 and May 1997.

calories and nutrients they need to grow properly and that dieting can retard growth. Stringent dieting may cause girls to stop menstruating, and will prevent boys from developing muscles, he says. If the diet doesn't provide enough calcium, phosphorus and vitamin D, bones may not lay down enough calcium. This may increase the risk of osteoporosis later in life, although more studies are needed to confirm this.

Instead of dieting because "everyone" is doing it or because you are not as thin as you want to be, first find out from a doctor or nutritionist whether you are carrying too much body fat for your age and height.

What If You Need to Lose Weight?

The flip side to feeling pressured to be thin is having legitimate concerns about overweight that adults dismiss by saying, "It's just baby fat" or "You'll grow into your weight." Most girls reach almost their full height once they start to menstruate, notes Kleinman. Although boys usually don't stop growing until age 18, data from a study suggest that adolescent obesity can carry serious lifelong health consequences for them.

The study, which followed the medical histories of 508 people from childhood to age 70, found that men who had been overweight teenagers were more likely to develop colon cancer and to suffer fatal heart attacks and strokes than their thinner classmates. Women who had been overweight teens had an increased tendency to develop clogged arteries (atherosclerosis) and arthritis. By age 70, these problems made it difficult for them to walk more than a quarter mile, lift heavy objects, or climb stairs.

While this study linked adolescent obesity to health problems decades down the road, some adverse effects show up much earlier. Sometimes teens develop high blood pressure, elevated cholesterol, and conditions that often precede diabetes. Also, as Kleinman points out, "The longer in adolescence you remain overweight, the greater the likelihood that the problem will persist into adulthood."

As with most everything else, there's a right way and a wrong way to lose weight. The wrong way is to skip meals, resolve to eat nothing but diet bread and water, take diet pills, or make yourself vomit. You may make it through the end of the week and maybe even lose a pound or two, but you're unlikely to keep the weight off for more than a few months—if that. And inducing vomiting can lead to an eating disorder called bulimia, which can result in serious health problems.

"The more you deprive yourself of the foods you love, the more you will crave those foods. Inevitably, you'll break down and binge," says

Jo Ann Hattner, a clinical dietitian at Packard Children's Hospital in Palo Alto, Calif. Then you'll not only gain those pounds back, you'll likely add a couple more.

Experts call this cycle of weight loss and weight gain "yo-yo" dieting. Obesity researchers believe that truly overweight people should continue to try to control their weight because studies are inconclusive on whether weight cycling is harmful, according to the National Institute of Diabetes and Digestive and Kidney Diseases. In contrast, the health risks from being overweight are well-known. Although the yo-yo effect may not hurt future weight-loss efforts, you need to make lifelong changes in eating behavior, diet, and physical activity.

Additionally, low-calorie diets that allow only a few types of foods can be bad for your health because they don't allow you to get enough vitamins and minerals. Kleinman warns that rapid weight loss from very-low-calorie "starvation diets" can cause serious effects in teenagers, such as gallstones, hair loss, weakness, and diarrhea.

Diet Pills

In 1992, The Food and Drug Administration (FDA) banned 111 ingredients in over-the-counter (OTC) diet products—including amino acids, cellulose, and grapefruit extract—after manufacturers were unable to prove that they worked. A number of products (Cal-Ban 3000, Cal-Lite 1000, Cal-Trim 5000, Perma Slim, Bodi Trim, Dictol 7 Plus, Medi Thin, Nature's Way, and East Indian Guar Gum) were also recalled because they posed serious health risks. The products contained guar gum, which supposedly swelled in the stomach to provide a feeling of fullness. However, the swelling from the guar gum caused blockages in the throat and stomach.

In February 1996, FDA also proposed new warning labels for OTC diet pills containing phenylpropanolamine (PPA), including the statement that the product is "For use by people 18 years of age and older."

PPA is an ingredient found not only in many OTC diet pills but also in cough-cold and allergy products as well. FDA is concerned PPA may possibly increase the risk of a type of stroke (hemorrhagic) caused by bleeding into the brain, as was suggested by some reports of bleeding in the brain among PPA users, typically young women. This possible risk could be further increased if a person took more than the recommended dose of PPA, which might occur inadvertently from also taking a cough-cold product with PPA.

While FDA agrees that studies have not shown a definite link between PPA and stroke, the agency believes data from a more comprehensive study are needed to confirm the ingredient's safety. As a result, the OTC drug industry began a five-year study in 1994.

Michael Weintraub, M.D, director of FDA's Office of Drug Evaluation V, says, "PPA is not recommended for use by teenagers also because they are still growing and if they suppress their appetite, they may not get proper nutrition." The author of studies on PPA published in scientific journals, Weintraub adds, "This is especially true of teens who don't need to lose weight but think that they do."

The Real Skinny on Weight Loss

If going to extremes won't do the trick, what will? Believe it or not, it's as simple as making a few changes in your eating habits to emphasize healthy foods and exercise—good advice even if you don't need to lose weight.

Hattner describes a good diet as one that has balance, variety and moderation in food choices. She suggests using the U.S. Department of Agriculture's "Food Pyramid." These guidelines call for six to 11 servings a day of grains (bread, cereal, rice and pasta), three to five servings of vegetables, two to four servings of fruit, and two to three servings each of dairy (milk, cheese and yogurt) and protein-rich foods (meat, eggs, poultry, fish, dry beans, and nuts).

"The most important dietary change you can make is to limit the amount of high-fat foods that you eat," she adds. "Balance your favorite foods [which are usually high in fat] with fruits and vegetables [which are almost always very low in fat]; eat a wide variety of foods to keep from getting bored and to make sure your diet is nutritionally sound; and keep portion sizes reasonable so that you can have your [thin] slice of cake and lose weight, too."

To keep fat intake down, Hattner recommends making simple lower fat substitutions for the foods that you eat: Switch to 1 percent or skim milk instead of whole milk, nonfat or low-fat frozen yogurt or nonfat or low-fat ice cream instead of regular ice cream, and pretzels instead of corn chips. High-fat foods such as french fries, candy bars, and milkshakes that have no low-fat substitutes should only be eaten once in a while or in very small amounts.

Move It and Lose It

Whether you are overweight or not, regular exercise (at least three times a week) is important to look and feel your best. If you do need to lose weight, stepping up your activity level will cause you to burn calories more quickly and help make weight loss easier.

"Exercise increases lean body weight. Also, you will appear slimmer as you develop your muscles because muscles give shape and form to your body," notes Hattner.

Fad or starvation diets and diet pills offer temporary solutions, at best. At worst, they may jeopardize your health. According to Weintraub, "The safest way for teenagers to control their weight is to eat a healthy, low-fat diet and get enough exercise."

—by Ruth Papazian

Ruth Papazian is a writer in Bronx, New York.

Chapter 25

Hope for Overweight Teens

Twenty-five percent of US children are overweight or at risk for becoming overweight, and that number is increasing rapidly, according to The National Institutes of Health. The city of Birmingham, Alabama serves as a microcosm: In Birmingham, 23 percent of African-American girls and 10 percent of Anglo girls are obese by age 5, and 13 percent of African-American boys and 6 percent of Anglo boys are obese at this same age, reports Reinaldo Figueroa-Colon, M.D. while studying increased blood pressure in elementary school-aged children. And kids often aren't losing their excess weight by adolescence.

"Teenage obesity is complex in that both the potential physical and psychosocial consequences of obesity at this age need to be taken into account," says Dianne Neumark-Sztainer, Chair of the Public Health Nutrition Program, School of Public Health, University of Minnesota.

It also hurts parents, such as New York City mom Laura Vik, to see their teens in physical or emotional distress. "My 17-year-old son is 6 feet tall and weights around 300 pounds," Vik says. "He's always tired and complaining about his bad knee hurting when he walks." Vik's overweight daughter, Kari, faced name-calling from teenaged peers. But more than just ridicule, teenage obesity can lead to increased risk for cardiovascular disease, diabetes, and other serious health disorders.

Kendeyl Johansen, TeenagersToday.com, http://teenagerstoday.com/resources/articles/overweight.htm, copyright 1999-2001 iParenting, LLC. Reprinted with permission.

How did this overweight epidemic start and how can parents fight it? Experts blame the rise in obesity on unhealthy food choices and increasingly sedentary lifestyles. A recent study published in the American Journal of Health Promotion found that students decreased their consumption of breakfast, fruits, vegetables, and milk as they moved from elementary to junior high and middle school. Between the third to the eighth grades, fruit consumption fell by 41 percent and vegetable consumption dropped by 25 percent. Soft drink consumption tripled, often at the expense of healthier alternatives, such as milk and fruit juice.

School Interventions

Neumark-Sztainer champions the need for effective weight control programs aimed at the prevention of obesity in children. She recently divided teens into several focus groups, asking hard questions such as: If you were designing a weight control program aimed at healthy weight control, healthy eating and increased exercise, what would you do? What activities? When? Where? She also asked if programs should include all kids or only overweight kids.

Teens across the board wanted fun, interactive activities—such as in-line skating, aerobics, and yoga—within a supportive environment. They asked for physical fitness facilities and programs to be available both during and after school hours and requested appealing, healthy foods. The teenagers recommended focusing on a healthy lifestyle instead of specific weight issues and offering programs to all students, regardless of weight, to avoid stigmatizing those with a problem. But some students did express concern over differences in athletic ability and perceived embarrassment between overweight and normal-weight teens.

"The focus group data will help us in planning programs that meet the needs of teenagers with weight concerns," says Neumark-Sztainer. Indeed, many of the above suggestions were incorporated into the "New Moves" program, currently undergoing a pilot test in Minneapolis. "New Moves" aims to help overweight girls function in a society that values thinness, to avoid unhealthy weight control practices and to maintain healthy eating and exercise habits. Researchers have implemented the program for overweight girls only, and for girls of mixed weights to assess the advantages and disadvantages of both programs.

How can parents get local schools to start programs such as "New Moves?" "The program is now being studied," Neumark-Sztainer says. "We hope that in the future it will be available to all schools."

Margaret Roiniotis of Chicago wants to see a program such as "New Moves" available for her overweight 11-year-old daughter. A nutritionist spoke at Roiniotis' parent/teacher organization last year but she feels her daughter's school could do more to help. "I really think there could be programs developed for kids who have a difficult time with sports," she says. "Maybe yoga, or something where you don't have to be a major athlete to compete. My daughter has asthma and she used to like swimming, but she is too self-conscious about how she looks in a swimsuit to do it very often now."

Linda Morris battles negative reinforcement from her son's high school. "My oldest son, who is a 6-foot, 4-inch sophomore and weighs 250 pounds, was recently told by the football coach that he would like to see him reach 275 to 300 pounds by the time he becomes a senior in high school." As a nurse, Morris was appalled by the coach's suggestion.

Eat Smart, but How?

"The development of permanent lifestyle changes is the main goal of pediatric weight management programs, not necessarily weight loss," says Deborah Bonnell, clinical nutritionist at Children's Hospital in Birmingham, Ala. "Adult weight management programs may be inappropriate for children, given their need for growth and development."

Bonnell encourages parents to set a positive example by practicing healthy living through diet and exercise. "A parent cannot expect their child to adhere to a healthy lifestyle if they, themselves, do not practice a healthy lifestyle." She adds that it's important to combat obesity in children early; obese adolescents often become obese adults.

Bonnell recommends that families stick to three meals and two or three snacks per day with age-appropriate serving sizes of food. Meals should consist of three to four food servings and snacks should be smaller portions of one or two servings. "No food is out of the question; it depends on how often and how much you consume a high-fat, high-sugary food. Moderation is the key," she says.

Bonnell offers several suggestions for teen-friendly snacks:

- non-starchy vegetables such as carrots, celery, and broccoli dipped in fat-free salad dressings

- sugar-free gelatin prepared with canned mixed fruit in its own juice

- half of a bagel with fat-free or light cream cheese or jelly

- baked chips with fat-free dip

- bagel pizza made with reduced-fat shredded cheeses and turkey pepperoni

Fight for Fitness

Losing weight and choosing a healthy lifestyle are difficult for teens who may feel defeated by obesity so early in life. But 16-year-old Kari Vik battled her weight and won. Kari walked, rode her bike and cut down on junk food consumption to drop from a size 14 to a size 7. She offers advice for parents who want to help their overweight kids: "Walk and exercise with them. Try to help them eat right. Give the support they need and tell them daily [that] they are doing good." She says she wants schools to teach the risks of being overweight in health classes and offer teenagers more healthy foods. She'd also like longer gym periods and exercise classes such as aerobics.

There are several ways parents can help teens slim down. Crystel Riggs of Clemson, South Carolina has taught her overweight daughter about fat grams, calories, and serving sizes, and she helps her daughter maintain a healthy diet. Roiniotis encourages her 11-year-old to exercise and eat healthy foods, resulting in weight loss by munching on carrots with low-calorie dressing, drinking peach iced-tea and participating in camp sports.

The changes shouldn't only happen in the home; parents can help fight childhood obesity by encouraging schools to offer a variety of physical activities, healthy food choices and weight intervention programs. Experts suggest parents lobby the local Parent-Teacher Association or pick up the phone and ask what the school is doing to help overweight kids. Also, they say, check with local health care organizations to find healthy lifestyle programs tailored to children.

—by Kendeyl Johansen

Kendeyl Johansen lives in Utah with her Norwegian husband, Lars. When not chasing her three sons, she's skiing on water or snow.

Chapter 26

Using Over-the-Counter Medications Wisely

Pharmacy shelves are filled with medicines you can buy without a prescription. But teens should be aware that just because a drug is available over the counter (often abbreviated OTC), that doesn't mean it's always free of side effects. On the contrary, you need to take OTC drugs with much the same caution as drugs prescribed by your doctor. Special care is necessary if you use more than one of these products at the same time, or if you take an OTC product while also being treated with a prescription product. And there are some OTC drugs that shouldn't be taken by people with certain medical problems. If possible, teens should ask a parent, pharmacist or physician for advice before taking any OTC product you haven't used before.

Besides getting expert advice, the most important thing teens can do before buying an OTC drug is to read the label. The name of the product isn't always the same as the name of the drug it contains, and some products contain more than one ingredient. For example, a product for coughs and one for colds might each contain pseudoephedrine. A person taking both products at the same time might get too much of this ingredient.

Judith Levine Willis, "On the Teen Scene: Using Over-the-Counter Medications Wisely," *FDA Consumer*, November 1991. The version below is from a reprint of the original article and contains revisions made in May 1995, Food and Drug Administration (FDA) Pub. No. 95-3199, http://www.fda.gov/opacom/catalog/ots_otc.html. Updated in January, 2001 by Dr. David A. Cooke, MD, Diplomate, American Board of Internal Medicine.

There are also many dietary supplements, herbs, and vitamins sold OTC. Treat these with the same caution you would use with any medicine. Even "natural" products are not necessarily safe, and they can have side effects and drug interactions just like any other medicine.

Aspirin and Other Fever Reducers

Reading the label becomes especially important for teens when it comes to products containing aspirin (acetylsalicylic acid) or their chemical cousins, other salicylates, which are used to reduce fever or treat headaches and other pain. Teenagers (as well as children) should not take products containing aspirin or salicylates when they have chickenpox, flu, or symptoms that might be the flu (this includes most colds). Children and teenagers who take aspirin and other salicylates during these illnesses may develop a rare but life-threatening condition called Reye syndrome. (Symptoms usually occur near the end of the original illness and include severe tiredness, violent headache, disorientation, belligerence, and excessive vomiting.)

Acetaminophen (sold under brand names such as Datril and Tylenol) can also reduce fever and relieve pain and has not been associated with Reye syndrome. Remember, though, because fevers in most colds don't normally go above 100 degrees Fahrenheit and don't cause much discomfort, you usually don't have to take any drug for the fever. If you think you have a cold but your temperature is running higher, consult your doctor because you might have flu or a bacterial infection.

Acetaminophen is a very safe medicine, and is usually the best choice for teens. Read the label carefully for dosing, however. Acetaminophen, if taken in overdose, can cause severe liver poisoning. Many teens each year die or need liver transplants from taking too much acetaminophen. As long as you don't exceed the maximum dose listed on the bottle, you shouldn't need to worry about problems from this very useful medicine.

Sniffle and Cough Combinations

OTC drugs to relieve stuffy noses often contain more than one ingredient. Some of these products are marketed for allergy relief and others for colds. They usually contain both an antihistamine and a nasal decongestant. The decongestant ingredient unstuffs nasal passages; antihistamines dry up a runny nose. But some of these products may also contain aspirin or acetaminophen, and some contain a decongestant alone. Some of these drugs are "extended-release" or "long-acting" preparations that continue to work for up to 12 hours. Others are immediate-release products and usually work for four to six hours. Again, it's important to read the label—and check with the pharmacist—to be sure you're getting the right product for your symptoms.

Most antihistamines can cause drowsiness, while many decongestants have the opposite effect. Still, it's hard to predict whether any one product will make you sleepy or keep you awake—or neither—because reactions to drugs can vary from one person to another. So it's best not to drive or operate machinery until you find out how the drug affects you. In addition, alcohol, sedatives and tranquilizers intensify the drowsiness effect of antihistamines, so it's best not to take them at the same time unless a doctor tells you to.

Some brand names of products containing both antihistamines and decongestants are Allerest, Actifed and Dimetapp. Brand names of products that contain only antihistamines include Dimetane, Chlor-Trimeton and Benadryl. But you should be aware that closely related products with similar names may have other ingredients—pointing up again the importance of reading the label so you'll know what you're getting. For example, Chlortrimeton Non-Drowsy Decongestant and Dimetapp Decongestant contain decongestants but no antihistamines, while Actifed Plus, Dimetapp Cold & Flu, and Benadryl Allergy Sinus Headache contain antihistamines, decongestants and acetaminophen.

If you decide you want to try to relieve nasal stuffiness without pills, there are other medications in the form of nasal drops and sprays sold OTC for this purpose. As with pills, some of these are long acting (up to 12 hours) and some are shorter acting. And, as with pills, most have some side effects. Many of the products contain a nasal decongestant such as oxymetazoline or phenylephrine. When used for more than three days or more often than directed by the label, these drops or sprays can sometimes cause a "rebound" effect, in which the nose gets more stuffy. Other nose drops and sprays are formulated with a saline (salt) solution and can be used for dry nose or to relieve clogged nasal passages.

As you can see, selecting a product to treat a stuffy nose can be tricky. So can choosing a product to treat a cough. In addition to one or more ingredients specifically for coughs, many cold or cough syrups contain the same ingredients that are in pills to treat allergies and colds. This means that if you're taking acetaminophen pills or cold pills, you'll want to read the label or consult the pharmacist to make sure that you're not getting a double dose of the ingredients by taking a cold or cough syrup.

There are several different types of ingredients to treat coughs, depending on the kind of cough you have. Some ingredients make it easier for you to bring up phlegm, while others suppress the cough. Before taking any kind of cough medicine, it's a good idea to first try drinking plenty of liquids and adding moisture to the air by using a vaporizer or boiling water. Sometimes just doing these things will reduce the cough enough that you won't have to take any medicine. If a cough lasts more than a few days, see your doctor.

Diet Pills

The FDA recently banned 111 ingredients in OTC weight control products because they had not been proven effective. Among the substances were alcohol, ascorbic acid (vitamin C), caffeine, several forms of sugar, guar gum, phenacetin (a pain reliever), sodium, and yeast.

In late 2000, the FDA also ordered all medications containing phenylpropanolamine (PPA) removed from store shelves. This was the result of studies showing that PPA can cause strokes and brain hemorrhages when taken by young, healthy people. PPA was used in many diet pills, such as Dexatrim, as well as many cold and sinus medicines. Check OTC medications in your house to make sure they do not contain PPA. If they do, throw them out.

Recently, diet pills containing ephedra (also called Ma Huang) have become popular. Some brand names include Metabolife, Metabolite, Metabolift, Herbalife, and many "Fat Burner" formulas. Ephedra is a stimulant, which may reduce appetite. However, its safety is very questionable. There have been many reports of high blood pressure, rapid heart beats, strokes, heart attacks, and sudden death in young people taking ephedra-containing medications. The FDA has issued warnings regarding ephedra use, and is closely studying its safety. Ephedra does not work well for weight loss, and is probably best avoided.

There are also a number of "fat trapper," "overnight weight loss," and "metabolic enhancers" being sold OTC. Unfortunately, none of them have ever been shown scientifically to work, and are probably frauds. Remember, if it sounds too good to be true, it probably is!

Stomach Help

When your stomach gets upset, it's understandable that you want the quickest relief possible. But unless the problem continues for several days or is severe, drugs are usually not necessary.

Heartburn is a common problem that may occur after eating certain foods. For fast relief, antacids such as Tums, Rolaids, and Maalox can help. For longer-lasting symptoms, there are now several OTC medicines which can help. These include cimetidine (Tagament HB), ranitidine (Zantac 75), famotidine (Pepcid AC), and nizatidine (Axid AR). They may be combined with antacids, if necessary. If heartburn symptoms are frequent, or last more than a week, you should see your doctor. There may be something more serious going on, such as a stomach ulcer.

If you're constipated, drinking more water, getting more exercise, and eating high-fiber foods, such as fruits and vegetables, will often solve the problem.

Though appropriate for some medical conditions, laxatives can be habit forming and can make constipation worse when overused. Not having a bowel movement every day does not necessarily mean that you're constipated—for some people it's normal.

If you have diarrhea, it's a good idea to rest, eat only small amounts of food at a time, and drink plenty of fluids to prevent dehydration. OTC products marketed to stop diarrhea may contain loperamide (Imodium A-D), or attapulgite (Diasorb, Kaopectate and others), or bismuth subsalicylate (Pepto-Bismol and others). Teens should avoid products with bismuth subsalicylate if they have flu or chickenpox symptoms because of the risk of Reye syndrome mentioned earlier.

If you're running a fever above 100 F, or if your upset stomach symptoms are severe or continue for more than a day or two, consult your doctor, who may recommend one of the many OTC products available for these problems.

Rash Action

Because rashes can be caused by so many different things—including allergies, funguses, and poison oak or ivy—it's often best to get a doctor's opinion about what's causing your rash before treating it.

There are topical OTC products that you apply directly to the skin available specifically to treat poison ivy and oak. Some of these products contain calamine, which protects the skin, and benzocaine, which dulls the pain or itching. Other products contain an antihistamine or hydrocortisone, which relieve itching.

Antihistamine creams, such as Benadryl, and hydrocortisone products, such as Cortaid and Caldecort, can also be used for rashes from allergies and insect bites, but you shouldn't use them for more than seven days without seeing a doctor.

Another type of skin problem, pimples or acne, can also be treated with topical OTC products. Many of these lotions (such as Clearasil products and Oxy-5 and -10) contain benzoyl peroxide in strengths of 2.5, 5, or 10 percent. It's best to try the lower dosage level first, to keep your skin from getting too dry.

FDA has called for more safety studies on benzoyl peroxide because of concern about what happens when skin treated with it is exposed to the sun. Until research can establish or disprove a possible skin cancer link to the use of benzoyl peroxide products, the agency plans to require an extra warning and directions on the labeling:

"When using this product, avoid unnecessary sun exposure and use sunscreen."

"If going outside, use a sunscreen. Allow [product name] to dry, then follow directions in the sunscreen labeling. If irritation or sensitivity develops, discontinue use of both products and consult a doctor."

Other products (including some Clearasil and Oxy products) contain sulfur, sulfur combined with resorcinol, or salicylic acid. (There is no known association between Reye syndrome and the use of topical acne products containing salicylates.) If your face doesn't clear up while using these products, or if your skin gets overly dry or breaks out in a rash, contact your doctor.

Expert Advice

These are just a few of the types of products available over the counter. Their number and uses can be confusing to adults and teens alike. Before buying any product you haven't already used, it's best to read the labeling and, if possible, ask the pharmacist how the product works and what it should be used for. And, if still in doubt, check with your doctor.

Products Containing Salicylates

The following products don't have aspirin in their brand names but they contain aspirin or other salicylates and shouldn't be taken by teens who have symptoms of flu or chickenpox unless told to do so by a doctor (ingestion of salicylates during these illnesses increases children's and teens' risk of Reye syndrome).

- Alka-Seltzer Effervescent Antacid and Pain Reliever (also the extra-strength version)
- Alka-Seltzer Plus Night-Time Cold Medicine

- Anacin Maximum Strength Analgesic Coated Tablets
- Ascriptin A/D Caplets (also the regular and extra-strength versions)
- BC Powder
- BC Cold Powder Multi-Symptom Formula
- BC Cold Powder Non-Drowsy Formula
- Bayer Children's Cold Tablets
- Bufferin (all formulations)
- Excedrin Extra-Strength Analgesic Tablets and Caplets
- Pepto-Bismol
- Ursinus Inlay-Tabs
- Vanquish Analgesic Caplets
- In addition, many products to treat arthritis contain aspirin.

(This list contains many common products, but isn't all-inclusive. So be sure to read the label before purchasing any OTC medication.)

— by Judith Levine Willis

Judith Levine Willis is editor of *FDA Consumer*.

Chapter 27

Facts about Adolescent Immunization

Are There Vaccines That Protect against Communicable Diseases?

Yes! Immunizations against hepatitis B, measles, mumps, rubella (German measles), tetanus (lockjaw), diphtheria and varicella (chickenpox) are available for all adolescents. In addition, vaccinations against hepatitis A, influenza (flu) and pneumococcal disease are needed by some adolescents.

Should All Adolescents Be Immunized?

Yes. All adolescents require measles, mumps, rubella, tetanus, and diphtheria immunizations. All adolescents with diabetes or chronic heart, lung, liver, or kidney disorders need protection against influenza and pneumococcal disease, and should consult their healthcare providers regarding their need for these shots. Varicella (chickenpox) vaccine is recommended for those not previously vaccinated and who have no reliable history of the disease. Hepatitis B vaccine is indicated for all adolescents aged 8–18 who have not been vaccinated previously. Hepatitis A vaccine is recommended for adolescents traveling

This chapter contains text from "Facts About Adolescent Immunization" National Coalition for Adult Immunization, http://www.nfid.org/factsheets/ adolncai.html, August 2001, and "Key Facts about Adolescent Immunization," National Foundation for Infectious Diseases, http://www.nfid.org/factsheets/ adolescent.html, August 1996, copyright 1997- 2000 National Foundation for Infectious Diseases. Documents reprinted with permission of copyright holders.

to or working in countries where the disease is common, and for those living in communities with outbreaks of the disease. It is also recommended for adolescents who have chronic liver disease or clotting-factor disorders, use illegal injection drugs, or are male and have sex with other males.

How Often Do I Need to Be Immunized?

Hepatitis B vaccine is generally administered in 3 doses. Adolescents not previously vaccinated with 2 doses of MMR (Measles, Mumps, and Rubella) vaccine require these. Immunization against tetanus and diphtheria (Td vaccine) should be supplemented with a booster shot at 11–12 years of age and every 10 years thereafter, although Td vaccine supply shortages during 2001 resulted in postponing adolescent and adult 10 year booster shots until 2002. One dose of chickenpox vaccine is recommended for adolescents 11–12 years of age, or 2 doses for those 13 or older, if there is no proof of prior chickenpox disease or immunization. The flu shot should be administered yearly to adolescents who have any medical condition that places them at high risk for complications associated with influenza. Immunization against pneumococcal disease is recommended for adolescents with certain chronic diseases who are at increased risk for this disease or its complications, and a booster dose is recommended 5 years after the initial dose for this group. Hepatitis A vaccine is administered in 2 doses.

Are There Side Effects to These Shots?

Vaccines are among the safest medicines available. Some common side effects are a sore arm or low fever. As with any medicine, there are very small risks that serious problems could occur after getting a vaccine. However, the potential risks associated with the diseases that these vaccines prevent are much greater than the potential risks associated with the vaccines themselves.

Should I Carry a Personal Immunization Record?

Yes! This record will help you and your healthcare provider ensure that you are protected against vaccine-preventable diseases. Ask your provider for this record, and be sure to take it with you every time you visit so it can be reviewed by your provider and updated each time you are immunized.

- Vaccines are among the safest medicines available.

- Approximately 340,000 children and adolescents aged 2–18 years have chronic illnesses, placing them at risk for influenza and pneumococcal diseases and their complications.

- More than 8 million children and adolescents aged 2–18 years have at least one medical condition placing them at high risk for complications of the flu.

- Although no longer a very common disease in the United States, diphtheria remains a large problem in other countries and can pose a serious threat to United States citizens who may not be fully immunized and who travel to other countries or have contact with immigrants or international travelers coming to the U.S.

- Forty to fifty cases of tetanus (lockjaw) occur each year, resulting in at least 5 deaths annually in the United States.

- The majority of the estimated 181,000 new cases of hepatitis B reported each year strike adolescents and young adults. The hepatitis B virus is 100 times more infectious than HIV, the virus that causes AIDS.

- The hepatitis B vaccine is recognized as the first anti-cancer vaccine because it can prevent primary liver cancer caused by hepatitis B infection.

- The highest rates of hepatitis A occur among children and adolescents 5–14 years old, and most cases can be attributed to person-to-person transmission.

- Of the 575 measles patients in 1996 for whom age was known, one-third were 10–19 years old.

- About one-fifth of people infected with the mumps virus do not have any symptoms.

Key Facts about Adolescent Immunization

Varicella-zoster virus (VZV) causes both varicella (chickenpox) and zoster (shingles). VZV is a member of the herpes virus family, closely related but distinct from herpes simplex virus.

In the United States, the incidence of hepatitis B virus (HBV) infection among persons 15 to 19 and 20 to 29 years old is 10 in 100,000 and 20 in 100,000, respectively. The proportion of reported cases of measles occurring among persons 10 years or older during 1990–1994 was 47 percent compared to 10 percent during 1960–1964. Two recent serological studies of protection against tetanus revealed, respectively, 18 percent of children 6 to 16 years and 15 percent to 35 percent of children 9 to 13 years of age lacked a protective level of tetanus antitoxin. Another serologic study noted that 28 percent of children vaccinated 6 to 10 years previously lacked tetanus immunity compared to 14 percent among children last vaccinated one to five years ago. Finally, an estimated 20 percent of children 11 to 12 years of age remain susceptible to varicella, and data indicate the rate of complications following varicella is greatest in persons 15 years of age or older.

Chapter 28

Mononucleosis:
Takes You out of the Action

Missed parties. Postponed exams. Sitting out a season of team sports. And loneliness. These are a few of the ways that the scourge of high school and college students known as "mono" can affect your life.

The disease whose medical name is infectious mononucleosis is most common in people 10 to 35 years old, with its peak incidence in those 15 to 17 years old. Only 50 people out of 100,000 in the general population get mono, but it strikes as many as 2 out of 1,000 teens and twenty-somethings, especially those in high school, college, and the military. While mono is not usually considered a serious illness, it may have serious complications. Without a doubt your lifestyle will change for a few months.

You've probably heard people call mono the "kissing disease." But if your social life is in a slump, you may wonder, "How did I get this 'kissing disease' when I haven't kissed anyone romantically recently?"

Here's how. Mono is usually transmitted though saliva and mucus—which is where the "kissing disease" nickname comes from. But the kissing or close contact that transmits the disease doesn't happen right before you get sick. The virus that causes mono has a long incubation period—30 to 50 days from the time you're exposed to it to the time you get sick. In addition, the virus can be transmitted in other ways, such as sipping from the same straw or glass as an in-

Willis, Judith Levine "On the Teen Scene: When Mono Takes You Out of the Action," *FDA Consumer*, http://www.fda.gov/fdac/features/1998/398_mono.html, May-June, 1998.

fected person—or even being close when the person coughs or sneezes. Also, some people can have the virus in their systems without ever having symptoms and you can still catch it from them.

Two viruses can cause mono: Epstein-Barr virus (EBV) and cytomegalovirus (CMV). Both viruses are in the herpes family, whose other members include viruses responsible for cold sores and chickenpox.

EBV causes 85 percent of mono cases. About half of all children are infected with EBV before they're 5, but at that young age, it usually doesn't cause any symptoms. If you don't become infected with EBV until you're a teen or older, you're more likely to develop mono symptoms. After you're infected, the virus stays with you for life, but usually doesn't cause any additional symptoms. Still, every now and then you may produce viral particles in your saliva that can transmit the virus to other people, even though you feel perfectly fine. By age 40, 85 to 90 percent of Americans have EBV antibodies, indicating they have the virus in their systems and are immune to further EBV infection.

CMV is also a very common virus. About 85 percent of the U.S. population is infected with it by the time they reach adulthood. As with EBV, CMV is frequently symptomless, and mono most often results when infection occurs in the teens and 20s. Sore throat is less common in people who have CMV mono than in those infected with EBV.

As another one of its nicknames—glandular fever—implies, perhaps the most distinguishing mono symptom is enlarged glands or lymph nodes, especially in the neck, but also in the armpit and groin.

Another common mono symptom is fever. A temperature as high as 39.5 degrees Celsius (103 degrees Fahrenheit) is not uncommon. Other symptoms include a tired achy feeling, appetite loss, white patches on the back of the throat, and tonsillitis.

"My tonsils got so swollen they were touching each other in back," says Heidi Palombo of Annandale, Va., who had mono when she was a senior in college. She recalls her throat being "so hot and swollen that the only thing that felt good was ice water."

Cold drinks and frozen desserts are both ways to relieve sore throat symptoms. Doctors also recommend gargling with saltwater (about half a teaspoon salt to 8 ounces of warm water) and sucking on throat lozenges available over the counter in pharmacies and other stores. If throat or tonsils are infected, a throat culture should be taken so the doctor can prescribe an appropriate antibiotic. Ampicillin is usually not recommended because it sometimes causes a rash that can be confused with the pink, measles-like rash that 1 out of 5 mono patients develops.

For fever and achiness, you can take acetaminophen (marketed as Tylenol, Datril and others) or ibuprofen (marketed as Advil, Motrin, Nuprin, and others). If you're under 20, don't take aspirin unless your doctor approves it. In children and teens, aspirin taken for viral illnesses has been associated with the potentially fatal disease Reye syndrome. Sometimes a person with mono may have trouble breathing because of swelling in the throat, and doctors have to use other medications and treatment. A person who has mono—or those caring for the person—should contact a doctor immediately if the person starts having breathing problems.

Some people with mono become overly sensitive to light and about half develop enlargement of the spleen, usually two to three weeks after they first become sick. Mild enlargement of the liver may also occur.

Whether or not the spleen is enlarged, people who have mono should not lift heavy objects or exercise vigorously—including participating in contact sports—for two months after they get sick, because these activities increase the risk of rupturing the spleen, which can be life-threatening. If you have mono and get a severe sharp, sudden pain on the left side of your upper abdomen, go to an emergency room or call 911 immediately.

Because its symptoms can be very similar to those of other illnesses, doctors often recommend tests to find out exactly what the problem is.

"I was misdiagnosed at first and told I was bit by a spider," writes John L. Gipson, of Kansas City, Mo., in a note he posted to a website. "That's what I thought because I had killed a spider in my room. I figured I'd been bitten by a spider in my sleep. A few days after... I had no energy, a fever... and those pea-sized bumps on the back of my neck." Gipson returned to his doctor, who did blood tests and diagnosed mononucleosis.

Other diagnostic problems can result because enlarged lymphocytes, a type of white cell, are common with mono, but can also be a symptom of leukemia. Blood tests can distinguish between the type of white cell seen in leukemia and that with mono.

If your throat is sore, having a throat culture is usually a good idea for several reasons. First, the symptoms of mono and strep infection (including that caused by Strep-A, a particularly serious form of strep) are very similar. Second, strep throat or other throat infections can develop anytime during or shortly after in the disease. In any case, it's important that throat infections be diagnosed as soon as possible and treated with antibiotics that can kill the organism responsible for the infection.

The test most commonly used to tell whether you have mono or some other ailment is the mononucleosis spot test. This blood test detects the antibodies (proteins) that the body makes to fight EBV or CMV. Because it takes a while for antibodies to develop after infection, your doctor may need to order or repeat the test one to two weeks after you develop symptoms. At that time the test is about 85 percent accurate.

Other tests your doctor might order include a complete blood count (CBC) to see if your blood platelet count is lower than normal and if lymphocytes are abnormal, and a chemistry panel to see if liver enzymes are abnormal.

Bed rest is the most important treatment for uncomplicated mono. It's also important to drink plenty of fluids. Mono is not usually a reason to quarantine students. Many people are already immune to the viruses that cause it. But if you have mono you'll want to stay in bed and out of classes for several days, until the fever goes down and other symptoms abate. Even when you've started to get better, you can expect to have to curtail your activities for several weeks, and it can take two to three months or more until you feel your old self again.

The author of this article had mono herself when she was 16. Though she didn't mind getting out of all that homework (or at least putting it off), having to delay finals only added to her anxiety about college applications that many high school juniors experience. And then there was that guy who never called again.

When you add the time spent recuperating to the fact that most people are not exactly anxious to get close to a person with mono, you can understand why some students find themselves combating loneliness on top of their other troubles.

Getting through mono may be both challenging and depressing—and seem to take forever. But if you rest when your body tells you to, you can lessen the chances of complications and get back your life.

—by Judith Levine Willis

Judith Levine Willis is a member of FDA's public affairs staff.

Chapter 29

Loud Music and Hearing Loss

Rock musician Kathy Peck had been playing bass guitar for several years. But when her three-piece band, The Contractions, opened for Duran Duran at the Oakland Coliseum in California in 1984, Peck, then in her mid-20s, heard more than the echo of applause.

"My ears were ringing for days afterward," she remembers. Eventually Peck found she had destroyed 40 percent of her hearing from years of playing loud music.

"I was basically deaf for three years. It was very frustrating, very isolating," Peck says. It took her several years to learn to manage her handicap with hearing aids and lip reading.

"People in the music industry told me not to let anyone know about my condition, because they wouldn't listen to my records or anything," she says. "People were afraid, like I had leprosy."

Peck is just one of 23.3 million Americans who have hearing loss, according to a 1990 survey by the National Center for Health Statistics. About 1.3 million of them are 18 or younger. Although statistics are lacking, anecdotal evidence suggests more young people are losing their hearing today than ever before.

According to the National Institutes of Health, one-third of all hearing loss cases stem at least in part from the loud noises of mod-

Rebecca D. Williams, "On the Teen Scene: Enjoy, Protect the Best years of Your Life," *FDA Consumer*, May 1992, Food and Drug Administration (FDA) Pub. No. 92-1195, http://www.fda.gov/bbs/topics/CONSUMER/CON00141.html. Updated in February 2001 by Dr. David A. Cook, MD, Diplomate, American Board of Internal Medicine.

ern life: power lawn mowers, jet engines, city traffic, loud appliances, rock music, stereo headsets, and car "kicker boxes."

Some 59 million Americans are exposed to urban traffic noise, 16 million to aircraft noise, and 3.1 million to highway noise, according to the US Environmental Protection Agency.

Loud noises destroy the tiny hair cells in the inner ear that signal the auditory nerve to send sound messages to the brain. Once those cells die, they never grow back.

The result is a kind of deafness called "sensorineural hearing loss." This affects both volume and clarity, first at high pitches, then later at lower pitches where speech is heard.

Noise may also cause "tinnitus," a ringing in the ears. Besides being a constant annoyance, tinnitus often signals impending hearing loss. Although both conditions are permanent and incurable, they can be improved with hearing aids.

The Food and Drug Administration (FDA) regulates those devices, as well as equipment to diagnose hearing loss. But the agency hopes you choose an easier path to better hearing—protecting your ears while they're young.

"One of the things that bothers me is that [young people] are aging their ears before their chronological time," says audiologist David Lipscomb, who has researched hearing loss in students at the University of Tennessee.

In the fall of 1969, he tested the hearing of entering freshmen and found about 60 percent of them had hearing loss. Fourteen percent of the young men tested had hearing similar to the average 65-year-old. By comparison, only 3.8 percent of sixth-graders had hearing loss, suggesting that something—probably noise—was damaging hearing during the teen years.

"We know that the average 70-year-old will have some impairment from aging," says Lipscomb. "But for young people [exposed to loud noises], the aging process is sped up. They're blowing their spare tires."

Modern Life: A Pain in the Ear

In the absence of loud noises, hearing doesn't appear to deteriorate much with age.

For example, deep in the Sudan bush, a primitive tribe lives in a quiet environment, surrounded by swamps and the White Nile River. A study done in the early 1960s found that people of any age in the tribe had hearing superior to that of a comparison group of American farmers. Furthermore, the old people heard as well as the young.

Modern life is much harder on hearing. According to the American Speech-Language-Hearing Association (ASHA), an estimated 20 million Americans are regularly exposed to noise at dangerous levels.

Noise is measured in decibels. Anything 80 decibels or louder, such as a loud buzzer alarm clock, is potentially dangerous, according to ASHA. The higher the decibel, the louder the noise. The accompanying noise scale shows the loudness of common sounds.

The louder the noise, the shorter the time it takes to hurt your hearing. Your ears can endure 90 decibels of noise, such as a lawn mower, for about eight hours before damage occurs. For every 5 decibels above that, it takes only half as much time for damage to begin.

A noise at 95 decibels will hurt your ears in four hours. An arcade full of video games could cause damage in two hours. The average rock concert or stereo headset set at full blast (about 110 decibels) could damage your ears in a half hour.

Like Peck, most people don't notice they've lost any hearing until they develop tinnitus or they can't understand speech. But the damage begins long before that. An individual concert, hunting trip, lawn mower, or power tool may not hurt your ears at the time, but added together over the years, they can be disastrous.

Have you ever walked away from a construction site or loud concert and everything sounds as if you're under water? Or you feel a fullness or buzzing in your ears?

That's called a "temporary threshold shift." Although it goes away, it's a signal that you've damaged some hair cells in your inner ear. The cells will probably heal, but additional damage may permanently destroy them.

Want Better Hearing? Shhhh!

The best way to safeguard your hearing is to avoid loud noises as much as possible. How do you know if you're in danger? Lipscomb gives four clues:

- if your ears are ringing

- if things sound muffled, as if you're in a barrel

- if sounds are distorted, as if they're coming through a poor-quality speaker

- if you find yourself shouting to communicate

The rule of thumb for listening to music is to keep it low enough so that you can hear other sounds above the tunes. If you're listening to a Walkman portable radio or similar headset, no one else should be able to hear your music.

Hearing Protection

When loud noise can't be avoided—such as when you're mowing the lawn, working in shop class, or attending a concert—guard your ears with hearing protection devices.

Stuffing cotton in your ears will not do the trick. Good hearing protection is available with a number of devices, the most common and least expensive of which are earplugs.

Earplugs are available at most drug, hardware, music, and sporting goods stores, and custom-made plugs are available through an audiologist. Made of foam rubber or plastic, earplugs come with a noise reduction rating on the label established by the Environmental Protection Agency.

The Occupational Safety and Health Administration (OSHA), which regulates hearing safety in the workplace, recommends using earplugs with a rating twice as strong as you need to ensure protection.

For instance, if you're going to be mowing the lawn (90 decibels), you'd need to reduce the noise by about 15 decibels to be in a safe range, so buy earplugs with a 30-decibel rating.

For a rock concert (110 decibels), you'd need 45-decibel plugs. These are usually only available from an audiologist. If you can't get them, buy the strongest rating available in a drugstore (about 30 decibels). The most important thing is that you wear something to block out the sound.

"Most people say that hearing protection devices distort sound," says John Steelnack, an industrial hygienist with OSHA. "They really don't," he says. "They just reduce the intensity."

Hearing Aids

For those who have already suffered damage, hearing aids can help, but they still cannot restore normal hearing.

People are rarely as satisfied with their hearing aids as with their eyeglasses because many older hearing aids can't clarify sounds. Newer hearing aids are better at picking up certain sound frequencies, screening out much unwanted background noise.

"Basically, a hearing aid is an audio amplifier that provides amplification in the frequency range where the patient has the greatest hearing loss," says Harry Sauberman, chief of the ear, nose and throat division at FDA's Office of Device Evaluation.

"One of the concerns about hearing aids is that many of them amplify ambient [background] noise. That may be the reason people leave them on the dresser. They just don't find them desirable."

Sound Advice

Rock musician Peck cherishes what's left of her hearing. To educate others about noise-induced hearing loss, she helped establish a nonprofit organization called HEAR, for Hearing Education and Awareness for Rockers, with the Haight-Ashbury Free Medical Clinic in San Francisco.

HEAR has garnered a lot of publicity and support in the music industry, including a $10,000 donation from musician Pete Townsend of The Who, who also has hearing loss.

HEAR sponsors free hearing screening in the San Francisco Bay area and has a 24-hour hot line for information about noise-induced hearing loss. For more information, write HEAR at P.O. Box 460847, San Francisco, CA 94146.

While Peck doesn't play in a band anymore, she is still a rock music fan. However, now when she goes to concerts, she wears custom-made earplugs. Some are decorated with dangling earring-like ornaments.

She encourages other music fans to take precautions as well. "We're not against music, we're not anti-rock 'n' roll," says Peck. "I just want them to protect their hearing."

A Range of Noises

Here, listed by category, are an assortment of noises and their decibel levels:

Painful

- 140—firearms, air raid siren
- 130—jackhammer
- 120—jet plane takeoff

Extremely Loud

- 110—rock music

- 100—snowmobile, chainsaw
- 90—lawnmower

Very Loud

- 80—alarm clock
- 70—busy traffic, vacuum cleaner
- 60—conversation, dishwasher

Moderate

- 50—moderate rainfall
- 40—quiet room

Faint

- 30—whisper

—by Rebecca D. Williams

Rebecca D. Williams is a staff writer for *FDA Consumer*.

Chapter 30

Caution: False Medical Advertising Targets Teens

Introduction

Quackery, an age-old business, costs Americans billions of dollars each year and immeasurable losses suffered from harmful products and delayed medical treatment. The quack's victims are usually thought of as the aged or chronically ill.

But quacks are quick to spot new markets, so it's not surprising that they have discovered teenagers. These youths and their impatience with the blossoming process are fertile ground for quacks. Teenagers are ready to experiment with products that promise to speed their development and ease growing pains.

And many of these junior and senior high school age children have money enough to do the experimenting. In fact, a study by Teenage Research Unlimited revealed that 27.6 million teenagers spent an average of $93 a month on personal items in 1989 for a total of nearly $31 billion.

Further, in families in which both parents work, teens take on more of the family shopping responsibilities. These young shoppers often have access to mom or pop's credit card. And, like their parents, they are buying more through the mail, a medium that offers a cloak of anonymity under which quacks thrive.

"Quackery Targets Teens," *FDA Consumer*, February 1988, Revised April 1990, Food and Drug Administration (FDA) Pub. No. 90-1147, http://vm.cfsan.fda.gov/~dms/wh-teen2.html. Reviewed and revised by David A. Cooke, M.D. February 2001.

The teen years often insecure years, filled with questions like: "Am I beautiful (or handsome)?" "Will my breasts ever develop?" "Shouldn't I be more muscular?" "Am I too fat?" "Would a tan give me more sex appeal?"

Quacks love such questions. And they're ready with answers that have been—according to them—"overlooked or ignored by the established scientific community."

Time is of such essence to the young that they grasp at straws and don't recognize the quack's deceptions for what they really are.

Take a look at some of the advertisements in teen magazines. There's a "space age diet" that allows you to "eat all day and still lose weight," a beauty cream that will ensure "gorgeous, proportioned breasts," and a pill to provide a tan overnight. Sound unlikely? Impossible is a better word. But, fond of superlatives and driven by desire, teenagers are ready to believe such ads.

In 1994, the United States Congress passed a bill loosening restrictions on products sold over-the-counter as "vitamins," "herbal remedies," and "dietary supplements." Unfortunately, many quacks have taken advantage of these legal changes to market their products, and this has become a prime area for medical fraud. Some are widely advertised on radio and television, because changes in the law have made it much harder for the Food and Drug Administration (FDA) to prove that some of these medications are frauds.

Here are some of the dubious products that teenagers today are asked to believe in:

Breast Developers

For decades, millions of dollars have been spent on devices, creams and lotions advertised as breast developers. All wasted. There is no device or system of exercise that will increase the size of the breasts. At best, devices promoted as breast developers merely strengthen and develop the muscles that support the breasts, and exercising these muscles will not appreciably increase breast size.

Creams and lotions advertised as breast developers don't work either. Some contain the hormone estrogen. Estrogen can increase breast size, but in order to be sold without a prescription these products must contain such a small amount of the hormone that its effect is insignificant. (Estrogen is used in birth control pills and to treat symptoms of menopause. FDA approval for estrogen does not include use for breast development.)

The only proven method of increasing breast size is breast augmentation surgery, which carries some risks and is hardly recommended for teenagers.

Weight Loss

Teenagers—especially girls—are not exempt from the American penchant for dieting. One expert says that as many as three-fourths of high school girls are on a diet at any one time. Dr. Kelly Brownell of the University of Pennsylvania School of Medicine said that some children begin dieting as early as the fourth grade.

Those figures may startle some people, but not the quacks. They know them well and have pounced on that audience, offering "magical" diets and pills to keep the pounds off. Most of the diets and virtually all of the pills are worthless; some are even dangerous. At times, some diets will achieve a temporary weight loss that is usually unrelated to the "magical" food or pill.

The dieting craze may be particularly questionable for adolescents, since a well-balanced diet is vital during the teen years when the body goes through dramatic change and growth. Depending on the ingredients, some pills promoted for weight loss can cause side effects such as nervousness, nausea and insomnia, and can also be addictive.

Until recently, the recognized active ingredient in most nonprescription diet pills is either phenylpropanolamine (PPA) or benzocaine. PPA was withdrawn from the market late in the year 2000 by the FDA. Studies had shown an increased risk of strokes and bleeding inside the brain in healthy young people when they took PPA for the first time. Benzocaine is supposed to work by numbing the inside of the mouth to make food less appetizing. However, the effectiveness of this medication for weight loss has never been proven.

In the last several years, nonprescription weight loss products containing ephedra have become very popular. Ephedra, also known as Ma Huang, is a stimulant. Many manufacturers claim that it is a "fat burner" or that it "accelerates your metabolism," but its main effect appears to be as an appetite suppressant. It is usually combined in a pill with large doses of caffeine. The effectiveness of these products for weight loss has never been proven, and ephedra-based medications are being closely studied by the FDA. There have been many disturbing reports of serious side effects from ephedra-containing pills, ranging from rapid heart beats and high blood pressure, to even strokes, heart attacks, and sudden death in young people.

There have also been several companies prosecuted by the FDA recently for selling weight loss medications. Unscrupulous manufacturers put substances such as thyroid hormone in these pills, which are regulated prescription drugs. Use of thyroid hormones without monitoring by a physician can cause severe injury and illness. However, teens who bought these pills had no idea what they were actually taking.

Most weight-loss products are sold as part of a diet-and-pill plan. The pills don't work, but the plan may. Of course, the plan would work just as well without the product, which is nothing more than a psychological crutch.

Some devices are also promoted for weight loss. Electrical muscle stimulators, for example, have a legitimate use for physical therapy treatment, but FDA has had to take a number of such devices off the market because they were promoted for weight loss and "body toning." These stimulators can be dangerous when used incorrectly. Hazards include electrical shocks and burns.

Body wraps are another favorite gimmick of the quacks. They're touted as a means of "burning fat." The wraps are worn around part or all of the body, sometimes preceded by the application of a cream or lotion. Temporary weight loss may occur as the result of sweating and loss of water in the tissues, but when the water content of the tissue returns to normal, the "lost" weight reappears. The wraps do not "burn" or dissolve fat. Furthermore, experts consider them dangerous because they can cause severe dehydration and circulatory problems.

There are no magic foods, pills, wraps, diets or wands for losing weight. The only way to lose weight is to consistently eat fewer calories than the body needs and uses. But teenagers should be cautioned about excessive dieting. Their growing bodies can't tolerate the nutrient loss that comes with eating too little.

Steroids and Growth Hormone

Our sports-loving nation loves a winner, and it's fair to say that most of the 5 million boys and girls who compete in high school sports love to win. Some of them will go to great lengths to do so. That may mean using performance-enhancing drugs such as anabolic steroids and human growth hormone.

Anabolic steroids—compounds similar to the male hormone testosterone—are too often used by athletes, both boys and girls, to build muscle. They are also used by young men who just want to look better. They are prescription drugs, but most of those who use them obtain them illegally, often from the black market. Steroids have a lot of unwanted side effects—that's why they are supposed to be sold only by prescription. They may well build muscle, but it's a losing proposition, because their use—particularly in the large doses that athletes take—can stunt growth, lead to cancer, ruin the liver, and bring on other complications, including enlarged breasts in boys. For girls, the side effects include developing masculine traits that may be irreversible.

Black-market steroids often are produced in another country or by clandestine domestic manufacturers under questionable conditions and may be contaminated. The quacks have also moved in with phony steroids and phony pills that they say—falsely—will counter some of the side effects of steroids.

In 1988, FDA warned that a counterfeit version of the hormone human chorionic gonadotropin, or HCG, was being sold to weight lifters and other athletes. The bogus hormones were contaminated with a substance that causes infections and fever.

A black market has also sprung up for human growth hormone. This prescription drug is legitimately given to children who suffer from pituitary dwarfism or growth hormone deficiency, but it, too, has dangerous side effects. Nevertheless, athletes seeking to benefit from added growth are buying the hormone on the black market. Quacks are also marketing "growth tablets" that, in fact, contain no hormones or any other ingredients that can promote growth.

Tanning and Tanning Pills

Tanning is never harmless, regardless of the source: the sun, a sunlamp, a tanning bed or a pill. Exposure to ultraviolet radiation from the sun or other sources leads to premature aging of the skin. It is also the number one cause of skin cancer.

Many teenagers get their tans a tanning parlors, where they may be told that the type of ultraviolet radiation from the lamps will not be harmful. That's not true. Ultraviolet radiation from any source can be harmful.

Other youths may turn to tanning pills. But they're not safe either. They generally contain a color additive that has not been approved by FDA for coloring the body. Advertisement claim that the pills produce "a rich, golden-bronze natural-looking tan that make one look healthy, energetic, and attractive all year." But the pills actually produce a distinct orange tinge on the skin. The pills may also leave fatty deposits in the blood, liver and skin, and on the eye's retina, where they may interfere with night vision. Further, the tan the pills produce is no protection against sunburn.

Hair Removal and Growth

The only effective way to remove hair permanently is with electrolysis a process by which hair roots are destroyed with an electrified needle. Electrolysis should only be performed by a physician or professional electrologist, according to the American Medical Association (AMA). While it is safe when done correctly, it can be tedious, painful and expensive, the AMA adds. Scarring may result and regrowth is possible.

Effective means of temporarily removing hair include shaving, tweezing, waxing, and using cream or lotion depilatories. But FDA cautions that there is no risk-free method of removing hair. Waxing for example can be painful, and creams can cause rashes and swelling.

Recently, the FDA did approve a cream which can slow the growth of facial hair. However, this is only available with a doctor's prescription.

There is limited good news about removing hair, however. According to the AMA hair removal does not make renewed growth thicker or stiffer, nor does it quicken regrowth.

While girls struggle to remove hair, some teenage boys worry that they won't be able to keep theirs. Since most baldness is hereditary, young men may take a look at their long-since bald fathers and fear that they will soon be watching the tops of their heads get smoother. There's currently no solution to this dilemma, a fact that bothers quacks not at all. The health fraud artists are ready with a variety of cures for baldness and their intended victims include those worried youngsters.

At present, there are only two medications which have been proven to help prevent hair loss and baldness. Minoxidil, which is marketed as Rogaine and other brands, is available over-the-counter as a lotion, cream, and a gel. Finasteride, also called Propecia, is a pill, and can only be bought with a prescription. Unfortunately, these medications only work for about half the people who try them, and it may take months to see the effects.

Anything else that claims to grow hair, especially any "sure-fire" cure for hair loss, is a fraud. Quack hair regrowers and hair tonics have been popular for over one hundred years, and show no sign of going away.

Look-Alike Drugs

The widespread use of illegal drugs among teenagers has helped generate a market for fake drugs. These look-alike drugs are intentionally made to look like amphetamines, barbiturates or other often-abused drugs. They are sold on the street and by mail order, and the seller often implies that they are the illegal drugs they resemble.

The look-alikes generally contain decongestants, caffeine, and other stimulants in what FDA has called dangerous illogical combinations. Some contain alarmingly high doses of one ingredient. For example, in the late 1990s the FDA banned a number of "herbal ecstacy" pills containing high doses of ephedra after several young people died. When taken in excess or mixed with alcohol, the look-alikes have caused strokes and death. They are extremely dangerous when mixed with, or replaced by real uppers or downers.

The availability and use of look-alikes make it harder for health professionals and law enforcement officials to combat the problem of illegal drug use. The AMA points out the following problems caused by look-alikes:

- School children and others who don't normally abuse drugs are told that the look-alikes are okay to use because they are legal and safe (in fact they are neither).

- Look-alike drugs may make youngsters believe that the illegal drugs they mimic aren't as potent and dangerous as they really are.

- Traditional drug abuse education programs are hampered by the wide availability of the imitation drugs.

- Physicians and poison centers are deceived by the fake drugs, which makes drug-related diagnoses difficult.

- The look-alikes make it even more difficult for law enforcement officials to stop illegal drug traffic.

Most states have banned the manufacture and marketing of look-alikes, and the federal government has taken action against some manufacturers. But the availability of look-alike drugs is still a threat to the health and safety of teenagers.

Recognizing Quackery

It is during the teenage years that people start to become serious consumers, and there's no better time to learn how to avoid quackery. Here are some tips:

- Be wary if immediate, effortless or guaranteed results are promised.

- Look for telltale words and phrases such as "breakthrough," "miracle," "secret remedy," "exclusive," and "clinical studies prove that..."

- Beware of promotions for a single product claimed to be effective for a wide variety of ailments.

- Ads that use many "testimonials" from people who have used the product are very suspicious. "Testimonials" are classic tools of quacks. The people quoted in the ads may not exist, or were paid to speak in favor of the product.

- Don't forget that, unlike scientists and health professionals, quacks do not subject their products to the scrutiny of scientific research. The quack simply thrusts a product onto the market in order to get your money.

- Be cautious of money-back guarantees, for a guarantee is only as good as the company that backs it.

- If it sounds too good to be true—it probably is.

For More Information

If you have questions about a product or company, or to get answers before you make a purchase, contact:

- the Better Business Bureau

- the nearest Food and Drug Administration (FDA) office

- your local consumer office or state attorney general's office

- your doctor

Part Three

Adolescent Sexual Health

Chapter 31

Puberty

What Is Puberty?

Puberty usually is defined as the age of sexual maturity, that stage of life when males and females undergo bodily changes that make it possible for them to have children. Puberty begins with the appearance of what are called "secondary sexual characteristics." Girls experience growth of the breasts and their first menstrual period. Boys have their first ejaculation (emission of semen from the penis) and the voice cracks and then deepens. A spurt in body growth is a very prominent part of puberty. These and many other physical changes underlie the emotional changes of adolescence. In sum, they signify a process of biological maturation that young people undergo when passing from childhood to adulthood.

The striking physical changes that mark puberty, and which occur in a relatively brief time, reflect a surge in secretion of the so-called "sex hormones." At the outset, brain activity triggers the release of hormones called gonadotropins by the pituitary gland, a small but very important "central station" for hormone secretion. In boys, gonadotropins cause the testicles to secrete testosterone, which in turn stimulates the formation of sperm cells. In girls the same hormones stimulate the ovaries to secrete estrogen, which in turn allows ovulation—the periodic release of eggs from the ovary.

Text in this chapter was written by Dr. David Cramer, a medical writer in Chicago, IL; © Omnigraphics 2001.

Is There a "Right" Age for Puberty?

In boys, puberty often begins with enlarging testicles and the sprouting of pubic hair, followed by a growth spurt. A "wet dream," with semen issuing unexpectedly from the penis, may be a surprising introduction to puberty. These changes can normally occur any time between ages 9 ½ and 13 ½ years. The time between the first sign of puberty and its completion can range from about 2 to 5 years. For all of these boys, puberty is "on time."

Girls usually enter puberty a year or two earlier than boys. The first changes tend to be breast budding and the growth of pubic hair, and the final event often is the first menstrual period. Today, the average age at first menstruation in the US and other western countries is about 12 ½ years, but any time between ages 10 and 16 is viewed as normal. The entire process of puberty can take from 18 months to 6 years to complete.

Puberty in Girls

- As the breasts begin to grow a girl notices small, sometimes tender lumps beneath one or both nipples, which will get progressively larger over the next few years. It is not uncommon for one breast to develop faster than the other or for the breasts to be asymmetrical. This can be embarrassing, but breast size usually evens out within a few months. Breast development is a noticeable event, and some girls who receive unwanted attention as a result may feel uncomfortable.

- A few soft, slightly pigmented pubic hairs will be succeeded in time by thick, curly hairs, and hair also may begin growing on the legs and under the arms. At the same time, changes in the skin glands that produce oil and sweat may lead to acne.

- One to two years after the first signs of puberty, at age 10 on average, a growth spurt can be expected. Your daughter's body will start building up fat; rounded hips and buttocks along with enlarging breasts create womanly contours. Her arms, legs, hands, and feet also will get bigger. Unfortunately different parts of the body grow at different rates, explaining why so many girls feel "gangly" and awkward. They also may be self-conscious at being taller than most boys at the very time they begin to notice them. Some girls— especially those who develop early—become very sensitive about gaining weight and may diet unnecessarily.

- The first menstrual period usually comes about a year after the breasts begin enlarging and at the peak of the growth spurt. It may follow a few months of increased whitish or yellow vaginal discharge. Although parents often believe that the first period means the onset of puberty, in fact it occurs quite late in the pubertal process. The first periods often are heavy and/or irregular, but within about a year they will be more "on schedule" (a 3- to 7-day period every 24 to 34 days is typical). Menstrual cramps are more common in adolescence than later in life.

- A girl's voice may deepen at puberty but not as much as a boy's.

Puberty in Boys

- The first signs of puberty often are enlarging testicles and the appearance of pubic hair. About half of boys have swelling or tenderness under the nipples, a temporary occurrence that nevertheless may cause a boy to panic. Usually this breast tissue disappears within about 6 months. In time, hair sprouts on the arms, legs, and face as well as at the base of the penis. The scrotum enlarges and becomes darker.

- The penis itself grows larger and erections become more frequent (although they are not anything new, occurring even during infancy). Your pubertal son may need to be reassured that the size of his penis at rest does not determine its size when erect. The first ejaculation typically is a result of either masturbation or a nocturnal emission ("wet dream").

- In boys, the growth spurt begins at an average age of 12 or 13, roughly 2 years later than in girls, and reaches its peak about 2 years later. At this stage boys may grow 3 to 4 inches a year. It is important for both boys and their parents to realize that there is no set timetable for body growth or other changes during puberty. Unlike girls, who accumulate mostly fat tissue, boys gain lean muscle and bone mass. Muscular development is most noticeable in the upper arms, thighs, and shoulders. Facial features become sharper as the adult appearance begins to emerge. The hands and feet are the first body parts to reach adult size. The arms and legs grow faster than the torso, creating feelings of awkwardness. The heart and lungs become larger and boys are able to use oxygen more efficiently, enabling them to exercise more vigorously.

- Growth of the larynx (the "voice box") deepens the voice. At the same time the "Adam's apple" becomes more prominent.

- Pubertal boys, like girls, are susceptible to developing oily skin and acne.

How Puberty Makes Children Feel

At the time of puberty, many children are uncomfortable with their self-image. They may resent looking the way they do, or they misinterpret how their peers and others see them. The profound physical changes of puberty tend to make children feel clumsy, shy, and insecure. Boys often are sensitive when the voice begins to crack. For many pubertal children, boys and girls alike, acne and pimples are a major source of embarrassment and can easily make social activities burdensome. Above all, young people at this stage of life want to be like everyone else their age. Consequently, a girl who has her first period before her classmates, or who develops breasts first (or last) may be very self-conscious. For boys, the growth of pubic hair can cause similar concerns.

During puberty your boy or girl cannot help shifting between how it feels to be a child, and the physical, mental, and emotional indicators that adulthood is fast approaching. Although children at this stage of life begin to feel liberated, they still require support from their parents. Forming close friendships with others of the same age may make a young teenager more self-confident. At the same time, feelings of insecurity may make a child want to imitate his or her peers.

Puberty is a time of physical changes and their emotional consequences. Reactions vary widely. Some girls, for instance, are excited about their new breasts while others feel that everyone is staring at them. Likewise, some boys are proud of having to shave while others are uncomfortable with the attention their new facial hair brings. Young teenagers must learn to wash each day and to use an antiperspirant or deodorant. A boy who doesn't know about wet dreams may be afraid that something serious has gone wrong. Masturbation is normal for boys and girls, but they often are confused by the new feelings they are experiencing and are not sure whether what they are doing is all right.

Puberty and Family Life

It is more the rule than the exception that the way a child feels about his or her parents changes, sometimes markedly, at the time of puberty. Developing children may feel that their parents are old-fashioned and annoying. The parents, in turn, may find that their child has suddenly become disrespectful and sullen. These altered attitudes can set the stage for ongoing parent-child conflicts. A good starting point is to recognize that tension and argument between young teenagers and their parents are an expected part of family life. In fact, the absence of all conflict may be an indication that a child is hiding problems. Because teenagers who suppress emotional difficulties may later have trouble forming normal relationships, the parents should welcome a chance to discuss with their child all of his or her concerns; no subject should be taboo.

It still is the case that some troubled adolescents engage in substance abuse, take part in violent acts, or experiment sexually. Parents, while not minimizing the importance of such behavior, must realize that adolescents naturally experiment with new ideas and behaviors, and tend to oppose their parents' traditional values. It is particularly at those times when both parties feel that they can't talk freely to one another that lines of communication must be kept open.

What Parents Can Do—Talking about Puberty

Parents of a pubertal child should not imagine that, just because so much can be found about sex and relationships on television and the Internet, this would be sufficient. Talking about issues surrounding puberty still is a critical task for parents. Do not wait for your boy or girl to start asking questions about physical changes; that time may never come. These discussions will be easier if the parents and child have addressed bodily changes since the toddler years. A child 8 years of age should know about the physical and emotional changes connected with puberty. A boy's first ejaculation or a girl's first period should not come as a surprise. Even if your child's school is providing sex education, boys and girls may be taught separately despite the importance of girls knowing about the changes boys go through, and vice versa. Planning talks to coincide with school lessons, however, may help ease into a meaningful conversation.

Parents should let their child know that they are available to talk any time, but they also should deliberately make time to talk. A child may hesitate to approach a parent who is obviously embarrassed, but knowing something about puberty can make this process easier for the parent. It's all right to let your child know that you may be a little uncomfortable, but that it is important to talk anyway. Rather than having a single major talk it is much better to have a series of discussions that ideally will start when the young child starts to ask questions. Any question that a child brings up should be answered right away. Deferring an answer until later may mean that the subject will not arise again.

Talking to Girls

Girls who enter puberty become very sensitive about the appearance of their face and body. Those who develop early are the most at risk for developing a poor body image and eating disorders. The most striking development experienced by pubertal girls is the start of menstruation. It is most important that parents talk about menstruation before the first period. A common question is when this will happen, and parents can reassure their child that this is quite variable and may not occur until age 17. A girl likely will also be concerned about when she will develop pubic hair. Again, parents should stress the broad variation in timing and the fact that this is an individual trait. Breast size is also a frequent concern. You may want to reassure your daughter that having attractive breasts does not depend on their size, and that breast size is unrelated to breast function.

A mother's own views about menstruation and womanhood can send subtle but unmistakable messages to her pre-pubertal or pubertal daughter. Probably the best way of promoting a positive body image is for the mother to model one by eating a healthy diet, exercising regularly, and having a positive attitude toward her own body.

Talking to Boys

In discussing puberty, girls tend to receive the most attention. Parents as well as educators too often fail to recognize the significance of pubertal development to boys. It is as important to boys as to girls that they be aware of the great variation in the physical changes that are taking place in their bodies and in when these changes occur. The first ejaculation is an event comparable in importance to the start of menstruation for girls. Boys will feel more comfortable about it and more positively about their bodies when prepared in advance by their parents and teachers.

The key for parents is to open channels of communication and keep them open. Your son's desire for privacy, which must be respected, may conflict with his need to know what is happening to him. Parents should realize that boys get mixed messages about what being a man means. The parent should be a good listener, and should let his or her son know that it is all right to talk about these matters. Among the most frequently asked questions by pubertal boys are those concerning penile size, when they will get pubic hair, and the presence of breast tissue.

When Puberty Comes Early

Premature puberty, or "precocious" puberty, occurs before age 8 in girls and age 9 in boys. It is rare—about 6 of every 1,000 otherwise normal children are affected. Early puberty may be a normal variation, but a disorder may also be responsible. If your child's primary care physician is concerned, he probably will ask you to consult with an endocrinologist specializing in hormonal abnormalities. Removal of a mass that is stimulating hormone secretion or treatment to suppress the production of sex hormones may solve the problem. Paradoxically, a child with precocious puberty may at first be taller than his peers, but without effective treatment growth may stop early and the child's growth will be stunted. It may be necessary to attend to the psychological problems that develop in some children who enter puberty at a very early age.

When Puberty Comes Late

More often than not, delayed puberty is simply due to a normal variation in pubertal development from child to child. Boys tend to be affected by this more often than girls. These boys may be very troubled by the contrast with their more powerful peers or embarrassed at showering with them. Because sex hormones affect the brain as well as the body, physical immaturity typically is accompanied by emotional immaturity. A large majority of children with delayed puberty will catch up over time without any treatment. If there is a family history of delayed puberty and the father shares this fact with his son, the boy will feel reassured that he will develop into a normal man in his own time. Effective treatment is available if some malfunction in the brain, pituitary gland, testes, or ovaries is responsible for delayed puberty. Boys can be given testosterone, and girls, an estrogen preparation. Some patients may require sex hormone replacement for an indefinite time.

Conclusion

Puberty is defined as the age of sexual maturity, but it is also a time of profound physical, emotional, mental, and social change. Parents can offer much needed support and preparation for their children during this time. Some children experience puberty earlier or later than others, and many youth need reassurance that their development is normal. If the lines of communication are kept open, puberty can be a positive experience for both parents and children.

Chapter 32

All about Menstruation

On the Teen Scene: A Balanced Look at the Menstrual Cycle

Some young women feel it coming days before they get it. Others are hardly aware they have it. Friends who compare notes about their periods will probably find that menstruation—the monthly shedding of the lining of the uterus, or womb—affects each of them a little differently, both physically and emotionally.

"The menstrual cycle has its ups and downs of hormones, and different people react differently to hormonal swings," says Lisa Rarick, MD, a gynecologist in FDA's (Food and Drug Administration) Center for Drug Evaluation and Research. She explains that just before and during menstruation, levels of the female hormones estrogen and progesterone are low. That's when some women feel bloated, irritable or blue, or "just crummy," she says.

"Just crummy" might mean cramps, sore breasts, backache, headache, nausea, and feeling tired.

This chapter contains text from Marian Segal, "On the Teen Scene: A Balanced Look at the Menstrual Cycle," *FDA Consumer*, December 1993, revised October 1994, Food and Drug Administration (FDA) Pub. No. 94-1215, updated in June 2001 by Dr. David A. Cooke, MD, Diplomate, American Board of Internal Medicine; and Charles Wibbelsman, MD, "Talking to Your Daughter about Menstruation," www.tnpc.com/parentalk/adolescence/teens29.html, The National Parenting Center, all rights reserved, www.tnpc.com, Dr. Wibbelsman's full bio can be found at www.tnpc.com/parentalk/bios2.html.

"A day or two after your period starts you begin to feel better. Hormone levels go back on the upswing and you get back to what you're accustomed to during the rest of your cycle," Rarick explains.

Cramps, a Common Complaint

More than half of menstruating women have cramp-like pain during their periods. The medical term for menstrual pain is dysmenorrhea. Cramps are usually felt in the pelvic area and lower abdomen, but can radiate to the lower back or down the legs.

"Many girls have cramps severe enough to keep them home from school," Rarick says. In fact, according to Danforth's Obstetrics and Gynecology, dysmenorrhea is the most frequent cause of absenteeism from school among younger women. Rarick says women seem to go through phases when cramps are severe, then get better for several years, and then maybe worsen again. She adds that most women find they have less menstrual pain after having children.

Mechanically, cramps are like labor pains. Just as the uterus contracts to open up the cervix (neck of the uterus) and push out a baby, it contracts to expel menstrual blood. Often, after several years of menstruating, or after childbirth, the cervical opening enlarges. The uterus doesn't have to contract as much to discharge the menstrual flow, so there is less cramping.

Menstrual pain may also come from the bleeding process itself. When the uterine lining separates from the wall, it releases chemicals called prostaglandins. Prostaglandins cause blood vessels to narrow, impeding the supply of oxygen to the uterus. Just as the pain of a heart attack comes from insufficient blood to the muscles of the heart, too little blood to the uterine muscle might cause the pain of menstrual cramps.

Menstrual pain can have other causes, although these are rare among teenagers. They include tumors, fallopian tube infection, and endometriosis, a condition in which fragments of the lining of the uterus become embedded elsewhere in the body.

Pain, Pain Go Away

Sometimes, simple measures are all that's needed to feel better. Cutting down on salt might help reduce fluid buildup, and support hose may alleviate swelling in the legs or ankles. Crawling into bed for some extra rest or sleep is one way to deal with fatigue, and taking along a heating pad or hot water bottle eases cramps for some.

Exercising also helps reduce pain in many young women, and may lift a blue mood as well.

Charles Debrovner, MD, associate clinical professor of obstetrics and gynecology at New York University School of Medicine, explains that exercising during menstruation lessens pain because it causes release of brain chemicals called endorphins, which are natural pain-killers. He says exercise may also decrease pain by affecting prostaglandin metabolism.

Rarick adds that exercise may also help because it increases blood flow, and because it "just makes a lot of people feel better in general."

If symptoms interfere with work, school or sleep, the American College of Obstetricians and Gynecologists recommends seeing a doctor, who may suggest taking one or more medicines. Certain anti-inflammatory drugs called NSAIDs (an abbreviation for nonsteroidal anti-inflammatory drugs) inhibit prostaglandin production, thus easing cramps. Prescription NSAIDs include naproxen (Naprosyn, Anaprox), ibuprofen (Motrin, IBU), indomethacin (Indocin), and mefenamic acid (Ponstel).

If needed, your doctor may prescribe stronger painkillers or even oral contraceptives. One side effect of birth control pills is relief of menstrual cramps.

"Birth control pills work two ways to lessen cramps," says Rarick. "They prevent the lining of the uterus from building up so much, so there's less bleeding. This means less prostaglandin production and blood vessel narrowing because there's less lining to separate, and fewer contractions because there's less tissue to push out."

Although frequently requested and prescribed for bloating or fluid retention around menstrual periods, most studies have not found diuretics (water pills) to be very effective for treating menstrual symptoms. These are generally best avoided, because they can deplete the body of essential minerals.

Over-the-Counter Relief

In 1984, FDA approved ibuprofen in over-the-counter (OTC) strengths to be sold without a prescription. It's the active ingredient in medicines such as Advil, Nuprin, and Motrin IB. In 1994, the agency approved naproxen for OTC marketing in lower doses than the prescription strength. OTC naproxen is sold under the brand name Aleve.

Like NSAIDs, aspirin also suppresses prostaglandins, but it's often not as effective as other NSAIDs for menstrual pain. Aspirin should never be used by children or teenagers who have chickenpox or flu symptoms before checking with a doctor. This is because Reye syndrome, a rare but sometimes deadly illness, may develop in children and teenagers who have taken aspirin or products that contain it while they were sick with chickenpox or flu.

Several OTC products, such as Midol and Pamprin, are specifically formulated for menstrual symptoms. Read the labels of these medicines before you buy them, because different formulations often contain different ingredients or strengths of ingredients. For example, Teen Formula Midol contains acetaminophen for pain and pamabrom (a mild diuretic) for fluid retention. Pamprin contains acetaminophen, pamabrom and pyrilamine maleate (an antihistamine) for tension and irritability. Cramp Relief Formula Midol IB contains as its sole ingredient ibuprofen. Manufacturers may change their products' ingredients from time to time, so it's a good idea to check the label each time you buy the product.

Plain acetaminophen products like Tylenol, Datril, and Aspirin-Free Anacin also may help menstrual pain. It takes time for pain relievers to work, so it's best to take them before the pain gets bad and continue for one or two days, as needed.

Some 20 to 40 percent of menstruating women have PMS, or premenstrual syndrome. Starting anywhere from mid-cycle to a few days before menstruation begins, women with PMS may have one or all of a virtual laundry list of physical and emotional symptoms. They include breast swelling and tenderness, fluid retention, increased thirst or appetite, craving for sweets and salty foods, headaches, anxiety, restlessness, irritability, depression, hostility, and loss of self confidence. Experts say PMS doesn't usually affect teenagers, though. It increases with age and is more prevalent in the 30s and 40s.

A closely related disorder is Premenstrual Dysphoric Disorder, or PMDD. Women with PMDD have marked mood swings, depression, or anxiety that relate to their menstrual period. This may coexist with PMS; it is usually diagnosed when the mood symptoms are particularly severe. Many women with PMDD respond to the use of antidepressants. One such medication has been FDA-approved for PMDD, and is marketed as Serafem. It contains the same medication as Prozac, but is only taken one week out of the month. Other antidepressants are also probably effective, although they do not yet have FDA approval for this indication.

From Menarche to Menopause

In the United States, the average age of menarche—a girl's first period—is 12 years, although it's normal to start as early as 10 or as late as 16. Menopause—when periods stop—usually occurs around age 50, although that, too, can vary by several years. Except perhaps for the first two years of menstruation—and barring pregnancy, nursing, and certain illnesses or other problems—the reproductive cycle repeats with predictable regularity every month.

Exercise, diet and stress can delay the onset of menstruation, Rarick says, or alter cycles once they've been established.

"Gymnasts, ballerinas and others who exercise strenuously can sometimes delay the onset of their periods, so you might not be surprised to find a 16- or 17-year-old in that group who hasn't started menstruating," she says. "Some experts believe the connection between exercise and amenorrhea [the absence of menstrual periods] is related to body fat content, because fat affects estrogen. Young women who are very thin from malnourishment may not start menstruating until they gain weight, with a certain portion of that weight being fat. So, girls who exercise a lot—who are all bone and muscle with no fat—may delay their periods."

Similarly, young women with severe eating disorders such as anorexia or bulimia often do not menstruate.

The American College of Obstetricians and Gynecologists recommends that a girl see her doctor if she hasn't started menstruating by age 16, or if by age 13 or 14 she hasn't begun to develop breasts or pubic and underarm hair.

Just Like Clockwork?

Many young women have very irregular periods the first couple years of menstruating—even skipping some months, until, as Rarick says, "the system is well-tuned."

In addition, she says, young women don't always ovulate every month when they first get their periods. She adds that there's no sure way for a young woman to know which month she is ovulating and which she is not. So, from the time her periods begin, a young woman should assume she can get pregnant each and every month, even if her periods are irregular.

Eventually, periods become regular, but even when they do, a missed or late period once a year—especially at a stressful time—is considered normal, according to Rarick.

Also, just as strenuous exercise and eating disorders can delay the onset of menstruation, they can also cause previously regular menstrual cycles to become irregular or stop completely.

Monthly Changes

Menstruation is just one part of the menstrual cycle, in which a woman's body prepares for pregnancy each month. A cycle is counted from the first day of one period to the first day of the next. An average cycle is 28 days, but anywhere from 23 to 35 days is normal.

Estrogen and progesterone levels are very low at the beginning of the cycle. During menstruation, levels of estrogen, made by the ovaries, start to rise and make the lining of the uterus grow and thicken. In the meantime, an egg (ovum) in one of the ovaries starts to mature. It is encased in a sac called the Graafian follicle, which continues to produce estrogen as the egg grows.

At about day 14 of a typical 28-day cycle, the sac bursts and the egg leaves the ovary, traveling through one of the fallopian tubes to the uterus. The release of the egg from the ovary is called ovulation. Some women know when they're ovulating, because at mid-cycle they have some pain—typically a dull ache on either side of the lower abdomen lasting a few hours. The medical word for this is mittelschmerz, from the German, meaning middle pain. Some women also have very light bleeding, or spotting, during ovulation.

After the egg is expelled, the sac—now called a corpus luteum—remains in the ovary, where it starts producing mainly progesterone. The rising levels of both estrogen and progesterone help build up the uterine lining to prepare for pregnancy.

The few days before, during and after ovulation are a woman's "fertile period"—the time when she can become pregnant. Because the length of menstrual cycles vary, many woman ovulate earlier or later than day 14. It's even possible for a woman to ovulate while she still has her period if that month's cycle is very short (stress and other things can sometimes cause a cycle to be shorter or longer). If a woman has sex with a man during this time and conception occurs (his sperm fertilizes the egg), she becomes pregnant.

The fertilized egg attaches to the uterus, and the corpus luteum makes all the progesterone needed to keep it implanted and growing until a placenta (an organ connecting the fetus to the mother) develops. The placenta then makes hormones and provides nourishment from the mother to the baby.

If an egg is not fertilized that month and the woman doesn't get pregnant, the corpus luteum stops making hormones and gets reabsorbed in the ovary. Hormone levels drop again, the lining of the uterus breaks down, menstruation begins, and the cycle repeats.

Menstrual Bleeding: What's Normal, What's Not

Most menstrual periods last from three to five days, but anywhere from two to seven days is normal. The amount of blood flow varies, too, but for most women, bleeding starts out light at first, followed by heavier flow for a day or two and then another light day or two. Sanitary pads or tampons, which are made of cotton or another absorbent material, are worn to absorb the blood flow. Sanitary pads are placed inside the panties; tampons are inserted into the vagina.

"The amount of bleeding varies from woman to woman because everybody's body has a different way of building up the lining of the uterus," says Lisa Rarick, MD "A lighter flow or heavier flow doesn't mean you can't get pregnant as easily or you're never going to get pregnant, or that your periods will always stay the same way. But if you're bleeding excessively—soaking one or more tampons or pads an hour—you should see a doctor to see if there's a problem."

Rarick, a gynecologist with FDA's Center for Drug Evaluation and Research, says teenagers often are concerned if they expel blood clots during their periods. She says this is not dangerous; they are clumps of pooled blood in the vagina. Sometimes, instead of flowing freely, blood drains from the uterus and stays in the vagina until there's a change in position—say, from sitting to standing.

Women who use tampons should be aware of toxic shock syndrome, or TSS, a rare but serious—and sometimes fatal—disease that's been associated with tampon use. Tampon packages carry information about TSS on the box or inside. Because TSS mostly affects 15- to 19-year-olds, it's especially important for teenagers to know what signs to look for. If you develop the following symptoms while menstruating, remove the tampon and get medical help right away:

- sudden fever over 102 degrees Fahrenheit
- vomiting
- diarrhea
- dizziness, fainting, or near fainting when standing up
- a rash that looks like a sunburn

Talking to Your Daughter about Menstruation

Girls need to know about menstruation well before "menarche," the first menstrual period, occurs. Too many parents wait until a girl is a certain age, say twelve, to discuss the subject, not realizing that many normal girls may begin menstrual periods as early as the age of nine or ten.

Signs that your daughter may be approaching menarche are breast development and pubic hair growth. Talk with her about all the normal changes of puberty, and the process of the menstrual cycle. Take this time to dispel any myths about menstruation.

Reassure your daughter that it is natural and that it doesn't have to keep her from her normal activities. While menstruation is certainly not a hygienic emergency, this may be a good time to discuss with your daughter how she can best care for her body with daily baths, use of a deodorant, and frequent changes of pads or tampons.

Contrary to prevailing myths, girls who are virgins can safely use tampons from menarche on, if they choose. Help your daughter to prepare emotionally and in practical terms for her first period with her own supply of sanitary products, ready in advance.

Feeling that menarche is a natural event can help a girl feel better about becoming a young woman.

—by Charles Wibblesman, MD

About the Author of this Section

A noted specialist in adolescent medicine, Dr. Wibblesman is a practicing physician at The Kaiser Foundation Hospital Department of Pediatrics in San Francisco. Wibblesman is also chief of The Teenage Clinic, at Kaiser Permanente's Medical Center and author of four books on the subject of adolescence including the best-selling *The New Teenage Body Book*.

Chapter 33

Teen Gynecologic Exams

A Teen's First Visit to the Gynecologist

A teenager's first internal exam can be as awkward for her parents as it is for her. Knowing what to expect and picking a gynecologist who can connect with a teenage girl can help alleviate some of the anxiety associated with that first visit.

"We recommend that girls between the ages of 13 and 15 see a gynecologist for a visit that does not include a pelvic exam unless there is a problem," says Owen C. Montgomery, MD, a Pennsylvania Hospital obstetrician/gynecologist, who also serves on the American College of Obstetrics and Gynecology's National Committee for Adolescent Health.

At that visit, Montgomery discusses any concerns the patient may have about changes in her body, her menstrual cycle, and other issues. "This helps to establish a good relationship for the future," he says. He also recommends that young women who are 18 or who are sexually active see a gynecologist for regular pelvic exams, Pap smears and birth control counseling.

A visit to the gynecologist provides teens with an opportunity to gain information that will help them to sort out confusing issues.

This chapter contains text from "A Teen's First Visit to the Gynecologist," http://www.uphs.upenn.edu/pahosp/pah_news/quill/gynecology/teen_gyn_visit. html, Pennsylvania Hospital, updated October 2001, reprinted with permission, and "Having a Pelvic Exam and Pap Test" an undated document from the National Cancer Institute (NCI), National Institutes of Health (NIH), http://cancernet.nci.nih.gov/peb/pelvic_exam/PELVIC_MAIN.htm, cited November 2001.

"These young women are exposed to a whirlwind of ideas about their bodies, peer relationships, independence, personal identity and, of course, sexuality," he says. "They need non-judgmental and well-informed medical guidance when it comes to their concerns."

It is up to parents to lay the groundwork for these discussions. "Every parent should talk directly and honestly with their kids about sex, relationships, and other key issues. If they don't, parents won't know what information their teens will get," says Montgomery. For example, a study by the Center for Disease Control (CDC) found that teens whose mothers talked with them about condoms before the first sexual encounter were three times more likely to use condoms than teens who either never discussed condoms with their mothers or did so only after initiating sexual activity. This reinforces the important role parents can play in HIV (human immunodeficiency virus) prevention, since half of those infections in the US occur in people under 25.

"Despite how teens act, the vast majority of them accept their parents' basic values," says Montgomery. "If you take the time to listen, be flexible, and trust your teenager, they will treat you with the same respect. And that will have long-term benefits when it comes to avoiding risky behaviors."

While parents are responsible for finding the right doctor for their teen-aged children, it is the adolescent's responsibility to follow through on the doctor's recommendations. The more active they are in their own care, the more likely they are to have a healthy lifestyle.

Here are some things to consider when selecting a gynecologist for a teenage daughter:

- The waiting room should have informational materials on puberty, sexually transmitted diseases and contraception to help teens feel that it's okay to talk about these subjects.

- The physician should have a good rapport with teens and enjoy working with them.

- The first interview with the teen should be private, unless she specifically asks to have a parent with her. She should be fully clothed and seated in a comfortable environment where she can raise her concerns or describe her needs.

- When she does have her first pelvic exam, she should be encouraged to feel in control of the situation and able to stop the exam at any time to ask questions.

- She should be reassured that her communications with the doctor are strictly confidential and will only be shared with her parent with her permission.

Having a Pelvic Exam and Pap Test

Getting Ready for the Pelvic Exam

- A nurse will ask you about your health.

- You will go into the exam room. You will have a paper gown to put on and a sheet to cover you.

- You will lie down on the table with a sheet over your legs and stomach. You will let your knees fall to the side and put your feet in holders called stirrups.

Here's Some Good Advice from Women Who Have Had This Exam

"If I start to feel embarrassed, I take some deep breaths and then I feel better."

"It feels funny to lie on the table with your knees up in the air, but you don't have to be there very long."

"The nurse told me not to have sex, use vaginal creams, or douche for 24 hours before the exam."

"She also told me not to have the Pap test when I am having my period."

Having the Exam

- The nurse or doctor will look at your vaginal area to see if you have any signs of infection or other problems.

- The nurse or doctor will slide a thin piece of plastic or metal that looks like a duck bill into your vagina to check inside.

- During the Pap test, the nurse or doctor will use a small brush to take a few cells from your cervix (the opening to the womb). A lab will check these cells for cancer or other problems. If cancer is found early, it is easier to cure.

- After the Pap test, the nurse or doctor will check your tubes, ovaries, and uterus (womb) by putting two gloved fingers inside your vagina. With her other hand, she will feel from the outside for any lumps or tenderness. This takes only a few minutes.

- When the exam is over you can get dressed.

- Be sure to ask any questions before the nurse or doctor leaves the room.

- Most Pap test results are normal.

- The doctor or clinic will contact you if yours is not.

Chapter 34

Diseases of the Female Reproductive Organs

Chapter Contents

Section 34.1

Bacterial Vaginosis

Centers for Disease Control and Prevention (CDC), Division of Sexually Transmitted Diseases, http://www.cdc.gov/nchstp/dstd/Fact_Sheets/ FactsBV.htm, September 2000.

What Is Bacterial Vaginosis?

Bacterial vaginosis (BV) is the most common vaginal infection in women of childbearing age, and it is sometimes accompanied by discharge, odor, pain, itching, or burning.

What Causes Bacterial Vaginosis?

The cause of BV is not fully understood. BV is associated with an imbalance in the bacteria that are normally found in a woman's vagina. The vagina normally contains mostly "good" bacteria, and fewer "harmful" bacteria. BV develops when there is a change in the environment of the vagina that causes an increase in harmful bacteria.

How Do Women Get Bacterial Vaginosis?

Not much is known about how women get BV. Women who have a new sex partner or who have had multiple sex partners are more likely to develop BV. Women who have never had sexual intercourse are rarely affected. It is not clear what role sexual activity plays in the development of BV, and there are many unanswered questions about the role that harmful bacteria play in causing BV. Women do not get BV from toilet seats, bedding, swimming pools, or from touching objects around them.

How Common Is Bacterial Vaginosis?

Scientific studies suggest that BV is common in women of reproductive age. In the United States, as many as 16% of pregnant women have BV. This varies by race and ethnicity from 6% in Asians and 9%

in whites to 16% in Hispanics and 23% in African Americans. BV is generally more commonly seen in women attending STD clinics than in those attending family planning or prenatal clinics.

What Are the Signs and Symptoms of Bacterial Vaginosis?

Women with BV often have an abnormal vaginal discharge with an unpleasant odor. Some women report a strong fish-like odor, especially after intercourse. The discharge is usually white or gray; it can be thin. Women with BV may also have burning during urination or itching around the outside of the vagina, or both. Some women with BV report no signs or symptoms at all.

How Is Bacterial Vaginosis Diagnosed?

A health care provider must examine the vagina for signs of BV (e.g., discharge) and perform laboratory tests on a sample of vaginal fluid to look for bacteria associated with BV.

Who Is at Risk for Bacterial Vaginosis?

Any woman can get BV. However, some activities or behaviors can upset the normal balance of bacteria in the vagina and put women at increased risk:

- having a new sex partner or multiple sex partners
- douching
- using an intrauterine device (IUD) for contraception
- pregnant women are at increased risk for complications of BV

What Are the Complications of Bacterial Vaginosis?

In most cases, BV causes no complications. But there are some serious risks from BV:

- Pregnant women with BV more often have babies who are born early or with low birth weight.

- The bacteria that cause BV can sometimes infect the uterus (womb) and fallopian tubes (egg canals). This type of infection is called pelvic inflammatory disease (PID). PID can cause infertility or damage the fallopian tubes enough to increase the future risk of ectopic pregnancy and infertility. Ectopic pregnancy is a life-threatening condition in which a fertilized egg grows outside the uterus, usually in a fallopian tube.

- BV can increase a woman's susceptibility to HIV (human immunodeficiency virus) infection if she is exposed to the virus.

- Having BV increases the chances that an HIV-infected woman can pass HIV to her sex partner.

- BV can increase a woman's susceptibility to other Sexually Transmitted Diseases (SDS), such as chlamydia and gonorrhea.

Who Should Be Treated for Bacterial Vaginosis?

Although BV will sometimes clear up without treatment, all women with symptoms of BV should be treate to avoid such complications as PID. Treatment is especially important for pregnant women. All pregnant women, regardless of symptos, who have ever had a premature delivery or low birth weight baby should be considered for a BV examination and be treated when necessary. All pregnant women who have symptoms of BV should be checked and treated. Male partners generally do not need to be treated. However, BV may spread between female sex partners.

What Is the Treatment for Bacterial Vaginosis?

BV is treatable with antimicrobial medicines prescribed by a health care provider. Two different medicines are recommended as treatment for BV: metronidazole or clindamycin. Either can be used with non-pregnant or with pregnant women, but the recommended dosages differ. Women with BV who are HIV-positive should receive the same treatment as those who are HIV-negative. BV can recur after treatment.

How Can Bacterial Vaginosis Be Prevented?

BV is not completely understood by scientists, and the best ways to prevent it are unknown. However, enough is known to show that BV is associated with having a new sex partner or having multiple sex partners. It is seldom found in women who have never had intercourse.

Some basic prevention steps can help reduce the risk of upsetting the natural balance in the vagina and developing BV:

- use condoms during sex

- limit the number of sex partners

- do not douche

- use all of the medicine prescribed for treatment of BV, even if the signs and symptoms go away

Section 34.2

Pelvic Inflammatory Disease

National Institute of Allergy and Infectious Diseases (NIAID), National Institutes of Health (NIH), http://www.niaid.nih.gov/factsheets/stdpid.htm, July 1998.

Introduction

Aside from AIDS (acquired immune deficiency syndrome), the most common and serious complication of sexually transmitted diseases (SDS) among women is pelvic inflammatory disease (PID), an infection of the upper genital tract. PID can affect the uterus, ovaries, fallopian tubes, or other related structures. Untreated, PID causes scarring and can lead to infertility, tubal pregnancy, chronic pelvic pain, and other serious consequences.

Each year in the United States, more than 1 million women experience an episode of acute PID, with the rate of infection highest among teenagers. More than 100,000 women become infertile each year as a result of PID, and a large proportion of the 70,000 ectopic (tubal) pregnancies occurring every year are due to the consequences of PID. In 1997 alone, an estimated $7 billion was spent on PID and its complications.

Cause

PID occurs when disease-causing organisms migrate upward from the urethra and cervix into the upper genital tract. Many different organisms can cause PID, but most cases are associated with gonorrhea and genital chlamydial infections, two very common SDS. Scientists have found that bacteria normally present in small numbers in the vagina and cervix also may play a role.

Investigators are learning more about how these organisms cause PID. The gonococcus, *Neisseria gonorrhea*, probably travels to the fallopian tubes, where it causes sloughing (casting out) of some cells and invades others. Researchers think it multiplies within and beneath these cells. The infection then may spread to other organs, resulting in more inflammation and scarring.

Chlamydia trachomatis and other bacteria may behave in a similar manner. Researchers do not know how other bacteria that normally inhabit the vagina (e.g., organisms such as *Gardnerella vaginalis* and *Bacteroides*) gain entrance into the upper genital tract. The cervical mucus plug and secretions may help prevent the spread of microorganisms to the upper genital tract, but it may be less effective during ovulation and menses. In addition, the gonococcus may gain access more easily during menses, if menstrual blood flows backward from the uterus into the fallopian tubes, carrying the organisms with it. This may explain why symptoms of PID caused by gonorrhea often begin immediately after menstruation as opposed to any other time during the menstrual cycle. It is noteworthy that the co-incidence of menses and chlamydial infection is not a prominent feature of chlamydial PID.

Symptoms

The major symptoms of PID are lower abdominal pain and abnormal vaginal discharge. Other symptoms such as fever, pain in the right upper abdomen, painful intercourse, and irregular menstrual bleeding can occur as well. PID, particularly when caused by chlamydial infection, may produce only minor symptoms or no symptoms at all, even though it can seriously damage the reproductive organs.

Risk Factors for PID

- Women with SDS—especially gonorrhea and chlamydial infection—are at greater risk of developing PID; a prior episode of PID increases the risk of another episode because the body's defenses are often damaged during the initial bout of upper genital tract infection.

- Sexually active teenagers are more likely to develop PID than are older women.

- The more sexual partners a woman has, the greater her risk of developing PID.

Recent data indicate that women who douche once or twice a month may be more likely to have PID than those who douche less than once a month. Douching may push bacteria into the upper genital tract. Douching also may ease discharge caused by an infection, so the woman delays seeking health care.

Diagnosis

PID can be difficult to diagnose. If symptoms such as lower abdominal pain are present, the doctor will perform a physical exam to determine the nature and location of the pain. The doctor also should check the patient for fever, abnormal vaginal or cervical discharge, and evidence of cervical chlamydial infection or gonorrhea. If the findings of this exam suggest that PID is likely, current guidelines advise doctors to begin treatment.

If more information is necessary, the doctor may order other tests, such as a sonogram, endometrial biopsy, or laparoscopy to distinguish between PID and other serious problems that may mimic PID. Laparoscopy is a surgical procedure in which a tiny, flexible tube with a lighted end is inserted through a small incision just below the navel. This procedure allows the doctor to view the internal abdominal and pelvic organs, as well as take specimens for cultures or microscopic studies, if necessary.

Treatment

Because culture of specimens from the upper genital tract are difficult to obtain and because multiple organisms may be responsible for an episode of PID, especially if it is not the first one, the doctor will prescribe at least two antibiotics that are effective against a wide range of infectious agents. The symptoms may go away before the infection is cured. Even if symptoms do go away, patients should finish taking all of the medicine. Patients should be re-evaluated by their physicians two to three days after treatment is begun to be sure the antibiotics are working to cure the infection.

About one-fourth of women with suspected PID must be hospitalized. The doctor may recommend this if the patient is severely ill; if she cannot take oral medication and needs intravenous antibiotics; if she is pregnant or is an adolescent; if the diagnosis is uncertain and may include an abdominal emergency such as appendicitis; or if she is infected with HIV (human immunodeficiency virus, the virus that causes AIDS).

Many women with PID have sex partners who have no symptoms, although their sex partners may be infected with organisms that can cause PID. Because of the risk of reinfection, however, sex partners should be treated even if they do not have symptoms.

Consequences of PID

Women with recurrent episodes of PID are more likely than women with a single episode to suffer scarring of the tubes that leads to infertility, tubal pregnancy, or chronic pelvic pain. Infertility occurs in approximately 20 percent of women who have had PID.

Most women with tubal infertility, however, never have had symptoms of PID. Organisms such as *C. trachomatis* can silently invade the fallopian tubes and cause scarring, which blocks the normal passage of eggs into the uterus.

a women who has had PID has a six-to-tenfold increased risk of tubal pregnancy, in which the egg can become fertilized but cannot pass into the uterus to grow. Instead, the egg usually attaches in the fallopian tube, which connects the ovary to the uterus. The fertilized egg cannot grow normally in the fallopian tube. This type of pregnancy is life-threatening to the mother, and almost always fatal to her fetus. It is the leading cause of pregnancy-related death in African-American women.

In addition, untreated PID can cause chronic pelvic pain and scarring in about 20 percent of patients. These conditions are difficult to treat but are sometimes improved with surgery.

Another complication of PID is the risk of repeated attacks of PID. As many as one-third of women who have had PID will have the disease at least one more time. With each episode of reinfection, the risk of infertility is increased.

Prevention

Women can play an active role in protecting themselves from PID by taking the following steps:

- Signs of discharge with odor or bleeding between cycles could mean infection. Early treatment may prevent the development of PID.

- If used correctly and consistently, male latex condoms will prevent transmission of gonorrhea and partially protect against chlamydial infection.

Research

Although much has been learned about the biology of the microbes that cause PID and the ways in which they damage the body, there is still much to learn. Scientists supported by the National Institute of Allergy and Infectious Diseases (NIAID) are studying the effects of antibiotics, hormones, and substances that boost the immune system. These studies may lead to insights about how to prevent infertility or other complications of PID. Topical microbicides and vaccines to prevent gonorrhea and chlamydial infection also are being developed. Clinical trials are in progress to test a suppository containing lactobacilli—the normal bacteria found in the vaginas of healthy women. These bacteria colonize the vagina and may be associated with reduced risk of gonorrhea and bacterial vaginosis, both of which can cause PID.

Rapid, inexpensive, easy-to-use diagnostic tests are being developed to detect chlamydial infection and gonorrhea. A recent study conducted by NIAID-funded researchers demonstrated that screening and treating women who unknowingly had chlamydial infection reduced cases of PID by more than 60 percent. Meanwhile, researchers continue to search for better ways to detect PID itself, particularly in women with "silent" or asymptomatic PID.

Section 34.3

Toxic Shock Syndrome

Dixie Farley, "On the Teen Scene: T.S.: Reducing the Risk," *FDA Consumer*, October 1991, Food and Drug Administration (FDA) Pub. No. 98-1196, http://www.fda.gov/bbs/topics/CONSUMER/con00116.html, revised September 1997 and January 1999.

Introduction

Women taking the necessary measures to prevent menstrually-related toxic shock syndrome (TSS) can be credited with much of the reduction in the number of cases in recent years. In 1997, there were only five confirmed menstrually-related TSS cases and no deaths.

TSS is a rare but potentially fatal disease that, when related to menstruation, occurs most frequently in young women aged 15 to 24, usually in association with tampon use.

The number of confirmed menstrually-related TSS cases peaked in 1980 at 814, with 38 deaths. At that time, the national Centers for Disease Control (CDC) found that 71 percent of women who developed the condition had been using Rely, a brand of highly absorbent tampons that had recently come on the market. These tampons were removed from the market, and the Food and Drug Administration and tampon manufacturers developed product labeling to help women avoid the life-threatening condition.

The incidence of menstrually-related TSS was reduced to 470, with 13 deaths, in 1981 and has continued to fall steadily since then.

TSS was first identified as a distinct disease in 1978 and also affects people who don't use tampons. It occurs in children, men, and non-menstruating women, most frequently in connection with wounds. Though scientists know there is a relationship between the development of TSS and the use of tampons, especially high-absorbency tampons, the exact connection remains unclear.

Scientists think that in order for the disease to develop, bacteria called *Staphylococcus aureus* must be present. These bacteria release one or more toxins (poisons) into the bloodstream. *S. aureus* bacteria commonly live in body areas such as the nose, skin, or vagina and usually cause no problem. But the bacteria also can lead to serious infection after a deep wound or surgery or, for reasons not fully understood, during tampon use.

Keeping Your Risk Low

If you've ever had TSS, get medical advice before using tampons.

You can reduce your risk of TSS by not using tampons or by alternating between tampons and pads. Whether the benefits of using tampons—particularly high-absorbency ones—are worth the increased risk of TSS is an individual decision.

Because the TSS risk increases with tampon absorbency, if you use tampons, you should use products with the lowest absorbency that meets your needs. There's usually less need for high absorbency at the end of a menstrual period. You can find what's best for you by experimenting with different sizes and different brands, beginning with the least absorbent.

To help women compare absorbency from brand to brand, The Food and Drug Administration (FDA) requires that manufacturers use a standard test to measure absorbency and that the absorbency be stated on the label using standard terminology. When shopping for tampons, look on the packages for the following absorbency terms and ranges and then compare brands before you make your selection.

Table 34.1. Tampon Absorbency Rating Scale.

if the package says:	The absorbency range is:
Junior Absorbency	6 grams and under
Regular Absorbency	6 to 9 grams
Super Absorbency	9 to 12 grams
Super Plus Absorbency	12 to 15 grams

It also helps to:

- follow the manufacturer's instructions.

- store tampons in a clean, dry place.

- wash hands with soap and water before and after inserting or removing a tampon.

- try a less absorbent variety if a tampon is irritating or difficult to remove.

FDA also requires manufacturers to give information about TSS on the tampon box or in a package insert. This information must include a warning about the association between TSS and high-absorbency tampons. You can stay up-to-date on TSS by reading the package information when you buy tampons and asking about TSS when you get a medical checkup.

Symptoms may not appear until the first few days after the end of your period. Be sure to explain to your doctor what your symptoms are, when your period began, and whether you've ever had TSS before. If you use tampons, mention what absorbency you use.

TSS symptoms appear quickly and are often severe. Not all cases are exactly alike, and you may not have all the symptoms. You may have aching muscles, bloodshot eyes, or a sore throat, making it seem like the flu. The sunburn-like rash may not develop until you're very ill; it may go unnoticed if it's only on a small area. Later, the skin on your palms and soles may flake or peel. A first episode may be so mild that you don't connect the symptoms with TSS, but the next time, the symptoms may be severe. Once you've had TSS, you're more likely to get it than someone who never has had it.

Deaths, though rare, tend to happen during the first week of illness. The danger lies in a sudden drop in blood pressure, which could lead to shock if not treated in time.

TSS is usually treated with antibiotics, and drugs to lower temperature, and large amounts of fluids and electrolytes (essential body chemicals) to raise lowered blood pressure. Blood and other specimens from the body are analyzed in a laboratory to identify bacteria. Antibiotics are given to help prevent recurrence. Patients often are hospitalized, and severe cases require intensive care. With proper treatment, patients generally recover within three weeks.

While TSS is rare, it's an important health concern for menstruating women, and especially young women. Knowing how to prevent it and recognizing its symptoms can do much to reduce its dangers and continue to keep its incidence low.

TSS Symptoms

Remove your tampon if you're using one and get medical help right away if you have the following symptoms during menstruation:

- sudden high fever—102 degrees Fahrenheit (38.9 degrees Celsius) or higher

- vomiting

- diarrhea

- muscle aches

- dizziness, fainting, or near fainting when standing up

- a rash that looks like a sunburn

Early diagnosis and speedy treatment are crucial to avoiding the most serious effects of TSS.

—by Dixie Farley

Dixie Farley is a staff writer for *FDA Consumer*. Judith Levine Willis also contributed to this article.

Section 34.4

Getting Rid of Yeast Infections

Judith Levine Willis, *FDA Consumer*, April 1996, Food and Drug Administration (FDA) Pub. No. 97-2301, (this article originally appeared under the title "On the Teen Scene: An Itch Like No Other."), http://www.fda.gov/fdac/features/396_yst.html, revised March 1997.

It's an itchy feeling you might hardly notice at first.

Maybe, you muse, it's just that your jeans are too tight.

Actually, tight jeans may have something to do with it. But if the itch keeps getting itchier, even when your jeans have been off for awhile, then there's something else involved.

That something else could very well be a fungus whose technical name is Candida, and which causes what is often called a "yeast" infection. Such infections are most common in teenage girls and women aged 16 to 35, although they can occur in girls as young as 10 or 11 and in older women (and less often, in men and boys as well). You do not have to be sexually active to get a yeast infection.

The Food and Drug Administration (FDA) now allows medicines that used to be prescription—only to be sold without a prescription to treat vaginal yeast infections that keep coming back. But before you run out and buy one, if you've never been treated for a yeast infection you should see a doctor. Your doctor may advise you to use one of the over-the-counter products or may prescribe a drug called Diflucan (fluconazole). FDA recently approved the drug, a tablet taken by mouth, for clearing up yeast infections with just one dose.

Though itchiness is a main symptom of yeast infections, if you've never had one before, it's hard to be sure just what's causing your discomfort. After a doctor makes a diagnosis of vaginal yeast infection, if you should have one again, you can more easily recognize the symptoms that make it different from similar problems. If you have any doubts, though, you should contact your doctor.

In addition to intense itching, another symptom of a vaginal yeast infection is a white cuddy or thick discharge that is mostly odorless. Although some women have discharges midway between their menstrual periods, these are usually not yeast infections, especially if there's no itching.

Other symptoms of a vaginal yeast infection include:

- soreness

- rash on outer lips of the vagina

- burning, especially during urination

It's important to remember that not all girls and women experience all these symptoms, and if intense itching is not present it's probably something else.

Candida is a fungus often present in the human body. It only causes problems when there's too much of it. Then infections can occur not only in the vagina but in other parts of the body as well—and in both sexes. Though there are four different types of *Candida* that can cause these infections, nearly 80 percent are caused by a variety called *Candida albicans*.

Many Causes

The biggest cause of Candida infections is lowered immunity. This can happen when you get run down from doing too much and not getting enough rest. Or it can happen as a result of illness.

Though not usual, repeated yeast infections, especially if they don't clear up with proper treatment, may sometimes be the first sign that a woman is infected with HIV (human immunodeficiency virus), the virus that causes AIDS (acquired immune deficiency syndrome).

FDA requires that over-the-counter (OTC) products to treat yeast infections carry the following warning:

"If you experience vaginal yeast infections frequently (they recur within a two-month period) or if you have vaginal yeast infections that do not clear up easily with proper treatment, you should see your doctor promptly to determine the cause and receive proper medical care."

Repeated yeast infections can also be caused by other, less serious illnesses, or physical and mental stress. Other causes include:

- use of antibiotics and some other medications, including birth control pills

- significant change in the diet

- poor nutrition

- diabetes

- pregnancy

Some women get mild yeast infections towards the end of their menstrual periods, possibly in response to the body's hormonal changes. These mild infections sometimes go away without treatment as the menstrual cycle progresses. Pregnant women are also more prone to develop yeast infections.

Sometimes hot, humid weather can make it easier for yeast infections to develop. And wearing layers of clothing in the winter that make you too warm indoors can also increase the likelihood of infection.

"Candida infections are not usually thought of as sexually transmitted diseases," says Renata Albrecht, MD, of FDA's division of anti-infective drug products. But, she adds, they can be transmitted during sex.

The best way not to have to worry about getting yeast infections this way is not to have sex. But if you do have sex, using a condom will help prevent transmission of yeast infections, just as it helps prevent transmission of more commonly sexually transmitted diseases, including HIV infection, and helps prevent pregnancy. Teens should always use a latex condom if they have sex, even if they are also using other forms of birth control.

If one partner has a yeast infection, the other partner should also be treated for it. A man is less likely than a woman to be aware of having a yeast infection because he may not have any symptoms. When symptoms do occur, they may include a moist, white, scaling rash on the penis, and itchiness or redness under the foreskin. As with females, lowered immunity, rather than sexual transmission, is the most frequent cause of genital yeast infections in males.

OTC Products

The OTC products for vaginal yeast infections have one of four active ingredients: butoconazole nitrate (Femstat 3), clotrimazole (Gyne-Lotrimin and others), miconazole (Monistat 7 and others), and tioconazole (Vagistat). These drugs are in the same anti-fungal family and work in similar ways to break down the cell wall of the Candida organism until it dissolves. FDA approved the switch of Femstat 3 from prescription to OTC status December 1996 and a similar switch for Vagistat in February 1997. The others have been available OTC for a few years.

When you visit the doctor the first time you have a yeast infection, you can ask which product may be best for you and discuss the advantages of the different forms the products come in: vaginal suppositories (inserts) and creams with special applicators. Remember to read the warnings on the product's labeling carefully and follow the directions.

Symptoms usually improve within a few days, but it's important to continue using the medication for the number of days directed, even if you no longer have symptoms.

Contact your doctor if you have the following:

- abdominal pain, fever, or a foul-smelling discharge

- no improvement within three days

- symptoms that recur within two months

OTC products are only for vaginal yeast infections. They should not be used by men or for yeast infections in other areas of the body, such as the mouth or under the fingernails.

Candida infections in the mouth are often called "thrush." Symptoms include creamy white patches that cover painful areas in the mouth, throat, or on the tongue. Because other infections cause similar symptoms, it's important to go to a doctor for an accurate diagnosis.

Wearing artificial fingernails increases the chance of getting yeast infections under the natural fingernails. Fungal infections start in the space between the artificial and natural nails, which become discolored. Treatment for these types of infections—as well as those that occur in other skin folds, such as underarms or between toes—require different products, most of which are available only with a doctor's prescription.

Knowing the causes and symptoms of yeast infections can help you take steps—such as giving those tight jeans a rest—to greatly reduce the chances of getting an infection. And, if prevention sometimes isn't enough, help is easily at hand from your doctor and pharmacy.

How to Avoid Infection

Here are some steps young women can take to make vaginal yeast infections less likely:

- Wear loose, natural-fiber clothing and underwear with a cotton crotch.

- Limit wearing of panty hose, tights, leggings, nylon underwear, and tight jeans.

- Don't use deodorant tampons and feminine deodorant sprays, especially if you feel an infection beginning.

- Dry off quickly and thoroughly after bathing and swimming—don't stay in a wet swimsuit for hours.

- It's better not to have sex in your teens, but if you're sexually active, always use a latex condom.

—by Judith Levine Willis

Judith Levine Willis is editor of *FDA Consumer*.

Section 34.5

Teen Endometriosis

Dixie Farley, "On the Teen Scene: Endometriosis: Painful, but Treatable," *FDA Consumer*, January 1995, Food and Drug Administration (FDA) Pub. No. 93-1205, http://www.fda.gov/opacom/catalog/ots_endo.html, revised January 1995 and September 1997.

"The pain was so sharp I thought I'd ruptured my appendix, but the doctor said, no, it wasn't that. It was between my periods, so I didn't connect it with menstruation. I was 16."

"Over the next 10 years, I had more and more of these 'pain attacks,' and my periods gradually became heavier and more painful."

"When I was pregnant with my first child, I was virtually pain-free. But shortly after he was born, each month around ovulation, I went to bed in tears from horrible pain. And I bled so much during menstruation I didn't dare leave the house. I went back to the doctor. It was endometriosis."

Introduction

Endometriosis is a mysterious, often painful, and disabling condition in which fragments of the lining of the uterus (womb) become embedded, or implanted, elsewhere in the body.

Of the more than 3,000 patients registered with the research program of the International Endometriosis Association in Milwaukee, 41 percent report having symptoms as teenagers. About 5 million American women and girls, some as young as 11, have endometriosis, according to the association.

"These girls have terrible pain," says Lyle Breitkopf, MD, a gynecologist in New York City. "Typically, they come to the school nurse month after month—maybe six to eight of their 12 menstrual cycles—needing something for pain or being sent home vomiting, writhing on the floor."

For a woman from Des Moines, Iowa, 25 years with endometriosis led to removal of her uterus, fallopian tubes, and ovaries a number of years ago. For many women today, new medicine and less drastic surgery reduce endometriosis symptoms and preserve reproductive organs. The Food and Drug Administration (FDA) has approved several drugs to treat endometriosis and regulates medical devices, such as lasers, used in surgical treatment.

A woman who thinks she may have endometriosis should be examined by a gynecologist. The sooner treatment begins, the better it is for the patients, says Breitkopf. "When we find them at an early stage, we can arrest the condition more easily and keep after it so it doesn't progress as far."

Doctors don't know why endometriosis only strikes certain women.

Some probably inherit it, says Breitkopf. "I've seen it in sisters, including identical twins, and in grandmother-mother-daughter situations."

According to Robert Badwey, MD, a gynecologist in suburban Washington, DC, "For whatever reason—greater incidence, better diagnostic techniques, or both—we're much more aware of endometriosis now than even a few years ago."

What's Happening in the Body?

Normally, an increased level of hormones each month triggers the release of an egg from the ovary. Finger-like tissues on one of the fallopian tubes grasp the egg, and tiny hair-like "cilia" inside the tube transport it toward the uterus. When the egg is not fertilized, the uterine lining breaks down and is shed during menstruation.

The abnormal implants of endometriosis are not in the uterus, but they respond to hormonal changes controlling menstruation. Like the uterine lining, these fragments build tissue each month, then break down and bleed. Unlike blood from the lining, however, blood from implants outside the uterus has no way to leave the body. Instead, it is absorbed by surrounding tissue, which can be painful.

As the cycle recurs month after month, the implants may get bigger. They may seed new implants and form scar tissue and adhesions (scarring that connects one organ to another). Sometimes, a collection of blood called a sac or cyst forms. If a cyst ruptures, it often causes excruciating pain.

Symptoms vary from patient to patient. Severity of symptoms frequently has little to do with the extent of the implants. For instance, some women with just a few implants have severe pain, while some with many implants have little or no pain.

For some, pain starts before or during menstruation and gets worse as the period progresses. Others report pain at a variety of times during the month. There may be a sharp pain at ovulation when the egg, trying to move into the fallopian tube, causes a cyst on the ovary to burst. (Many women normally feel a twinge of pain at ovulation. Pain caused by a ruptured endometriosis cyst is severe.)

Patients whose implants affect the bladder or intestines often report painful urination or bowel movements and, sometimes, blood in the urine or stool.

Endometriosis sometimes causes premenstrual staining and, as the period progresses, heavy menstrual flow.

Often, endometriosis remains hidden a long time. A symptom such as pain at menstruation may not be seen as unusual, explains Mary Lou Ballweg, executive director of the Endometriosis Association.

"Perhaps a young woman is told by Mom, who had the same problems, that menstrual pain is normal," Ballweg says. "So she just lives with it and doesn't see a doctor until the symptoms become unbearable. Some young women with endometriosis have apparently normal menstrual periods for years before having discomfort and pain. Others report they've nearly always had difficult periods."

As many as 30 percent of women who report infertility problems have endometriosis.

Severe endometriosis can lead to infertility in various ways. In the ovaries, it can produce cysts that prevent the egg's release. In the fallopian tubes, implants can block the passage of the egg. Also, adhesions can fix ovaries and tubes in place so that projections on the tubes can't grasp the egg and move it into the tube. The effect of mild endometriosis on infertility is less clear.

Women with endometriosis may have a higher rate of "ectopic" pregnancy, a potentially life-threatening condition in which the fertilized egg begins to develop outside the womb.

The most common way to see whether a woman has endometriosis is by surgical examination using laparoscopy, a fairly simple procedure usually done without an overnight hospital stay. The doctor makes a tiny incision and inserts a lighted, flexible, telescope-like device called a laparoscope that allows a close look at the pelvis and internal organs. However, sometimes the implants themselves can only be seen through microscopic evaluation of biopsy specimens.

Drug Treatment

Drugs for endometriosis should not be taken by women who are, or who may be, pregnant.

The earliest drug approved to treat endometriosis was Danocrine (danazol), a synthetic steroid related to the hormone testosterone.

Taken orally, in pill form, Danocrine changes endometrial tissue, shrinking and eliminating implants in some cases. Side effects include fluid retention, weight gain, and masculinizing effects such as voice change, hairiness, and reduction of breast size. Other side effects include menstrual irregularities, hot flashes, and vaginal dryness.

Other drugs, related to gonadotropin-releasing hormone (GnRH), act in a different way to decrease the hormones that make abnormal implants grow. One version is a nasal spray called Synarel (nafarelin acetate). In clinical studies, Synarel, at 400 or 800 micrograms a day (within the prescribed dosage range), was comparable to Danocrine at 800 milligrams a day (the recommended dosage) in relieving the clinical symptoms of endometriosis (such as pain) and in reducing the size of implants. Side effects include non-menstrual vaginal bleeding or ovarian cysts during the first two months of use, cessation of menstruation, hot flashes, headaches, decreased sex drive, vaginal dryness, acne, reduction in breast size, and a small loss in bone density. In clinical trials, about 10 percent of the patients experience nasal irritation from the spray.

Other drugs approved for treatment of endometriosis that are chemically related to Synarel include Lupron Depot (leuprolide acetate), a drug injected monthly into muscle, and Zoladex (goserelin acetate implant), which is injected under the skin of the upper abdomen. These drugs don't cause nasal irritation, but otherwise their side effects are similar to those of Synarel, and their effectiveness is also similar.

Women taking endometriosis drugs need to watch for problems such as difficulty breathing or chest or leg pain, which may indicate a blood clot and should be reported to the doctor immediately. Other possible severe side effects include irregular heart rhythms. Frequent checkups are needed to monitor effects such as possible thinning of the bones. A patient should immediately report any new or worsened symptoms to the doctor. However, it's normal for endometriosis symptoms to temporarily worsen when a woman begins taking medicine.

Surgery

Sometimes medicine is not enough. Surgery may be needed to remove diseased tissue or to correct misaligned organs.

One method to remove diseased tissue combines laparoscopy with laser surgery. The laser is connected to the laparoscope and positioned so that its intense light beam is directed through the laparoscope onto the tissue to destroy it. The procedure usually is done without an overnight hospital stay and requires only about a week's recovery time at home.

Recurrence rates after treatment need further study, Ballweg says.

The monthly pain and heavy menstrual periods of chronic endometriosis can be frustrating and painful, and can lead to conceiving and infertility problems. But today, with prompt diagnosis and treatment, a young woman's life can often return to normal.

—by Dixie Farley

Dixie Farley is a staff writer for *FDA Consumer*.

Chapter 35

Testicular Cancer

What Is Testicular Cancer?

Testicular cancer is a disease in which cells become malignant (cancerous) in one or both testicles.

The testicles (also called testes or gonads) are a pair of male sex glands. They produce and store sperm, and are also the body's main source of male hormones. These hormones control the development of the reproductive organs and male characteristics. The testicles are located under the penis in a sac-like pouch called the scrotum.

Testicular cancer can be broadly classified into two types: seminoma and nonseminoma. Seminomas make up about 30 percent of all testicular cancers. Nonseminomas are a group of cancers that include choriocarcinoma, embryonal carcinoma, teratoma, and yolk sac tumors. A testicular cancer may have a combination of both types.

Although testicular cancer accounts for only 1 percent of all cancers in men, it is the most common form of cancer in young men between the ages of 15 and 35. Any man can get testicular cancer, but it is more common in white men than in black men.

"Questions and Answers about Testicular Cancer," National Cancer Institute (NCI), National Institutes of Health (NIH), http://cis.nci.nih.gov/fact/6_34.htm, reviewed February 2000.

What Are the Risk Factors for Testicular Cancer?

The causes of testicular cancer are not known. However, studies show that several factors increase a man's chance of developing testicular cancer.

- Undescended testicle (cryptorchidism): Normally, the testicles descend into the scrotum before birth. Men who have had a testicle that did not move down into the scrotum are at greater risk for developing the disease. This is true even if surgery is performed to place the testicle in the scrotum.

- Abnormal testicular development: Men whose testicles did not develop normally are also at increased risk.

- Klinefelter's syndrome: Men with Klinefelter's syndrome (a sex chromosome disorder that may be characterized by low levels of male hormones, sterility, breast enlargement, and small testes) are at greater risk of developing testicular cancer.

- History of testicular cancer: Men who have previously had testicular cancer are at increased risk of developing cancer in the other testicle.

How Is Testicular Cancer Detected?
What Are Symptoms of Testicular Cancer?

Most testicular cancers are found by men themselves. Also, doctors generally examine the testicles during routine physical exams. Between regular checkups, if a man notices anything unusual about his testicles, he should talk with his doctor. When testicular cancer is found early, the treatment can often be less aggressive and may cause fewer side effects.

Men should see a doctor if they notice any of the following symptoms:

- A painless lump or swelling in either testicle

- Any enlargement of a testicle or change in the way it feels

- A feeling of heaviness in the scrotum

- A dull ache in the lower abdomen or the groin (the area where the thigh meets the abdomen)

- A sudden collection of fluid in the scrotum

- Pain or discomfort in a testicle or in the scrotum

These symptoms can be caused by cancer or by other conditions. It is important to see a doctor to determine the cause of any symptoms.

How Is Testicular Cancer Diagnosed?

To help find the cause of symptoms, the doctor evaluates a man's general health. The doctor also performs a physical exam and may order laboratory and diagnostic tests. If a tumor is suspected, the doctor will probably suggest a biopsy, which involves surgery to remove the testicle.

- *Blood tests* measure the levels of tumor markers. Tumor markers are substances often found in higher-than-normal amounts when cancer is present. Tumor markers such as alpha-fetoprotein (AFP), human chorionic gonadotropin (HCG), and lactase dehydrogenase (LDH) may detect a tumor that is too small to be detected during physical exams or imaging tests.

- *Ultrasound* is a diagnostic test in which high-frequency sound waves are bounced off tissues and internal organs. Their echoes produce a picture called a sonogram. Ultrasound of the scrotum can show the presence and size of a mass in the testicle. It is also helpful in ruling out other conditions, such as swelling due to infection.

- *Biopsy.* Microscopic examination of testicular tissue by a pathologist is the only sure way to know whether cancer is present. In nearly all cases of suspected cancer, the entire affected testicle is removed through an incision in the groin. This procedure is called inguinal orchiectomy. In rare cases (for example, when a man has only one testicle), the surgeon performs an inguinal biopsy, removing a sample of tissue from the testicle through an incision in the groin and proceeding with orchiectomy only if the pathologist finds cancer cells. (The surgeon does not cut through the scrotum to remove tissue, because if the problem is cancer, this procedure could cause the disease to spread.)

If testicular cancer is found, more tests are needed to find out if the cancer has spread from the testicle to other parts of the body.

Determining the stage (extent) of the disease helps the doctor to plan appropriate treatment.

How Is Testicular Cancer Treated?
What Are the Side Effects of Treatment?

Most men with testicular cancer can be cured with surgery, radiation therapy, and/or chemotherapy. The side effects depend on the type of treatment and may be different for each person.

Seminomas and nonseminomas grow and spread differently, and each type may need different treatment. Treatment also depends on the stage of the cancer, the patient's age and general health, and other factors. Men are often treated by a team of specialists, which may include a surgeon, a medical oncologist, and a radiation oncologist.

Surgery to remove the testicle through an incision in the groin is called a radical inguinal orchiectomy. Men may be concerned that losing a testicle will affect their ability to have sexual intercourse or make them sterile (unable to produce children). However, a man with one remaining healthy testicle can still have a normal erection and produce sperm. Therefore, an operation to remove one testicle does not make a man impotent (unable to have an erection) and seldom interferes with fertility (the ability to produce children). Men can also have an artificial testicle, called a prosthesis, placed in the scrotum. The implant has the weight and feel of a normal testicle.

Some of the lymph nodes located deep in the abdomen may also be removed (lymph node dissection). This type of surgery does not change a man's ability to have an erection or an orgasm, but it can cause sterility because it interferes with ejaculation. Patients may wish to talk with the doctor about the possibility of removing the lymph nodes using a special nerve-sparing surgical technique that may protect the ability to ejaculate normally.

Radiation therapy, also called radiotherapy, uses high-energy rays to kill cancer cells and shrink tumors. Radiation therapy is a local therapy; it affects cancer cells only in the treated areas. Radiation therapy for testicular cancer comes from a machine outside the body (external beam radiation) and is usually aimed at lymph nodes in the abdomen. Seminomas are highly sensitive to radiation. Nonseminomas are less sensitive to radiation, so men with this type of cancer usually do not undergo radiation.

Radiation therapy affects normal as well as cancerous cells. The side effects of radiation therapy depend mainly on the treatment dose. Common side effects include fatigue, skin changes at the site where the treatment is given, loss of appetite, nausea, and diarrhea. Radiation therapy interferes with sperm production, but most patients regain their fertility within a matter of months.

Chemotherapy is the use of anticancer drugs to kill cancer cells throughout the body. Chemotherapy is given to destroy cancerous cells that may remain in the body after surgery. The use of anticancer drugs following surgery is known as adjuvant therapy. Chemotherapy may also be the initial treatment if the cancer is advanced; that is, if it has spread outside the testicle. Most anticancer drugs are given by injection into a vein (IV).

Chemotherapy is a systemic therapy, meaning that drugs travel through the blood stream and affect normal as well as cancerous cells all over the body. The side effects depend largely on the specific drugs and the dose. Common side effects may include nausea, loss of hair, fatigue, diarrhea, vomiting, fever, chills, coughing/shortness of breath, mouth sores, or skin rash. Other common side effects are dizziness, numbness, loss of reflexes, or difficulty hearing. Some anticancer drugs interfere with sperm production. Although the reduction in sperm count is permanent for some patients, many others recover their fertility.

Men with testicular cancer should discuss their concerns about sexual function and fertility with the doctor. If a man is to have treatment that might lead to infertility, he may want to ask the doctor about sperm banking (freezing sperm before treatment for use in the future). This procedure can allow some men to produce children after loss of fertility.

Is Follow Up Treatment Necessary? What Does It Involve?

Regular followup exams are extremely important for men who have been treated for testicular cancer. Like all cancers, testicular cancer can recur. Men who have had testicular cancer should see their doctor regularly and should report any unusual symptoms right away. Followup may vary for different types and stages of testicular cancer. Generally, patients are checked frequently by a doctor and have regular blood tests to measure tumor marker levels. They also have regular x-rays and computed tomography, also called CT scans or CAT scans (detailed pictures of areas inside the body created by a computer linked to an x-ray machine). Men who have had testicular cancer have an increased likelihood of developing cancer in the remaining testicle. They also have an increased risk of certain types of leukemia, as well as other types of cancers. Regular followup care ensures that any changes in health are discussed, and any recurrent cancer can be treated as soon as possible.

Are Clinical Trials (Research Studies) Available for Men with Testicular Cancer?

Yes. Participation in clinical trials is an important treatment option for many men with testicular cancer. To develop new, more effective treatments, and better ways to use current treatments, the National Cancer Institute (NCI) is sponsoring clinical trials in many hospitals and cancer centers around the country. Clinical trials are a critical step in the development of new methods of treatment. Before any new treatment can be recommended for general use, doctors conduct clinical trials to find out whether the treatment is safe for patients and effective against the disease.

Patients who are interested in learning more about participating in clinical trials can access NCI's cancer trials Web site at http://cancertrials.nci.nih.gov/ on the Internet.

Chapter 36

Communicating about Sex

Chapter Contents

Section 36.1

Talking with Your Teen about Sexuality

Excerpted from William W. Mallory, Gary L. Hansen, Ph.D. "Talking with Your Teen about Sexuality," National Network for Family Resilience, http://www.nnfr.org/adolsex/fact/adolsex_talkteen.html, cited November 2001. Reprinted with permission.

Sex. Like all children, your children are going to be curious about it. They're going to be thinking about it. They're going to be exposed to it in the media. They're going to be talking to friends about it. They're going to be learning about it. Are you going to be involved? Are you going to be a source of information for them? Are your children going to come to you with their questions? Are they going to come to you with their problems?

How well you communicate with your children about sexuality determines how much you're involved in this important part of their lives. This chapter is designed to help. If you haven't been talking about sexuality with your child, it may help you get started. If you have been talking about sexuality, it may help you communicate better.

Sexuality and the Reluctance to Talk

It's important to realize that your children's sexuality encompasses far more than the physical acts of sex. It also includes how their bodies develop and respond sexually. It includes how they feel about those responses. It includes what they think is right and wrong related to sexuality. As you can see, there's a lot to talk about.

If you're a typical parent or guardian, you have a thousand and one things you'd like to share with your children. You realize how difficult it is for young people to grow up today and you don't want your children to make irresponsible sexual decisions that could have life-threatening results. Despite a desire to talk with your children about sexuality, you're probably not doing it as often or as well as you would like. There are a number of reasons why that may be the case.

- You don't know what to say or how to say it. Many of today's parents were raised in families where sexuality was seldom, if ever, discussed. Since they didn't talk about sexuality with their parents, they don't have a model of what parents should say to their children or how they should say it. They may also worry about being asked questions they can't answer. If this describes you, there are a number of things you can do. First, you can fill the gaps in your own sexual knowledge. Your local library or bookstore should have a number of good books on sexuality. Look for them. Remember, however, that your child doesn't expect you to be an "expert" who knows all the facts. It's far more important for you to be caring, concerned, supportive and available. Second, you can learn some of the techniques for communicating about sexuality that have worked for other parents. This chapter should be helpful. Third, you can simply "take the plunge." Like the first time you ever dived off the diving board at a swimming pool, sooner or later you've simply got to overcome your anxiety and fear and start talking. Like that first dive, you'll survive, and it will get easier and easier the more you do it.

- You're afraid talking about sexuality will encourage your children to be sexually active. This belief is the basis for much of the opposition to any sexuality education. While it may seem logical, it simply isn't true. There is no concrete evidence that providing a young person valid sexual information increases sexual activity. If anything, it delays it.

- You're sure your children don't need to talk about sexuality since they're neither sexually active now nor likely to be in the foreseeable future. While most parents want to believe this, can you really be sure? One study has found that only 10 percent of teens tell their parents the full extent of their sexual activity. According to the Centers for Disease Control, 54 percent of all American high school students have had sexual intercourse. Among high school seniors, the figure is 70 percent. Even if your teen isn't sexually active now, there's a good chance he or she will be active before long. Furthermore, providing your teen with the facts may help him or her avoid becoming a victim of sexual exploitation. Also, your teen may become a valuable source of sexuality information for his or her peers.

- Your children don't want to talk to you. While this may appear to be true, most children really want to talk with their parents.

They want to know what their parents think. They want and need to be able to turn to parents for information, advice and support. You've simply got to be approachable. Your child has to feel comfortable talking with you. You've also got to take advantage of the "teachable moments" that come along.

Getting Ready

Talking about sexuality is going to be easier if you're prepared. You can start getting ready by completing the following exercise suggested by Jay Gale in his book *A Parent's Guide to Teenage Sexuality*.

Take a piece of paper and write eight statements that represent messages about sexuality you would like to communicate to your child at this time. (If you're having trouble coming up with eight, reading the list titled "Your Teen Needs to Know" may help you think of issues you'd like to talk about.) After you develop your list, visualize yourself discussing each topic, one at a time, with your teen. Think about what you would say and how you would say it. Think about what he or she is likely to say. Imagine the facial expressions both of you are likely to have. Now, think about how comfortable you feel about discussing each of the eight topics. Put two checks by the messages you're totally comfortable with, one check by those you're somewhat comfortable with and no checks by those you're uncomfortable with.

Your Teen Needs to Know

- what you think about sexual issues and what moral values or ethical standards you hold
- how to resist sexual pressure, coercion and exploitation
- how and why his or her body is developing
- about sexual expression, conception, and pregnancy
- about contraception
- about AIDS and other sexually transmitted diseases and how to prevent them
- how to act with sexual integrity

This exercise should give you some idea of what you really want to communicate to your teen and how comfortable you are likely to feel doing it. Since your communication probably won't be very effective if you're extremely uncomfortable, begin with the messages you're most comfortable with. Don't forget about the difficult topics, however. If you think the message is important, develop a strategy for communicating it. Would seeking more information help you feel more comfortable? Would giving your teen written material help introduce the message and make conversation easier?

If you have a partner who is actively involved in raising your teen, ask him or her to complete this exercise. Compare and discuss your results. Do the two of you want to send the same messages? If not, do the messages actually conflict with each other or do they simply focus on different aspects of sexuality? If they conflict, discuss your differences. While teens can benefit from hearing different viewpoints, receiving contradictory messages from parents or guardians can produce confusion and anxiety.

In addition to comparing the content of the messages you want to send, discuss your comfort levels. It may help you decide whether one or both of you should take the lead in discussing specific topics. It's important for the two of you to develop a joint strategy for talking with your teen and to periodically check with each other to see how it's going.

Getting Started

Talking with your teen about sexuality doesn't always need to consist of lectures or situations where you sit your child down to "talk about sex." There are many "teachable moments" that you can take advantage of to initiate a relaxed discussion. The average television viewer sees 14,000 references to sex in the course of one year. Use some of them as springboards for discussion. Ask your teen what he or she thinks about or would do in the situation being portrayed. Give your own opinion. Videos, tabloid, and magazine headlines at the check-out line of the supermarket or your teen's own comments and questions also can serve as conversation starters.

You also can use written materials to start discussions. Bring books about sexuality home from the public library and share them with your teen. Be sure to discuss the material after you both have read it. The simple act of bringing such material home is important. It lets your teen know that it's okay to talk about sexuality at home. It lets her or him know that you're open to talking about it.

While many of your discussions about sexuality will be in response to everyday experiences, there will be times when you want to sit down and discuss a specific topic. Simply invite your teen to talk. Say, "I've been wanting to talk with you. How about after you finish your homework tonight?" When the time comes, you might want to begin with a general statement like, "I've seen a lot of stories about AIDS lately and thought we ought to discuss it ourselves." Such statements are less likely to make your teen defensive or uncomfortable than ones about his or her own personal behavior.

Practicing these techniques will hopefully make talking about sexuality an ongoing process. Communication is most effective when discussions about sexuality become a natural and normal part of conversation. When this happens, both the parent and the teen can bring up topics for discussion at any time.

Effective Communication

While getting to the point of routinely discussing sexuality with your teen is never easy, practicing effective communication increases your chances of being successful. The following guidelines adapted from Gale's *A Parent's Guide to Teenage Sexuality* may help:

- Eliminate distractions. Pay attention to what your teen is saying. Shut off any distractions and make eye contact. If the time is inconvenient for either of you, arrange an alternative time to talk.

- Clarify what you've heard. Clarifying assures your teen that you've listened and understood what she or he said. It also gives him or her a chance to try again if you've misunderstood. The best way to clarify is to briefly summarize in your own words what you think your teen is saying.

- Don't interrupt. Listening without interrupting lets your teen know you want to know what he or she is thinking. Besides, interrupting shows a lack of respect.

- Use positive methods of communication. Since many teens are insecure and uncomfortable with sexuality, using positive communication techniques are particularly important when discussing it. Let your teen know she or he can be open and honest and be sure to be open and honest yourself. Provide truthful and direct information. If you do not know an answer to a question, don't guess or make something up. Admit you don't know and promise to try to find out more.

- Use "I" statements. Start your sentences with "I" or "I feel" instead of with "you." Starting a sentence with "you" is likely to put your teen on the defensive because is sounds accusatory or threatening. Tell your daughter, "I'm concerned that you and

Jason are so involved that you'll get careless and wind up pregnant." Don't tell her, "You're getting too involved with Jason."

- Clearly state what you want. It's more effective than stating what you don't want. For example, say "I want you home by 11:00." Don't say, "I don't want you staying out late."

- If possible, rephrase questions as statements that reflect your feelings. Many times questions are not used to elicit information. They're used to trap someone. Say, "I don't think someone your age should be dating just one person." Don't say, "Why don't you date other people?"

- Avoid using "absolutes" when in any kind of disagreement. Words like "always," "never," "every time," and "whenever" drag up the past. Sticking to the present usually results in more effective communication.

Following these guidelines will increase your odds of being able to communicate effectively with your teen. They will not guarantee it, however. Don't be overly concerned if your teen doesn't immediately share your enthusiasm for talking about sexuality. That may take time and there may be setbacks along the way. Don't give up. The important thing is that you're making the effort.

Difficult Issues

If you're like most parents, you will have to confront some difficult issues as you discuss sexuality with your teen. While we can't cover all, or even most, of them in a chapter like this, there are a few you should begin thinking about now.

Masturbation. Many parents are particularly embarrassed and uncomfortable talking about masturbation. It may have been a taboo subject when you were growing up and, because of religious or moral beliefs, you may think it's wrong. Realize that many teens practice it, however. One study of 15- and 16-year-olds found that three quarters of the boys and over half of the girls have masturbated.

Even if you have objections to masturbation, try to let your teen know that it is normal and natural to be interested in exploring your own body. Then you can go on to explain your own values. Try not to use shame or guilt, however. They're far more likely to produce fear and confusion than change behavior.

Resisting sexual pressure. This may sound like an easy issue but it's not. While it's easy to tell your teen to "just say no" to sex, she or he needs to hear more. Your teen needs to hear how to say "no." He or she needs to develop and practice the skills necessary for resisting unwanted sexual pressure. Talk with your teen about specific ways of countering the pressure. Talk about ways to show love besides having sex.

If both of you feel comfortable doing it, try role-playing situations where one of you resists pressure from the other to have sex. It's okay if the two of you start giggling. Laughter is a great way to reduce tension. You can have fun and your teen can learn some valuable skills at the same time. Role-playing works best when you and your teen develop your "script" together using your teen's own words. The goal is to have your teen prepare some ways to politely, but firmly, decline sexual propositions. Hopefully, they will be ways that are not likely to prompt an argument or result in coercion.

Contraception and "safer" sex. Most parents want their teens to postpone sexual involvement. In addition to simply feeling uncomfortable talking about contraception and "safer" sex, many feel that all sex outside of marriage is wrong. They worry that providing teens such information sends the message that they expect them to be sexually active and that it's okay if they are.

Obviously, you're the only person who can decide what's best for you to talk about and teach your teen. There are a couple of things you need to consider as you make that decision, however. First, teens who are informed tend to delay sexual involvement longer than those who are not. Second, your teen may not choose your values. Despite your best efforts, he or she may decide to try sexual intercourse. It's foolish to compound the problem by getting pregnant or catching a sexually transmitted disease (STD). A sexually active teen needs to know the risks and benefits of different contraceptive techniques and how to reduce the risk of AIDS and other STDs.

If you decide that you want your teen to know about contraception and safer sex, you'll need to see that he or she receives the information. Since some of it is fairly technical, a combination of talking and providing printed material may be the best strategy. Talking can emphasize the importance of reducing the risks of pregnancy and STDs for sexually active teens. Having printed material can provide time for your teen to digest the information. There are a variety of good books, as well as a number of leaflets, available. Don't just give them to your teen. Read them yourself and be ready for questions or discussion. In addition to simply learning the facts about contraception and "safer" sex, your teen needs to develop the skills necessary to always use or practice them. He or she needs to know how to obtain condoms and other contraceptives as well as ways to encourage a potentially reluctant partner to use them.

As you can see, you're going to confront some difficult issues as you talk with your teen about sexuality. Having your teen exposed to factual, comprehensive information outside the home will help you deal with them. Support efforts to provide such information in your teen's school and other community organizations and encourage your teen to participate.

Sexual Integrity and Talking with Your Teen

Honesty, sincerity and ethics are the hallmarks of sexual integrity. One of the best ways to encourage your teen to develop those characteristics is to be sure they characterize your communication with her or him. Always be honest and sincere and be sure to communicate your own ethics or moral values. Don't just state your values, however. Give your reasons. This will help your teen understand why you think the value is important. It doesn't guarantee he or she will accept it, however. Ultimately, your teen will choose a value system that seems right for him or her. Both of you are entitled to your own opinions. Both of you need to respect each other. If you do, you'll keep the lines of communication open.

Section 36.2

Talking with Your Teen about Sexual Abstinence

Excerpted from "Talking to Kids about Sex," from *Unlocking the Secret*, http://www.notmenotnow.org/talking.cfm, Not Me Not Now, copyright 2000 by Monroe County. Reprinted with permission.

Starting a Conversation about Sex

Sometimes starting a conversation with your child about sex is the hardest part of all. Parents often say that if they only could think of a good opening line, they would be better able to help their kids. Here are some good strategies to break the ice:

- The direct approach is usually the best approach. For example, if you think your 11-year old is wearing too much make-up, in a calm, direct voice say, "I have a problem with the amount of make-up you're wearing and I'd like to talk about it." If your child becomes too emotional, don't overreact. At least it's out in the open and you can come back to it later.

- State how you feel. Most kids are used to lectures and being told what to do. But when adults talk about their feelings, it puts them more at ease. For example, if your grandson uses dirty language to describe a girl in school, you could say, "It really disappoints me to hear you talk about another person like that. Do you know what I mean?"

- Start with a comfortable subject. Once you've broken the ice, you can then gradually move toward more difficult or embarrassing topics. For example, if you're worried that one of your child's friends is a bad influence, start by talking about what his or her friends are up to in general and then move on to the more difficult subject.

- Start by sharing an experience you had at their age. For example, you might say, "When I was in fifth grade there was a boy in my class who said he already had sex. Nobody believed him though."

- Start by telling a story and ask them what they think. Here's an example: "Yesterday I read a story in a magazine about a teen-age girl who got pregnant and was having a baby. The story said she had lots of problems. What do you think some of her problems would be?"

Helping Your Kids Say "Not Me Not Now"

How can you keep your kids from becoming sexually active too soon? As parents well know, you can't keep them locked in their rooms and you can't follow them around all day. In other words, you can influence your kids' lives but you can't control them. The best way to help them is to be open and honest about how you feel about sex and give them the skills to say, "Not Me, Not Now" to early sexual activity.

- Keep the lines of communications open. If you can't talk with your child, it will be hard to influence his or her behavior.

- Start communicating early. Most parents think that sex education starts when their kids are physically mature and have started dating. Ideas about healthy, respectful relationships will stick with your kids better if you start talking early on about friendships and other kinds of relationships. Even pre-schoolers can understand these ideas.

- Respect privacy. Sex is a very serious subject to young people. Don't make the mistake of talking about sex or your child's relationships in front of someone else. Don't share your conversations with your child with anyone else unless you get your child's permission.

- Tell your kids you want them to abstain from sex. Believe it or not, some parents just don't bother to tell their children that they don't want them to become sexually active. Kids are influenced by their parents' opinions.

- Share your reasons for not wanting them to have sex. Tell them why you think it's a good idea if they abstain from sex until they're older. Discuss the consequences of sexual activity and pregnancy. Talk about the dangers of AIDS and other sexually-transmitted diseases.

- Acknowledge peer pressure. Teens are experiencing peer pressure to become sexually active at a younger and younger age. Don't make light of it or brush it off by merely saying, "ignore it." The influence of peers is important in your child's life and affects self-esteem. Young teens are afraid that if they say "no" they won't be popular. By getting to know your child's friends, parents can use peer pressure in positive ways.

An Example

Laura is getting ready for her junior high prom when her mom notices she doesn't seem very excited. Laura's mom asks her daughter if she has a problem.

Laura: Well, this is kind of embarrassing, but tonight is John and my six-month anniversary of dating and, well, I think he might "expect something" from me.

Mom: I take it you don't mean a gift...has John been pressuring you to have sex?

Laura: Well, a little... I just don't know what to do.

Mom: I can understand how you feel, but I strongly believe you are too young to become sexually active. You could risk becoming pregnant or get a sexually transmitted disease. I just don't think it's worth the consequences you might face.

Laura: I think you're right, Mom, but how do I tell him no?

Mom: Try to explain your feelings to him. But if he keeps pressuring you, look him in the eye and say, "no" in a loud and firm voice. Be confident...tell him that it makes you angry when he doesn't listen. If that doesn't work, walk away. If he really cares, he'll respect your feelings.

Laura: I never knew you felt this strongly about it, Mom. I'm glad we talked.

What Worked

Laura's mom took the initiative in asking her daughter what was wrong. When Laura asked her mom's opinion about getting involved in a sexual relationship, she told her straight out what her views were and why. She also gave Laura some concrete, practical ways to deal with the situation.

Chapter 37

Teen Pregnancy

Chapter Contents

Section 37.1

Ten Tips for Parents to Help Their Children Avoid Teen Pregnancy

Excerpted from "Ten Tips for Parents to Help Their Children Avoid Teen Pregnancy," undated document from the National Campaign to Prevent Teen Pregnancy, http://www.teenpregnancy.org/tips.html, cited November 2001.

The National Campaign to Prevent Teen Pregnancy has reviewed recent research about parental influences on children's sexual behavior and talked to many experts in the field, as well as to teens and parents themselves. From these sources, it is clear that there is much parents and adults can do to reduce the risk of kids becoming pregnant before they've grown up.

Presented here as "ten tips," many of these lessons will seem familiar because they articulate what parents already know from experience—like the importance of maintaining strong, close relationships with children and teens, setting clear expectations for them, and communicating honestly and often with them about important matters. Research supports these common sense lessons: not only are they good ideas generally, but they can also help teens delay becoming sexually active, as well as encourage those who are having sex to use contraception carefully.

Finally, although these tips are for parents, they can be used by adults more generally in their relationships with teenagers. Parents—especially those who are single or working long hours—often turn to other adults for help in raising their children and teens. If all these caring adults are on the same "wavelength" about the issues covered here, young people are given more consistent messages.

So, What to Do?

Be clear about your own sexual values and attitudes. Communicating with your children about sex, love, and relationships is often more successful when you are certain in your own mind about these issues.

Talk with your children early and often about sex, and be specific. Kids have lots of questions about sex, and they often say that the source they'd most like to go to for answers is their parents. Start the conversation, and make sure that it is honest, open, and respectful. If you can't think of how to start the discussion, consider using situations shown on television or in movies as conversation starters. Tell them candidly and confidently what you think and why you take these positions; if you're not sure about some issues, tell them that, too. Be sure to have a two-way conversation, not a one-way lecture. Ask them what they think and what they know so you can correct misconceptions. Ask what, if anything, worries them.

Age-appropriate conversations about relationships and intimacy should begin early in a child's life and continue through adolescence. Resist the idea that there should be just one conversation about all this—you know, "the talk." The truth is that parents and kids should be talking about sex and love all along. This applies to both sons and daughters and to both mothers and fathers, incidentally. All kids need a lot of communication, guidance, and information about these issues, even if they sometimes don't appear to be interested in what you have to say. And if you have regular conversations, you won't worry so much about making a mistake or saying something not quite right, because you'll always be able to talk again.

Many inexpensive books and videos are available to help with any detailed information you might need, but don't let your lack of technical information make you shy. Kids need as much help in understanding the meaning of sex as they do in understanding how all the body parts work. Tell them about love and sex, and what the difference is. And remember to talk about the reasons that kids find sex interesting and enticing; discussing only the "downside" of unplanned pregnancy and disease misses many of the issues on teenagers' minds.

In addition to being an "askable parent," be a parent with a point of view. Tell your children what you think.

By the way, research clearly shows that talking with your children about sex does not encourage them to become sexually active. And remember, too, that your own behavior should match your words. The "do as I say, not as I do" approach is bound to lose with children and teenagers, who are careful and constant observers of the adults in their lives.

Supervise and monitor your children and adolescents. Establish rules, curfews, and standards of expected behavior, preferably through an open process of family discussion and respectful communication. If your children get out of school at 3 pm and you don't get home from work until 6 pm, who is responsible for making certain that your children are not only safe during those hours, but also are engaged in useful activities? Where are they when they go out with friends? Are there adults around who are in charge? Supervising and monitoring your kids' whereabouts doesn't make you a nag; it makes you a parent.

Know your children's friends and their families. Friends have a strong influence on each other, so help your children and teenagers become friends with kids whose families share your values. Some parents of teens even arrange to meet with the parents of their children's friends to establish common rules and expectations. It is easier to enforce a curfew that all your child's friends share rather than one that makes him or her different—but even if your views don't match those of other parents, hold fast to your convictions. Welcome your children's friends into your home and talk to them openly.

Discourage early, frequent, and steady dating. Group activities among young people are fine and often fun, but allowing teens to begin steady, one-on-one dating much before age 16 can lead to trouble. Let your child know about your strong feelings about this throughout childhood—don't wait until your young teen proposes a plan that differs from your preferences in this area; otherwise, he or she will think you just don't like the particular person or invitation.

Take a strong stand against your daughter dating a boy significantly older than she is. And don't allow your son to develop an intense relationship with a girl much younger than he is. Older guys can seem glamorous to a young girl—sometimes they even have money and a car to boot! But the risk of matters getting out of hand increases when the guy is much older than the girl. Try setting a limit of no more than a two- (or at most three-) year age difference. The power differences between younger girls and older boys or men can lead girls into risky situations, including unwanted sex and sex with no protection.

Help your teenagers to have options for the future that are more attractive than early pregnancy and parenthood. The chances that your children will delay sex, pregnancy, and parenthood are significantly increased if their futures appears bright. This means helping them set meaningful goals for the future, talking to them about what it takes to make future plans come true, and helping them reach their goals. Tell them, for example, that if they want to be a teacher, they will need to stay in school in order to earn various degrees and pass certain exams. It also means teaching them to use free time in a constructive way, such as setting aside certain times to complete homework assignments. Explain how becoming pregnant—or causing pregnancy—can derail the best of plans; for example, child care expenses can make it almost impossible to afford college. Community service, in particular, not only teaches job skills, but can also put teens in touch with a wide variety of committed and caring adults.

Let your kids know that you value education highly. Encourage your children to take school seriously and set high expectations about their school performance. School failure is often the first sign of trouble that can end in teenage parenthood. Be very attentive to your children's progress in school and intervene early if things aren't going well. Keep track of your children's grades and discuss them together. Meet with teachers and principals, guidance counselors, and coaches. Limit the number of hours your teenager gives to part-time jobs (20 hours per week should be the maximum) so that there is enough time and energy left to focus on school. Know about homework assignments and support your child in getting them done. Volunteer at the school, if possible. Schools want more parental involvement and will often try to accommodate your work schedule, if asked.

Know what your kids are watching, reading, and listening to. The media (television, radio, movies, music videos, magazines, the Internet) are chock full of material sending the wrong messages. Sex rarely has meaning, unplanned pregnancy seldom happens, and few people having sex ever seem to be married or even especially committed to anyone. Is this consistent with your expectations and values? If not, it is important to talk with your children about what the media portray and what you think about it. If certain programs or movies offend you, say so, and explain why. Be "media literate"—think about what you and your family are watching and reading. Encourage your kids to think critically: ask them what they think about the programs they watch and the music they listen to.

You can always turn the TV off, cancel subscriptions, and place certain movies off limits. You will probably not be able to fully control what your children see and hear, but you can certainly make your views known and control your own home environment.

Strive for a relationship that is warm in tone, firm in discipline, and rich in communication, and one that emphasizes mutual trust and respect. There is no single way to create such relationships, but the following habits of the heart can help:

Express love and affection clearly and often. Hug your children, and tell them how much they mean to you. Praise specific accomplishments, but remember that expressions of affection should be offered freely, not just for a particular achievement. Listen carefully to what your children say and pay thoughtful attention to what they do. Spend time with your children engaged in activities that suit their ages and interests, not just yours. Shared experiences build a "bank account" of affection and trust that forms the basis for future communication with them about specific topics, including sexual behavior. Be supportive and be interested in what interests them. Attend their sports events; learn about their hobbies; be enthusiastic about their achievements, even the little ones; ask them questions that show you care and want to know what is going on in their lives. Be courteous and respectful to your children and avoid hurtful teasing or ridicule. Don't compare your teenager with other family members (i.e., why can't you be like your older sister?). Show that you expect courtesy and respect from them in return. Help them to build self-esteem by mastering skills; remember, self-esteem is earned, not given, and one of the best ways to earn it is by doing something well. Try to have meals together as a family as often as possible, and use the time for conversation, not confrontation.

Section 37.2

What Mothers and Daughters Should Know about Birth Control

Excerpted from Carma Haley, "What Mothers and
Daughters Should Know about Birth Control,"
Teenagers Today/iParenting, http://teenagerstoday.com/
resources/articles/birthcontrol.htm, 2001.

When discussing sex, contraception, and protection with a teen, parents should remember to cover all bases and allow the child to ask questions along the way. Discussing sex is not offering a child an open invitation to participate or become sexually active; it is a parent's way of ensuring that a teen has accurate information to make an educated decision when the time comes—and it will come.

Most experts agree that abstinence is definitely the best option for teens. But if your child is sexually active—and many are—you can help your teen to be safe with the best method of protection.

Availability

Especially for teens, availability may decrease the number of choices of contraceptive methods. If a teen is taking on the responsibility alone, this can increase the difficulty of the task. "The number one aspect of choosing a contraception method is access," says Carol Carrozza, Vice President of Marketing for Ansell Healthcare, which manufactures LifeStyle condoms. "Access has to be fairly easy. A teen's access might be limited to what they can get, whether it is because of money, time, a parent's knowledge, etc., so the options may be limited on what methods they can get legally and over the counter." Teenaged girls may not know that they must visit a clinic or an OB/GYN to get fitted for a diaphragm or IUD or to get oral contraceptives. Or they may not have the money to pay for such service. A parent's involvement and support will broaden a teen girl's resources as well as her options for methods of contraception.

Lifestyle

"Next in importance of factors to consider would be lifestyle," Carrozza says. "If a teen has already decided to become sexually active she will need to consider the other aspects involved with her decision. For example, is her partner inclined to share in the responsibility? If so, there are simple methods available that either party can obtain. If he refuses, then she will have to look at the alternative methods that she's in control of and offer her the best protection." In addition, if a female is only sexual active once a month, resorting to a method of contraception that offers protection all month long may not be worth the time, effort or money. However, if a female is more sexually active, ensuring extended protection may be the better alternative.

Cost

Each method of contraception has some cost involved. As a young teen may not have money readily available, the price of obtaining contraception could be an important factor in deciding what method to use. "Is a 15- or 16-year-old girl going to be able to afford $20 a month [for a] supply of birth control pills or $7 dollar [for a] box of condoms, which may last longer than a month?" Carrozza asks. "It all depends upon what they have available to spend. Again, if a parent is involved, the alternatives are more readily available as the parent's medical insurance may cover the visit to the OB/GYN for the pill, IUD, diaphragm or contraceptive injections."

Methods of Contraception

Abstinence

The only method of birth control that is 100 percent effective each and every time it is used is abstinence. Abstinence is free, there is no medical exam needed and this method of contraception protects against both pregnancy and sexually transmitted diseases. Both males and females can practice abstinence for birth control.

"For an unmarried teenager, I believe that the best form of birth control is abstinence," says Marie Geiger, a freelance writer from western Pennsylvania. "Do I think it is the most realistic option? Not for everyone. Abstinence will only work for a teen [who] believes in the benefits of waiting to have sex. I wish someone had really emphasized this with me. My daughter is only 4 now, but I think about these things a lot. Based on my experience and from a women's health viewpoint, I will make sure that she is aware both of how her reproductive system works and what the options are that are available for preventing pregnancy once she is in a position to be worried about that. She will know her options—all of them."

The Pill

One of the most popular forms of contraception, the birth control pill—more commonly called "the Pill"—is an oral contraceptive that must be taken each day to prevent pregnancy. The Pill offers no protection against STDs and is 95 to 99.9 percent effective.

Taking the Pill will offer a constant and consistent amount of protection against pregnancy when taken regularly and as prescribed. Other advantages include more regularity in menstrual periods and a decrease in menstrual cramping. The Pill has also been shown to decrease the risk of osteoporosis, cervical cancer and pelvic inflammatory disease. Remember, though, that the Pill offers no protection against any sexually transmitted diseases. Other disadvantages of the Pill include the fact that it must be taken daily—regardless of the amount of sexual activity—to provide proper protection, and it may cause weight gain or depression. Women older than 35 or women who smoke are at greater risk of developing blood clots, heart attack and stroke while using the Pill as their means of contraception. The average cost of the pill ranges from $15 to $35 for one month's supply and additional costs are required for a medical exam before the Pill can be prescribed. All of these advantages and disadvantages must be weighed carefully when considering the Pill as the method of birth control.

The IUD

The Intrauterine Device—also known as the IUD—is a small plastic device that contains either copper or hormones and is implanted directly into the uterus by an OB/GYN. The IUD offers protection against pregnancy but will not prevent STDs from being transmitted from one partner to another. The IUD is 97.4 to 99.2 percent effective in protecting against pregnancy. "With the IUD, a woman must be educated in order for it to be effective," Carrozza says. "Women who use or have an IUD must learn the warning signs of when it has slipped out of place as well as what pain or discomfort associated with the device is cause for alarm. The IUD is beginning to gain popularity again as it offers constant protection against pregnancy. If a woman is educated on its use, the IUD could be ideal for her lifestyle."

The advantages of the IUD are that it provides consistent protection against pregnancy and can be forgotten—providing no complications arise. But teens may not be able to consider the IUD as a method of birth control, since the uterus may be too small for proper placement of the device. In addition, there are various conditions that can prevent the use of IUDs for both adults and teens, including various pelvic infections; vaginal infections; copper allergy; abnormality of the cervix, uterus or ovaries; Wilson's Disease; AIDS; or Leukemia. The cost of the IUD can be moderate to high, ranging from $95 to $300. There are also additional costs for office visits to an OB/GYN for fitting and placement, as well as costs for removal if complications arise. If the IUD is chosen as the method of birth control, the woman should feel comfortable with the risks involved and be well informed about the signs and symptoms of complications.

Norplant

One of the newer methods of birth control is Norplant. The protection of Norplant comes from the insertion of six match-stick-sized capsules placed under the skin of the upper arm. These capsules deliver a constant level of progesterone—a female hormone—into the body, which prevents an egg from being released and thickens the cervical tissue layer, preventing pregnancy. Norplant offers no protection against STDs and is 99.95 percent effective in protecting against pregnancy. The Norplant device, once inserted, is effective for up to five years. The cost of the Norplant is $500 to $600 for an exam, the implants and insertion. Cost of removing the implants upon evidence of complications can be as much as $200.

Complications of Norplant can include headache, dizziness, discoloration or discomfort at the insertion site, irregular menstrual periods or absence of flow, and weight gain. Woman who have diabetes, high cholesterol or blood pressure, heart disease, seizures that require medication, serious depression, conditions that may be aggravated by fluid retention, serious liver disease, breast cancer, or are breast-feeding should use caution when considering the Norplant as their method of birth control.

Barrier Methods

This category includes condoms, spermicidal creams, gels, suppositories and foams, the diaphragm, and the cervical cap. Barrier methods offer protection by not allowing the sperm access to the uterus where it would fertilize the egg and result in a pregnancy. These methods offer protection against pregnancy but—with the exception of the condom—do not protect against STDs. The effectiveness of the barrier methods ranges from 74 to 98 percent in protecting against pregnancy. The cost for barrier methods of birth control can be as little a $3 to as much as $50. With the exception of the cervical cap and the diaphragm, all of these barrier methods can be purchased over the counter with no need to seek professional instruction or direction for their use. Both the cervical cap and diaphragm must be fitted by an OB/GYN physician for proper protection.

"Latex condoms are not impervious to everything," Carrozza says. "They are not 100 percent. Nothing is 100 percent, which is why abstinence is still so important. It's best to be sure that it is a condom that is approved by the FDA (Food and Drug Administration). There are tons of novelty condoms out there but none are approved and will not offer the protection against pregnancy or STDs. The easiest way to know that the condom that is approved by the FDA is to look for an expiration date and a lot control number. Only use a condom within the expiration date and use it properly."

To make the task of discussing sex with their teen easier, parents should educate themselves and keep up to date with new methods of contraception and protection. An educated parent is more likely to have the answers that their child needs and wants. Also, it's probably a good idea to tell a child "I don't know" when that's the case.

Section 37.3

Communicating with Your Pregnant Teen

Excerpted from Megan Potter, "Mom, Dad, I'm Pregnant," Teenagers Today/iParenting, http://teenagerstoday.com/resources/articles/pregnant.htm, 2001.

"I don't want someone else to go through what I'm going through... You need a family. You need to be stable. I'm alone except for my baby."

This young mother's plight is a common one for teenagers who have found themselves in the unfortunate predicament of being pregnant. When the words "I'm pregnant" come out of a teen's mouth, parents are often at a loss for what to do. They react emotionally, not logically, and the resulting confrontations often leave the teens alone without the support of their parents and other family members.

So, what should you do if your teen tells you she is pregnant? The most important thing is to stay calm. Tracy Underwood, a licensed psychologist at Children's Medical Center of Dallas advises that parents "recognize that your child is likely frightened and confused and looking to you for guidance."

As one teen told the National Campaign to Prevent Teen Pregnancy, "I would like it if [parents] came out and said what they meant. The unhelpful thing is when they start to lecture." If all else fails, ask your son or daughter to leave you with time for yourself before you react to the shock.

When you do talk to them, remember to be honest about your feelings. There is no point in chastising them or lecturing them; the damage is already done. But that doesn't mean you can't tell your child just how disappointed you are in the behavior. Being supportive does not mean you have to be—or pretend to be—happy about the situation. Being supportive simply means that you help them through it.

Now that your child is in an adult situation, you'll want to make him or her aware of that by treating them like adults. When you talk to them, tell them why you feel the way you feel. Don't simply insist they use a particular option; explain your reasoning for it. Your kids may not follow your advice but they are more likely to consider it if it comes as advice and not as an order.

Some things you should be sure to discuss with your son or daughter include the choices (abortion, adoption, parenting), finances, responsibility, and your role in the situation. Tell your teen what you think of each of the options available to them, why you feel that way about each one, and which option you would prefer they chose. At the same time, offer to go with them to look into each of the options so they can make informed decisions. Talk to them about the financial issues, and be frank. Will your insurance cover the medical care? Who will be responsible for covering any extra expenses that might arise? What role will the other teen be taking in the finances? Whether they choose to parent or not, you should be aware that there are costs involved in all decisions, mainly medical and counseling.

"A plan needs to be generated Your plan of action should include—among others—finding a doctor, one who preferably works with young mothers," Underwood says.

Be sure to talk to your teen about what you can or will do to help out. Not all parents are willing to take on the same role. Some feel their children should be forced to accept the responsibility for their actions while others choose to shield their children as much as possible. Your options range from adopting the child yourself, allowing your child and the baby to live with you, asking them to pay room and board, or simply being a full- or part-time babysitter. Your ethics and other more practical issues—like money and space—can be influences in your decisions. Tell your child why you are willing to do what you are willing to do. Then discuss what they will have to work out. Remember they are children in an adult situation, offer your guidance in finding a place to live, buying groceries and anything else they may need you for.

"Parents need to play a leading force for the child," Underwood says. "Remember, they are still a child."

While you are talking to your son or daughter, there are other things you can be doing. Be sure to make the effort to meet the parents of the other teen involved and to talk about the same issues you discussed with your own teen. It may turn out that the other parents refuse to have anything to do with the situation. But you may find by meeting with them that you can come to agreements that will give your child and their child the best possible futures. Educate yourself about teen pregnancy and the options involved. When deciding about abortion look into the benefits and the consequences of the decision. Speak to both doctors and organizations that advise against abortion. Take the teens to visit adoption centers or lawyers. See if there is a way that your teen can talk to others who have chosen adoption. Go to places that serve pregnant teens and arrange to meet with those who have chosen to parent, and find out what they have to say. The Internet is also a great source of information on all three options.

Try to remain unbiased in your education. Learn everything you can and share it with your teens. There are nine months of pregnancy in which to make a final decision, so make sure that you have encouraged an informed decision and that everyone is prepared to handle the possible consequences of that decision. But remember: in the end, it is their decision and there may be nothing you can do to change it.

Most importantly, get counseling. Arrange for you and your spouse to speak to a professional. If you have other children, you may want to involve them, too. Be sure that your child is seeing some kind of counselor who will address the many emotional issues involved in teen pregnancy. Encourage the other teen and the teen's family to seek a counselor or to take part in some of your sessions.

"Parents need to recognize their own fear and uncertainty," Underwood says, "...acknowledge that it is a real thing."

Counseling provides a way to deal with fears and to come to grips with the situation. You can seek a counselor or therapist who does family work. You can turn to a local church for referral or you can ask a hospital how to contact your local crisis pregnancy center. All centers differ somewhat, but all are there to help pregnant teens (though some counsel others, too). Your teen will find knowledgeable support, group events and assistance with food, money, health, and more at one of these centers. They may or may not provide family counseling. If they do, consider taking part. Most municipalities will have a crisis pregnancy support group or center; it's simply a matter of locating it.

It's never too late for sex education. The statistics aren't readily available, but an inordinate amount of teen parents have more children before they are out of their teen years and have a stable base. Whether this is because they have given up hope for success, or they simply have neglected to take precautions, it remains that pregnancy doesn't always shock kids straight. Take advantage of the new relationship this situation has fostered and talk to your teen about having sex. Ask whether they plan to continue to have sex. Talk to them about contraception, what they did before and what they should be doing now. Be open and honest and encourage them to believe that one mistake doesn't make life a failure. Continue to be supportive of them and make it clear that they can always come to you with questions about sex now that the issue is in the open.

It is a devastating thing to find your teens have been irresponsible enough to get pregnant. But it's also a devastating thing to destroy a relationship in a few moments, or months, of anger and disappointment.

"When push comes to shove and families are not there for you, you start to feel like a failure. Then you start to act like one," says Fremor Williams, executive director of the Grimsby Life Centre.

If you are supportive and open, your kids might make the right decisions and be more likely to look forward to a bright and hopeful future. Without you, they may be doomed to fall in among the statistics of depression, poverty, abuse, neglect, and to have children with equally dim futures. Be the best parent you can be and stand by your teen—no matter what.

What You Should Not Say!

- Don't accuse them of being stupid or promiscuous—it will only cause anger and resentment.

- Don't threaten or force them to follow your decision—they might not do it and might not talk to you anymore if they feel threatened.

- Don't take it sitting down—they need to know you care enough to be upset by it.

- Don't kick them out. Statistics for teen parents and children on the street are grim. You'll regret the decision later.

- Don't play, "do what I say, not what I do." Help your kids with your actions and your words.

- Don't loose your temper. What's done is done. Move on and make the most of the situation.

Chapter 38

Sexually Transmitted Diseases (STDs) and Teens

Chapter Contents

Section 38.1

Preventing STDs

Excerpted from Judith Levine Willis, "On the Teen Scene: Preventing STDs," *FDA Consumer*, June 1993, Food and Drug Administration (FDA) Pub. No. 98-1210, http://www.fda.gov/opacom/catalog/ots_stds.html, the version below contains revisions made in February 1995 and April 1998.

You don't have to be a genius to figure out that the only sure way to avoid getting sexually transmitted diseases (STDs) is to not have sex.

But in today's age of acquired immunodeficiency syndrome (AIDS), it's smart to also know ways to lower the risk of getting STDs, including human immunodeficiency virus (HIV), the virus that causes AIDS.

Infection with HIV is spreading among teenagers. According to the Centers for Disease Control and Prevention (CDC), as of June 30, 1997, 2953 people had been diagnosed with HIV or AIDS when they were in their teens and 107,281 when in their twenties. Because it can be many years from the time a person becomes infected to when the person develops symptoms and is diagnosed with HIV infection, many people diagnosed in their 20s likely contracted HIV in their teens.

You may have heard that birth control can also help prevent AIDS and other STDs. This is only partly true. The whole story is that only one form of birth control currently on the market—latex condoms (thin rubber sheaths used to cover the penis)—is highly effective in reducing the transmission (spread) of HIV and many other STDs.

The Food and Drug Administration (FDA) has approved the marketing of male condoms made of polyurethane for people allergic to latex (see "Information on Labels"). Reality Female Condom, another form of birth control made of polyurethane, may give limited protection against STDs, but it is not as effective as male latex condoms.

So people who use other kinds of birth control, such as the pill, diaphragm, Norplant, Depo-Provera, cervical cap, or Intrauterine Device (IUD), also need to use condoms to help prevent STDs.

Here's why: Latex condoms work against STDs by keeping blood, a man's semen, and a woman's vaginal fluids—all of which can carry bacteria and viruses—from passing from one person to another. For many years, scientists have known that male condoms (also called safes, rubbers, or prophylactics) can help prevent STDs transmitted by bacteria, such as syphilis and gonorrhea, because the bacteria can't get through the condom. More recently, researchers discovered that latex condoms can also reduce the risk of getting STDs caused by viruses, such as HIV, herpes, and hepatitis B, even though viruses are much smaller than bacteria or sperm.

After this discovery, FDA, which regulates condoms as medical devices, worked with manufacturers to develop labeling for latex condoms. The labeling tells consumers that although latex condoms cannot entirely eliminate the risk of STDs, when used properly and consistently they are highly effective in preventing STDs. FDA also provided a sample set of instructions and requested that all condoms include adequate instructions.

Make the Right Choice

Male condoms now sold in the United States are made either of latex (rubber), polyurethane or natural membrane (called "lambskin," but actually made of sheep intestine). Scientists found that natural skin condoms are not as effective as latex condoms in reducing the risk of STDs because natural skin condoms have naturally occurring tiny holes or pores that viruses may be able to get through. Only latex condoms labeled for protection against STDs should be used for disease protection, unless one of the partners is allergic to latex. In that case, a polyurethane condom can be used.

Some condoms have lubricants added and some have spermicide (a chemical that kills sperm) added. The package labeling tells whether either of these has been added to the condom.

Lubricants may help prevent condoms from breaking and may help prevent irritation. But lubricants do not give any added disease protection. If an unlubricated condom is used, a water-based lubricant (such as K-Y Jelly), available over-the-counter (without prescription) in drugstores, can be used but is not required for the proper use of the condom. Do not use petroleum-based jelly (such as Vaseline), baby oil, lotions, cooking oils, or cold creams because these products can weaken latex and cause the condom to tear easily.

Some condoms have added spermicide. An active chemical in spermicides, nonoxynol-9, kills sperm. But spermicides alone (as sold in creams and jellies over-the-counter in drugstores) and spermicides used with the diaphragm or cervical cap do not give adequate protection against HIV and other STDs. For the best disease protection, a latex condom should be used from start to finish every time a person has sex.

FDA requires condoms to be labeled with an expiration date. Condoms should be stored in a cool, dry place out of direct sunlight. Closets and drawers usually make good storage places. Because of possible exposure to extreme heat and cold, glove compartments of cars are not a good place to store condoms. For the same reason, condoms shouldn't be kept in a pocket, wallet or purse for more than a few hours at a time. Condoms should not be used after the expiration date, usually abbreviated EXP and followed by the date.

Condoms are available in almost all drugstores, many supermarkets, and other stores. They are also available from vending machines. When purchasing condoms from vending machines, as from any source, be sure they are latex, labeled for disease prevention, and are not past their expiration date. Don't buy a condom from a vending machine located where it may be exposed to extreme heat or cold or to direct sunlight.

How to Use a Condom

- Use a new condom for every act of vaginal, anal, and oral (penis-mouth contact) sex. Do not unroll the condom before placing it on the penis.

- Put the condom on after the penis is erect and before any contact is made between the penis and any part of the partner's body.

- If the condom does not have a reservoir top, pinch the tip enough to leave a half-inch space for semen to collect. Always make sure to eliminate any air in the tip to help keep the condom from breaking.

- Holding the condom rim (and pinching a half inch space if necessary), place the condom on the top of the penis. Then, continuing to hold it by the rim, unroll it all the way to the base of the penis. If you are also using water-based lubricant, you can put more on the outside of the condom.

- If you feel the condom break, stop immediately, withdraw, and put on a new condom.

- After ejaculation and before the penis gets soft, grip the rim of the condom and carefully withdraw.

- To remove the condom, gently pull it off the penis, being careful that semen doesn't spill out.

- Wrap the condom in a tissue and throw it in the trash where others won't handle it (don't flush condoms down the toilet because they may cause sewer problems). Afterwards, wash your hands with soap and water.

Latex condoms are the only form of contraception now available that human studies have shown to be highly effective in protecting against the transmission of HIV and other STDs. They give good disease protection for vaginal sex and should also reduce the risk of disease transmission in oral and anal sex. But latex condoms may not be 100 percent effective, and a lot depends on knowing the right way to buy, store and use them.

New Information on Labels

Information about whether a birth control product also helps protect against sexually transmitted diseases (STDs), including HIV infection, is emphasized on the labeling of these products, because a product that is highly effective in preventing pregnancy will not necessarily protect against sexually transmitted diseases.

Labels on birth control pills, implants such as Norplant, injectable contraceptives such as Depo-Provera, intrauterine devices (IUDs), and natural skin condoms will state that the products are intended to prevent pregnancy and do not protect against STDs, including HIV infection (which leads to AIDS). Labeling of natural skin condoms will also state that consumers should use a latex condom to help reduce risk of many STDs, including HIV infection.

Laboratory tests show that organisms as small as sperm and the HIV virus cannot pass through polyurethane condom. But the risks of STDs, including HIV infection, have not been well studied in actual use with polyurethane condoms. So unless one or both partners is allergic to latex, latex condoms should be used.

Labeling for latex condoms states that if used properly, latex condoms help reduce risk of HIV transmission and many other STDs. This statement, a modification from previous labeling, now appears on individual condom wrappers, on the box, and in consumer information.

Besides highlighting statements concerning sexually transmitted diseases and AIDS on the consumer packaging, manufacturers will add a similar statement to patient and physician leaflets provided with the products.

Looking at a Condom Label

Like other drugs and medical devices, FDA requires condom packages to contain certain labeling information. When buying condoms, look on the package label to make sure the condoms are:

- made of latex

- labeled for disease prevention

- not past their expiration date (EXP followed by the date).

STD Facts

- Sexually transmitted diseases affect more than 12 million Americans each year, many of whom are teenagers or young adults.

- Using drugs and alcohol increases your chances of getting STDs because these substances can interfere with your judgment and your ability to use a condom properly.

- Intravenous drug use puts a person at higher risk for HIV and hepatitis B because IV drug users usually share needles.

- The more partners you have, the higher your chance of being exposed to HIV or other STDs. This is because it is difficult to know whether a person is infected, or has had sex with people who are more likely to be infected due to intravenous drug use or other risk factors.

- Sometimes, early in infection, there may be no symptoms, or symptoms may be confused with other illnesses.

- You cannot tell by looking at someone whether he or she is infected with HIV or another STD.

STDs can cause:

- pelvic inflammatory disease (PID), which can damage a woman's fallopian tubes and result in pelvic pain and sterility

- tubal pregnancies (where the fetus grows in the fallopian tube instead of the womb), sometimes fatal to the mother and always fatal to the fetus

- cancer of the cervix in women

- sterility—the inability to have children—in both men and women

- damage to major organs, such as the heart, kidney and brain, if STDs go untreated

- death, especially with HIV infection.

See a doctor if you have any of these STD symptoms:

- discharge from vagina, penis or rectum

- pain or burning during urination or intercourse

- pain in the abdomen (women), testicles (men), or buttocks and legs (both)

- blisters, open sores, warts, rash, or swelling in the genital or anal areas or mouth

- persistent flu-like symptoms—including fever, headache, aching muscles, or swollen glands—which may precede STD symptoms.

—by Judith Levine Willis

Judith Levine Willis is a member of FDA's Public Affairs Staff.

Section 38.2

Chlamydia

Excerpted from "Some Facts about Chlamydia,"
National Center for HIV, STD, and TB Prevention,
Centers for Disease Control and Prevention (CDC),
http://www.cdc.gov/nchstp/dstd/chlamydia_facts.htm,
page last reviewed August 07, 2000.

What Is Chlamydia?

Chlamydia is a sexually transmitted disease (STD) that is caused by the bacterium *Chlamydia trachomatis*. Because approximately 75% of women and 50% of men have no symptoms, most people infected with chlamydia are not aware of their infections and therefore may not seek health care.

When diagnosed, chlamydia can be easily treated and cured. Untreated, chlamydia can cause severe, costly reproductive and other health problems which include both short- and long-term consequences, including pelvic inflammatory disease (PID), which is the critical link to infertility, and potentially fatal tubal pregnancy.

Up to 40% of women with untreated chlamydia will develop PID. Undiagnosed PID caused by chlamydia is common. Of those with PID, 20% will become infertile; 18% will experience debilitating, chronic pelvic pain; and 9% will have a life-threatening tubal pregnancy. Tubal pregnancy is the leading cause of first-trimester, pregnancy-related deaths in American women.

Chlamydia may also result in adverse outcomes of pregnancy, including neonatal conjunctivitis and pneumonia. In addition, recent research has shown that women infected with chlamydia have a 3–5 fold increased risk of acquiring human immunodeficiency virus (HIV), if exposed.

Chlamydia is also common among young men, who are seldom offered screening. Untreated chlamydia in men typically causes urethral infection, but may also result in complications such as swollen and tender testicles.

What Is the Magnitude of the Problem?

Chlamydia is the most frequently reported infectious disease in the United States. Though 526,653 cases were reported in 1997, an estimated 3 million cases occur annually. Severe under reporting is largely a result of substantial numbers of asymptomatic persons whose infections are not identified because screening is not available. Highlights of reported data are as follows:

- From 1984 through 1997, reported rates of chlamydia increased from 3.2 to 207.0 cases per 100,000 population. This trend primarily reflects increased screening, recognition of asymptomatic infection (mainly in women), and improved reporting capacity rather than a true increase in disease incidence.

- In 1997, the reported rate of chlamydia for women (335.8) substantially exceeded the rate for men (70.4), due mainly to increased detection of asymptomatic infection in women through screening. Low rates of reported chlamydia among men suggest that many of the partners of women with chlamydia are not screened or treated.

- As in previous years, 1997 rates of chlamydia were highest in the West and the Midwest, where substantial resources have been committed for organized screening programs.

How Are Adolescents and Young Women Affected?

- As many as 1 in 10 adolescent girls tested for chlamydia is infected.

- Based on reports to the Centers for Disease Control and Prevention (CDC) provided by states that collect age-specific data, teenage girls have the highest rates of chlamydial infection. In these states, 15- to 19-year-old girls represent 46% of infections and 20- to 24-year-old women represent another 33%. These high percentages are consistent with high rates of other STDs among teenagers.

- Among women entering the Job Corps in 1997, chlamydia rates ranged from 4–14% by state (20,000 entrants are screened annually). Chlamydial infection is widespread geographically and highly prevalent among these economically disadvantaged young women between 16 and 24 years old.

What Does Chlamydia Cost?

The annual cost of chlamydia and its consequences in the United States is more than $2 billion. The CDC estimates screening and treatment programs can be conducted at an annual cost of $175 million. Every dollar spent on screening and treatment saves $12 in complications that result from untreated chlamydia.

What Is Being Done to Address the Problem?

In 1993, Congress appropriated funds to begin a national STD-related infertility prevention program. Through a cooperative effort between CDC and the Office of Population Affairs, the program involves strong collaboration among family planning, STD and primary health care programs, and public health laboratories. Significant progress has been made where screening programs have been fully implemented.

- A 65% decline in infection was demonstrated in family planning clinics in Federal Region X (Alaska, Idaho, Oregon, and Washington) in the first 8 years of screening, from 1988 to 1995. These declines have occurred across all age groups since testing began in 1988, although adolescents continue to have the highest rates of disease.

- A 31% decline in infection was indicated for females under age 20 during the first 2–1/2 years of initial large-scale screening in Region III (Delaware, the District of Columbia, Maryland, Pennsylvania, Virginia, and West Virginia), from 7.8% in 1994 to 5.4% during January–June 1996.

- A 16% decline in infection was indicated for females under age 20 during the first 2.5 years of initial large-scale screening in Region VIII (Colorado, Montana, North Dakota, South Dakota, Utah, and Wyoming), from 5.5% in 1994 to 4.6% during January–June 1996.

- Strong evidence is now available that chlamydia screening and treatment not only reduces the prevalence of lower genital tract infection, but also decreases the incidence of costly complications, such as PID. A randomized trial of chlamydia screening and treatment in a health maintenance organization demonstrated a 56% reduction in the incidence of PID in the screened group in the 12 months following the trial.

Due to resource constraints, the program continues only as demonstration projects in most parts of the country. CDC estimates that nearly 75% of women at risk reside in 30 states that are only just beginning to screen for chlamydia. For example, in California, Florida, Georgia, Illinois, New York, and Texas, more than 200,000 women in each state who attend publicly funded family planning and STD clinics currently do not have access to screening and treatment.

Since these programs have focused on prevention efforts in women, many men with chlamydia are not diagnosed and treated, thus continuing the cycle of infection.

CDC has developed recommendations for the prevention and management of chlamydia for all providers of health care. These recommendations call for screening of all sexually active females under 20 years of age at least annually, and annual screening of women ages 20 and older with one or more risk factors for chlamydia (i.e., new or multiple sex partners and lack of barrier contraception). All women with infection of the cervix and all pregnant women should be tested.

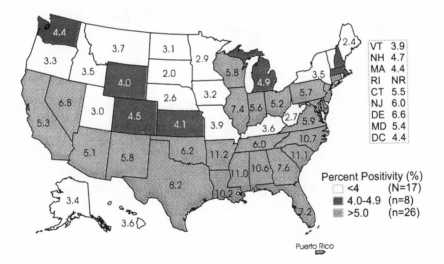

Figure 38.1. Positivity among 15- to 24-year-old women tested for Chlamydia in family planning clinics by state, 1997.

What Still Needs to Be Done?

Programs to provide testing for infection through screening and subsequent treatment are needed nationwide. A successful program must include comprehensive screening and treatment not only for women but also for men. Recent research advances have made available extremely accurate urine tests which make testing of males more feasible and less uncomfortable than older tests. In addition, single-dose antibiotic therapy promises to substantially enhance the likelihood of successful treatment—especially in adolescents—as compared to commonly used 7-day oral medication.

Section 38.3

Gonorrhea

Excerpted from "Gonorrhea," National Center for HIV, STD, and TB Prevention, Centers for Disease Control and Prevention (CDC), http://www.cdc.gov/nchstp/dstd/Fact_Sheets/FactsGonorrhea.htm, September 2000.

What Causes Gonorrhea?

Gonorrhea is caused by *Neisseria gonorrhoeae*, a bacterium that can grow and multiply easily in mucous membranes of the body. Gonorrhea bacteria can grow in the warm, moist areas of the reproductive tract, including the cervix (opening to the womb), uterus (womb), and fallopian tubes (egg canals) in women, and in the urethra (urine canal) in women and men. The bacteria can also grow in the mouth, throat, and anus.

How Do People Get Gonorrhea?

Gonorrhea is spread through sexual contact (vaginal, oral, or anal). This includes penis-to-vagina, penis-to-mouth, penis-to-anus, mouth-to-vagina, and mouth-to-anus contact. Ejaculation does not have to occur for gonorrhea to be transmitted or acquired. Gonorrhea can also be spread from mother to child during birth.

Gonorrhea infection can spread to other unlikely parts of the body. For example, a person can get an eye infection after touching infected genitals and then the eyes. Individuals who have had gonorrhea and received treatment may get infected again if they have sexual contact with persons infected with gonorrhea.

How Common Is Gonorrhea?

Gonorrhea is a very common infectious disease. Each year approximately 650,000 people in the United States are infected with gonorrhea. In 1998, the rate of reported gonorrhea infections was 132.9 per 100,000 persons.

What Are the Signs and Symptoms of Gonorrhea?

When initially infected, about 50% of men have some signs or symptoms. Symptoms and signs include a burning sensation when urinating and a yellowish white discharge from the penis. Sometimes men with gonorrhea get painful or swollen testicles.

In women, the early symptoms of gonorrhea are often mild, and many women who are infected have no symptoms of infection. Even when a woman has symptoms, they can be so non-specific as to be mistaken for a bladder or vaginal infection. The initial symptoms and signs in women include a painful or burning sensation when urinating and a vaginal discharge that is yellow or bloody. Women with no or mild gonorrhea symptoms are still at risk of developing serious complications from the infection. Untreated gonorrhea in women can develop into pelvic inflammatory disease (PID). Please see below for the complications of gonorrhea.

Symptoms of rectal infection include discharge, anal itching, soreness, bleeding, and sometimes painful bowel movements. Infections in the throat cause few symptoms.

When Do Symptoms Appear?

In males, symptoms usually appear 2 to 5 days after infection, but it can take as long as 30 days for symptoms to begin. Regardless of symptoms, once a person is infected with gonorrhea, he or she can spread the infection to others if condoms or other protective barriers are not used during sex.

How Is Gonorrhea Diagnosed?

Several laboratory tests are available to diagnose gonorrhea. A health care provider can obtain a sample of fluid from the infected mucus membrane (cervix, urethra, rectum, or throat) and send the specimen to a laboratory for analysis. Gonorrhea that is present in the male or female genital tract can be diagnosed in a laboratory by using a urine specimen from an infected person. A quick laboratory test for gonorrhea that can be done in the clinic or doctor's office is a Gram stain. The Gram stain allows the doctor to see the gonorrhea bacteria under a microscope. This test works better for men than for women.

Who Is at Risk for Gonorrhea?

Any sexually active person can be infected with gonorrhea. In the United States, approximately 75% of all reported gonorrhea is found in younger persons aged 15 to 29 years. The highest rates of infection are usually found in 15- to 19-year-old women and 20- to 24-year-old men. In 1998, approximately 1 of every 30 African American youths aged 15 to 24 had gonorrhea.

What Is the Treatment for Gonorrhea?

Many of the currently used antibiotics can successfully cure uncomplicated gonorrhea in adolescents and adults. Penicillin is a common antibiotic that is no longer used to treat gonorrhea, because many strains of the gonorrhea bacterium have become resistant to penicillin. Because many people with gonorrhea also have chlamydia, antibiotics for both infections are usually given together. Persons with gonorrhea should also be screened for other sexually transmitted diseases (STDs).

It is important to take all of the medication prescribed to cure gonorrhea, even if the symptoms or signs stop before all the medication is gone. Although medication will stop the infection, it will not repair any permanent damage done by the disease. Persons who have had gonorrhea and have been treated can also get the disease again if they have sexual contact with an infected person.

What Are the Complications of Gonorrhea?

Untreated gonorrhea can cause serious and permanent problems in both women and men.

In women, gonorrhea is a common cause of pelvic inflammatory disease (PID). About 1 million women each year in the United States develop PID. Women with PID do not necessarily have symptoms or signs. When symptoms or signs are present, they can be very severe and can include strong abdominal pain and fever. PID can lead to internal abscesses (pus pockets that are hard to cure), long-lasting pelvic pain, and infertility. PID can cause infertility or damage the fallopian tubes (egg canals) enough to increase the risk of ectopic pregnancy. Ectopic pregnancy is a life-threatening condition in which a fertilized egg grows outside the uterus, usually in a fallopian tube.

In men, gonorrhea can cause epididymitis, a painful condition of the testicles that can sometimes lead to infertility if left untreated. Without prompt treatment, gonorrhea can also affect the prostate and can lead to scarring inside the urethra, making urination difficult.

Gonorrhea can spread to the blood or joints. This condition can be life-threatening. Also, persons with gonorrhea can more easily contract human immunodeficiency virus (HIV), the virus that causes acquired immunodeficiency syndrome (AIDS). Persons with HIV infection and gonorrhea are more likely than persons with HIV infection alone to transmit HIV to someone else.

How Does Gonorrhea Affect a Pregnant Woman and Her Baby?

Gonorrhea in a pregnant woman can cause premature delivery or spontaneous abortion. The infected mother may give the infection to her infant as the baby passes through the birth canal during delivery. This can cause blindness, joint infection, or a life-threatening blood infection in the baby. Treatment of gonorrhea as soon as it is detected in pregnant women will lessen the risk of these complications. Pregnant women should consult a health care provider for appropriate medications.

How Can Gonorrhea Be Prevented?

Practice sexual abstinence, or limit sexual contact to one uninfected partner.

Use latex condoms correctly every time you have sex. Persons who choose to engage in sexual behaviors that can place them at risk for sexually transmitted diseases (STDs) should use latex condoms every time they have sex. A condom put on the penis before starting sex and worn until the penis is withdrawn can help protect both the male and the female partner from gonorrhea. When a male condom cannot be used appropriately, sex partners should consider using a female condom.

Condoms do not provide complete protection from all STDs. Sores and lesions of other STDs on infected men and women may be present in areas not covered by the condom, resulting in transmission of infection to another person.

Limit the number of sex partners, and do not go back and forth between partners.

If you think you are infected, avoid sexual contact and see a health care provider immediately. Any genital symptoms such as discharge or burning during urination or unusual sore or rash should be a signal to stop having sex and to consult a health care provider immediately. If you are told you have gonorrhea or any other STD and receive treatment, you should notify all of your recent sex partners so that they can see a health care provider and be treated.

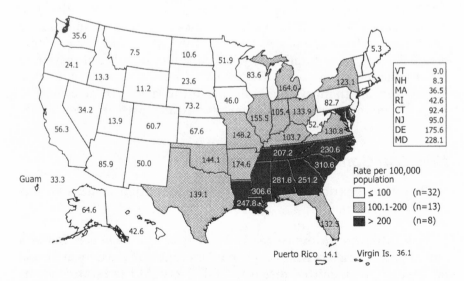

Figure 38.2. Gonorrhea: Rates by state.

This will reduce the risk that your partners will develop serious complications from gonorrhea and will reduce your own risk of becoming reinfected.

References

CDC. 1998 guidelines for treatment of sexually transmitted diseases. *Morbidity and Mortality Weekly Report* 1998;47(RR-1).

Hook, E.W. III and Handsfield, H.H. In: K. Holmes, P. Markh, P. Sparling et al (eds). *Sexually Transmitted Diseases, 3rd Edition*. New York: McGraw-Hill, 1999, 451–466.

Section 38.4

Genital Herpes

Excerpted from "Some Facts about Genital Herpes," National Center for HIV, STD, and TB Prevention, Centers for Disease Control and Prevention (CDC), http://www.cdc.gov/nchstp/dstd/Fact_Sheets/facts_Genital_Herpes.htm, page last reviewed August 07, 2000.

What Is Genital Herpes?

Herpes is a sexually transmitted disease (STD) caused by the herpes simplex virus (HSV). HSV-type 1 commonly causes fever blisters on the mouth or face (oral herpes), while HSV-type 2 typically affects the genital area (genital herpes). However, both viral types can cause either genital or oral infections. Most of the time, HSV-1 and HSV-2 are inactive, or "silent," and cause no symptoms, but some infected people have "outbreaks" of blisters and ulcers. Once infected with HSV, people remain infected for life.

How Is Genital Herpes Spread?

HSV-1 and HSV-2 are transmitted through direct contact, including kissing, sexual contact (vaginal, oral, or anal sex), or skin-to-skin contact.

Genital herpes can be transmitted with or without the presence of sores or other symptoms. It often is transmitted by people who are unaware that they are infected, or by people who do not recognize that their infection can be transmitted even when they have no symptoms.

How Common Is Genital Herpes?

Results of a recent, nationally representative study show that genital herpes infection is common in the United States. Nationwide, 45 million people ages 12 and older, or one out of five of the total adolescent and adult population, is infected with HSV-2.

HSV-2 infection is more common in women (approximately one out of four women) than in men (almost one out of five). This may be because male to female transmission is more efficient than female to male transmission. HSV-2 infection is also more common in blacks (45.9%) than in whites (17.6%). Race and ethnicity in the United States are risk markers that correlate with other more fundamental determinants of health such as poverty, access to quality health care, health care seeking behavior, illicit drug use, and living in communities with high prevalence of STDs.

Since the late 1970s, the number of Americans with genital herpes infection has increased 30%. Prevalence is increasing most dramatically among young white teens; HSV-2 prevalence among 12- to 19-year-old whites is now five times higher than it was 20 years ago. And young adults ages 20 to 29 are now twice as likely to have HSV-2.

Is Genital Herpes Serious?

HSV-2 usually produces mild symptoms, and most people with HSV-2 infection have no recognized symptoms. However, HSV-2 can cause recurrent painful genital ulcers in many adults, and HSV-2 infection can be severe in people with suppressed immune systems. Regardless of severity of symptoms, genital herpes frequently causes psychological distress among people who know they are infected.

In addition, HSV-2 can cause potentially fatal infections in infants if the mother is shedding virus at the time of delivery. It is important that women avoid contracting herpes during pregnancy, because a first episode during pregnancy creates a greater risk of transmission to the newborn. If a woman has active genital herpes at delivery, a cesarean-section delivery is usually performed. Fortunately, infection of an infant is rare among women with HSV-2 infection.

In the United States, HSV-2 may play a major role in the heterosexual spread of human immunodeficiency virus (HIV), the virus that causes acquired immunodeficiency syndrome (AIDS). Herpes can make people more susceptible to HIV infection, and can make HIV-infected individuals more infectious.

What Happens When Someone Is Infected with Genital Herpes?

Most people infected with HSV-2 are not aware of their infection. However, if symptoms occur during the primary episode, they can be quite pronounced. The primary episode usually occurs within two weeks after the virus is transmitted, and lesions typically heal within two to four weeks. Other symptoms during the primary episode may include a second crop of lesions, or flu-like symptoms, including fever and swollen glands. However, some individuals with HSV-2 infection may never have lesions, or may have very mild symptoms that they don't even notice or that they mistake for insect bites or a rash.

Most people diagnosed with a primary episode of genital herpes can expect to have several symptomatic recurrences a year (average four or five); these recurrences usually are most noticeable within the first year following the first episode.

How Is Genital Herpes Diagnosed?

The signs and symptoms associated with HSV-2 can vary greatly among individuals. Health care providers can diagnose genital herpes by visual inspection, by taking a sample from the sore(s) and by testing it to see if the herpes virus is present.

Is There a Cure for Herpes?

There is no treatment that can cure herpes, but antiviral medications can shorten and prevent outbreaks for whatever period of time the person takes the medication.

How Can People Protect Themselves against Infection?

The consistent and correct use of latex condoms is the best protection. However, condoms do not provide complete protection, because a herpes lesion may not be covered by the condom and viral shedding may occur. If you or your partner has genital herpes, it is best to abstain from sex when symptoms are present, and to use latex condoms between outbreaks.

References

Aral SO, Wasserheit JN. 1995. "Interactions among HIV, other sexually transmitted diseases, socioeconomic status, and poverty in women." In: O'Leary A, Jemmott LS, editors. *Women at Risk: Issues in the Primary Prevention of AIDS*. New York: Plenum Press.

Fleming DT, McQuillan GM, Johnson RE, Nahmias AJ, Aral SO, Lee FK, St. Louis ME. "Herpes Simplex Virus Type 2 in the United States, 1976 to 1994." *NEJM* 1997; 16:1105–1111.

Laumann EO, Gagnon JH, Michael RT, Michaels S. 1994a. "The number of partners." In: *The Social Organization of Sexuality: Sexual Practices in the United States*. Chicago: University of Chicago Press, pp. 174–224.

Laumann EO, Gagnon JH, Michael RT, Michaels S. 1994b. "Sexual networks." In: *The Social Organization of Sexuality: Sexual Practices in the United States*. Chicago: University of Chicago Press, pp. 225–268.

Section 38.5

Genital Warts and Human Papillomavirus

Excerpted from "Human Papillomavirus and Genital Warts," National Institute of Allergy and Infectious Diseases (NIAID), National Institutes of
Health (NIH), http://www.niaid.nih.gov/factsheets/stdhpv.htm, July 1998.

Introduction

Human papillomavirus (HPV) is one of the most common causes
of sexually transmitted disease (STD) in the world. Experts estimate
that as many as 24 million Americans are infected with HPV, and the
frequency of infection and disease appears to be increasing. More than
60 types of HPV have been identified by scientists. Some types of the
virus cause common skin warts. About one-third of the HPV types are
spread through sexual contact and live only in genital tissue. Low-
risk types of HPV cause genital warts, the most recognizable sign of
genital HPV infection. Other high-risk types of HPV cause cervical
cancer and other genital cancers.

Like many sexually transmitted organisms, HPV usually causes
a silent infection, that is, one that does not have visible symptoms.
One study sponsored by the National Institute of Allergy and Infectious Diseases (NIAID) reported that almost half of the women infected with HPV had no obvious symptoms. Because the viral infection
persists, individuals may not be aware of their infection or the potential risk of transmission to others and of developing complications.

Genital Warts

Genital warts (*condylomata acuminata* or venereal warts) are
caused by only a few of the many types of HPV. Other common types
of HPV infections, such as those that cause warts on the hands and
soles of the feet, do not cause genital warts. Genital warts are
spread by sexual contact with an infected partner and are very
contagious. Approximately two-thirds of people who have sexual
contact with a partner with genital warts will develop warts, usually within three months of contact. Scientists estimate that as many

as 1 million new cases of genital warts are diagnosed in the United States each year.

In women, the warts occur on the outside and inside of the vagina, on the cervix (the opening to the uterus), or around the anus. In men, genital warts are less common. If present, they are seen on the tip of the penis; however, they also may be found on the shaft of the penis, on the scrotum, or around the anus. Rarely, genital warts also can develop in the mouth or throat of a person who has had oral sexual contact with an infected person. Genital warts often occur in clusters and can be very tiny or can spread into large masses on genital tissues. Left untreated, genital warts often disappear. In other cases, they eventually may develop a fleshy, small raised growth with a cauliflower-like appearance. Because there is no way to predict whether the warts will grow or disappear, however, people who suspect that they have genital warts should be examined and treated, if necessary.

Diagnosis

A doctor usually can diagnose genital warts by direct visual examination. Women with genital warts also should be examined for possible HPV infection of the cervix. The doctor may be able to identify some otherwise invisible changes in the tissue by applying vinegar (acetic acid) to areas of suspected infection. This solution causes infected areas to whiten, which makes them more visible, particularly if a procedure called colposcopy is performed. During colposcopy, a magnifying instrument is used to view the vagina and uterine cervix. In some cases, it is necessary to do a biopsy of cervical tissue. This involves taking a small sample of tissue from the cervix and examining it under the microscope.

A Pap smear test also may indicate the possible presence of cervical HPV infection. A Pap smear is a microscopic examination of cells scraped from the uterine cervix in order to detect cervical cancer. Abnormal Pap smear results are associated with HPV infection. Women with abnormal Pap smears should be examined further to detect and treat cervical problems.

Treatment

Depending on factors such as their size and location, genital warts are treated in several ways. Although treatments can eliminate the warts, none eradicate the virus, and warts often reappear after treatment. Patients should consult their doctors to determine the best treatment for them.

The U.S. Food and Drug Administration (FDA) has approved imiquimod cream, which the patient can apply to the affected area, to treat genital warts. Other treatments include a 20 percent podophyllin solution, which the patient can apply to the affected area and later wash off, and a 0.5 percent podofilox solution, which also is applied to the affected area, but is not washed off. Pregnant women should not use podophyllin or podofilox because they are absorbed by the skin and may cause birth defects in babies. The doctor may also prescribe 5 percent 5-fluorouracil cream, which also should not be used during pregnancy, or trichloroacetic acid (TCA).

Small warts can be removed by cryosurgery (freezing), electrocautery (burning), or laser treatment. Occasionally, surgery is needed to remove large warts that have not responded to other treatment.

Some doctors use the antiviral drug alpha interferon, which they inject directly into the warts, to treat warts that have recurred after removal by traditional means. The drug is expensive, however, and does not reduce the rate of recurrence.

Complications

Low-risk papilloma viruses cause warts but not cervical cancer. High-risk viruses, however, cause cervical cancer and also are associated with vulvar cancer, anal cancer, and cancer of the penis (a rare cancer). Although most HPV infections do not progress to cancer, it is particularly important for women who have cervical dysplasia to have regular Pap smears. Potentially pre-cancerous cervical disease is readily treatable.

Genital warts may cause a number of problems during pregnancy. Sometimes they enlarge during pregnancy, making urination difficult. If the warts are on the vaginal wall, they can make the vagina less elastic and cause obstruction during delivery.

Rarely, infants born to women with genital warts develop laryngeal papillomatosis (warts in the throat). Although uncommon, it is a potentially life-threatening condition for the child, requiring frequent laser surgery to prevent obstruction of the airways. Research on the use of interferon therapy in combination with laser surgery indicates that this drug may show promise in slowing the course of the disease.

Prevention

The only way to prevent HPV infection is to avoid direct contact with the virus, which is transmitted by skin-to-skin contact. If warts are visible in the genital area, sexual contact should be avoided until the warts are treated. Using a latex condom during sexual intercourse may provide some protection.

Researchers are working to develop two types of HPV vaccines. One type would be used to prevent infection or disease (warts or precancerous tissue changes); another type would be used to treat cervical cancers. Clinical trials are in progress for both types of vaccines.

Section 38.6

HIV Infection and AIDS

This chapter contains text from "HIV Infection and AIDS: an Overview," http://www.niaid.nih.gov/factsheets/hivinf.htm, and "HIV Infection in Adolescents," http://www.niaid.nih.gov/factsheets/hivadolescent.htm, National Institute of Allergy and Infectious Diseases (NIAID), National Institutes of Health (NIH), May 2000.

HIV Infection and AIDS: an Overview

AIDS—acquired immunodeficiency syndrome—was first reported in the United States in 1981 and has since become a major worldwide epidemic. AIDS is caused by the human immunodeficiency virus (HIV). By killing or damaging cells of the body's immune system, HIV progressively destroys the body's ability to fight infections and certain cancers. People diagnosed with AIDS may get life-threatening diseases called opportunistic infections, which are caused by microbes such as viruses or bacteria that usually do not make healthy people sick.

More than 700,000 cases of AIDS have been reported in the United States since 1981, and as many as 900,000 Americans may be infected with HIV. The epidemic is growing most rapidly among minority populations and is a leading killer of African American males. According to the US Centers for Disease Control and Prevention (CDC), AIDS affects six times more African Americans than whites and three times more Hispanics than whites.

Transmission

HIV is spread most commonly by having sex with an infected partner. The virus can enter the body through the lining of the vagina, vulva, penis, rectum, or mouth during sex.

HIV also is spread through contact with infected blood. Before blood was screened for evidence of HIV infection and before heat-treating techniques to destroy HIV in blood products were introduced, HIV was transmitted through transfusions of contaminated blood or blood components. Today, because of blood screening and heat treatment, the risk of getting HIV from such transfusions is extremely small.

HIV frequently is spread among injection drug users by the sharing of needles or syringes contaminated with very small quantities of blood from someone infected with the virus. It is rare, however, for a patient to give HIV to a health care worker or vice-versa by accidental sticks with contaminated needles or other medical instruments.

Women can transmit HIV to their babies during pregnancy or birth. Approximately one-quarter to one-third of all untreated pregnant women infected with HIV will pass the infection to their babies. HIV also can be spread to babies through the breast milk of mothers infected with the virus. If the mother takes the drug Azidothymidine (AZT) during pregnancy, she can reduce significantly the chances that her baby will be infected with HIV. If doctors treat mothers with AZT and deliver their babies by cesarean section, the chances of the baby being infected can be reduced to a rate of 1 percent.

A study sponsored by the National Institute of Allergy and Infectious Diseases (NIAID) in Uganda found a highly effective and safe drug regimen for preventing transmission of HIV from an infected mother to her newborn that is more affordable and practical than any other examined to date. Interim results from the study show that a single oral dose of the antiretroviral drug nevirapine (NVP) given to an HIV-infected woman in labor and another to her baby within three days of birth reduces the transmission rate by half compared with a similar short course of AZT.

Although researchers have detected HIV in the saliva of infected individuals, no evidence exists that the virus is spread by contact with saliva. Laboratory studies reveal that saliva has natural properties that limit the power of HIV to infect. Research studies of people infected with HIV have found no evidence that the virus is spread to others through saliva such as by kissing. No one knows, however, whether so-called "deep kissing," involving the exchange of large amounts of saliva, or oral intercourse increase the risk of infection.

351

Scientists also have found no evidence that HIV is spread through sweat, tears, urine, or feces.

Studies of families of HIV-infected people have shown clearly that HIV is not spread through casual contact such as the sharing of food utensils, towels and bedding, swimming pools, telephones, or toilet seats. HIV is not spread by biting insects such as mosquitoes or bed-bugs.

HIV can infect anyone who practices risky behaviors such as:

- sharing drug needles or syringes

- having sexual contact with an infected person without using a condom or with someone whose HIV status is unknown.

Having a sexually transmitted disease such as syphilis, genital herpes, chlamydial infection, gonorrhea, or bacterial vaginosis appears to make people more susceptible to acquiring HIV infection during sex with infected partners.

Early Symptoms

Many people do not develop any symptoms when they first become infected with HIV. Some people, however, have a flu-like illness within a month or two after exposure to the virus. This illness may include fever, headache, tiredness, and enlarged lymph nodes (organs of the immune system easily felt in the neck and groin). These symptoms usually disappear within a week to a month and are often mistaken for those of another viral infection. During this period, people are very infectious, and HIV is present in large quantities in genital fluids.

More persistent or severe symptoms may not surface for a decade or more after HIV first enters the body in adults, or within two years in children born with HIV infection. This period of "asymptomatic" infection is highly individual. Some people may begin to have symptoms as soon as a few months, while others may be symptom-free for more than 10 years. During the asymptomatic period, however, the virus is actively multiplying, infecting, and killing cells of the immune system. HIV's effect is seen most obviously in a decline in the blood levels of CD4+ T cells (also called T4 cells)—the immune system's key infection fighters. At the beginning of its life in the human body, the virus disables or destroys these cells without causing symptoms.

As the immune system deteriorates, a variety of complications start to take over. For many people, their first sign of infection is large lymph nodes or "swollen glands" that may be enlarged for more than three months. Other symptoms often experienced months to years before the onset of AIDS include:

- lack of energy
- weight loss
- frequent fevers and sweats
- persistent or frequent yeast infections (oral or vaginal)
- persistent skin rashes or flaky skin
- pelvic inflammatory disease in women that does not respond to treatment
- short-term memory loss

Some people develop frequent and severe herpes infections that cause mouth, genital, or anal sores, or a painful nerve disease called shingles. Children may grow slowly or be sick a lot.

AIDS

The term AIDS applies to the most advanced stages of HIV infection. The CDC in Atlanta, GA, develops official criteria for the definition of AIDS and is responsible for tracking the spread of AIDS in the United States.

CDC's definition of AIDS includes all HIV-infected people who have fewer than 200 CD4+ T cells per cubic millimeter of blood. (Healthy adults usually have CD4+ T-cell counts of 1,000 or more.) In addition, the definition includes 26 clinical conditions that affect people with advanced HIV disease. Most of these conditions are opportunistic infections, which rarely cause harm in healthy people. In people with AIDS, these infections are often severe and sometimes fatal because the immune system is so ravaged by HIV that the body cannot fight off certain bacteria, viruses, fungi, parasites, and other microbes.

Opportunistic infections common in people with AIDS cause symptoms such as:

- coughing and shortness of breath
- seizures and lack of coordination
- difficult or painful swallowing
- mental symptoms such as confusion and forgetfulness

- severe and persistent diarrhea
- fever
- vision loss
- nausea, abdominal cramps, and vomiting
- weight loss and extreme fatigue
- severe headaches
- coma

Although children with AIDS may get the same opportunistic infections as adults with the disease, they also experience severe forms of the bacterial infections which all children may get, such as conjunctivitis (pink eye), ear infections, and tonsillitis.

People with AIDS are particularly prone to developing various cancers, especially those caused by viruses such as Kaposi's sarcoma and cervical cancer, or cancers of the immune system known as lymphomas. These cancers are usually more aggressive and difficult to treat in people with AIDS. Signs of Kaposi's sarcoma in light-skinned people are round brown, reddish, or purple spots that develop in the skin or in the mouth. In dark-skinned people, the spots are more pigmented.

During the course of HIV infection, most people experience a gradual decline in the number of CD4+ T cells, although some may have abrupt and dramatic drops in their CD4+ T-cell counts. A person with CD4+ T cells above 200 may experience some of the early symptoms of HIV disease. Others may have no symptoms even though their CD4+ T-cell count is below 200.

Many people are so debilitated by the symptoms of AIDS that they cannot hold steady employment or do household chores. Other people with AIDS may experience phases of intense life-threatening illness followed by phases in which they function normally.

A small number of people (fewer than 50) initially infected with HIV 10 or more years ago have not developed symptoms of AIDS. Scientists are trying to determine what factors may account for their lack of progression to AIDS, such as particular characteristics of their immune systems or whether they were infected with a less aggressive strain of the virus, or if their genes may protect them from the effects of HIV. Scientists hope that understanding the body's natural method of control may lead to ideas for protective HIV vaccines and use of vaccines to prevent the disease from progressing.

Diagnosis

Because early HIV infection often causes no symptoms, a doctor or other health care worker usually can diagnose it by testing a person's blood for the presence of antibodies (disease-fighting proteins) to HIV. HIV antibodies generally do not reach levels in the blood which the doctor can see until one to three months following infection, and it may take the antibodies as long as six months to be produced in quantities large enough to show up in standard blood tests.

People exposed to the virus should get an HIV test as soon as they are likely to develop antibodies to the virus. By getting tested early, they can get the right treatment at a time when their immune systems are most able to combat HIV and thus prevent the emergence of certain opportunistic infections (see "Treatment" below). Early testing also alerts HIV-infected people to avoid high-risk behaviors that could spread the virus to others.

Most doctors' offices or health clinics can do HIV testing and will usually offer counseling to the patient at the same time. Of course, individuals can be tested anonymously at many sites if they are concerned about confidentiality.

Doctors diagnose HIV infection by using two different types of antibody tests, enzyme-linked immunosorbent assay (ELISA) and Western Blot. If a person is highly likely to be infected with HIV and yet both tests are negative, a doctor may look for HIV itself in the blood. The person also may be told to repeat antibody testing at a later date, when antibodies to HIV are more likely to have developed.

Babies born to mothers infected with HIV may or may not be infected with the virus, but all carry their mothers' antibodies to HIV for several months. If these babies lack symptoms, a definitive diagnosis of HIV infection using standard antibody tests cannot be made until after 15 months of age. By then, babies are unlikely to still carry their mothers' antibodies and will have produced their own, if they are infected. New technologies to detect HIV itself are being used to more accurately determine HIV infection in infants between ages 3 months and 15 months. A number of blood tests are being evaluated to determine if they can diagnose HIV infection in babies younger than 3 months.

Treatment

The Food and Drug Administration has approved a number of drugs for treating HIV infection. The first group of drugs used to treat HIV infection, called nucleoside reverse transcriptase (RT) inhibitors, interrupts an early stage of the virus making copies of itself. Included in this class of drugs (called nucleoside analogs) are AZT (also known as azidothymidine, zidovudine or ZDV), ddC (zalcitabine), ddI (dideoxyinosine), d4T (stavudine), and 3TC (lamivudine). These drugs may slow the spread of HIV in the body and delay the onset of opportunistic infections.

Non-nucleoside reverse transcriptase inhibitors (NNRTIs), such as delvaridine (Rescriptor) and nevirapine (Viramune), are also available for use in combination with other antiretroviral drugs.

More recently, a second class of drugs has been approved for treating HIV infection. These drugs, called protease inhibitors, interrupt virus replication at a later step in its life cycle. They include ritonavir (Norvir), saquinivir (Invirase), indinavir (Crixivan), amprenivir (Agenerase), and nelfinavir (Viracept). Because HIV can become resistant to both classes of drugs, combination treatment using both is necessary to effectively suppress the virus.

Currently available antiretroviral drugs do not cure people of HIV infection or AIDS, however, and they all have side effects that can be severe. Some of the nucleoside RT inhibitors may cause a depletion of red or white blood cells, especially when taken in the later stages of the disease. Some may also cause an inflammation of the pancreas and painful nerve damage. Other complications, including lactic acidosis and severe hepatomegaly (enlarged liver) with steatosis (fatty liver) that may result in liver failure and death, have also been reported with the use of antiretroviral nucleoside analogs alone or in combination, including AZT, ddI, ddC, 3TC, and abacavir.

The most common side effects associated with protease inhibitors include nausea, diarrhea, and other gastrointestinal symptoms. In addition, protease inhibitors can interact with other drugs resulting in serious side effects.

Researchers have credited highly active antiretroviral therapy, or HAART, as being a major factor in reducing the number of deaths from AIDS in this country by 47 percent in 1997. HAART is a combination of several drugs to treat patients. These drugs include reverse transcriptase inhibitors and protease inhibitors. Patients who are newly infected with HIV as well as AIDS patients can take the combination.

HAART is not a cure. The health of HIV and AIDS patients has benefitted dramatically by combining protease inhibitors with other AIDS drugs, but there are drawbacks. Also, though HIV may not be found in the patients successfully treated with HAART, researchers know that it is still present, lurking in hiding places such as the lymph nodes, the brain, testes, and the retina of the eye.

A number of drugs are available to help treat opportunistic infections to which people with HIV are especially prone. These drugs include foscarnet and ganciclovir, used to treat cytomegalovirus eye infections, fluconazole to treat yeast and other fungal infections, and trimethoprim/sulfamethoxazole (TMP/SMX) or pentamidine to treat Pneumocystis carinii pneumonia (PCP).

In addition to antiretroviral therapy, adults with HIV whose CD4+ T-cell counts drop below 200 are given treatment to prevent the occurrence of PCP, which is one of the most common and deadly opportunistic infections associated with HIV. Children are given PCP preventive therapy when their CD4+ T-cell counts drop to levels considered below normal for their age group. Regardless of their CD4+ T-cell counts, HIV-infected children and adults who have survived an episode of PCP are given drugs for the rest of their lives to prevent a recurrence of the pneumonia.

HIV-infected individuals who develop Kaposi's sarcoma or other cancers are treated with radiation, chemotherapy or injections of alpha interferon, a genetically engineered naturally occurring protein.

Prevention

Because no vaccine for HIV is available, the only way to prevent infection by the virus is to avoid behaviors that put a person at risk of infection, such as sharing needles and having unprotected sex.

Many people infected with HIV have no symptoms. Therefore, there is no way of knowing with certainty whether a sexual partner is infected unless he or she has repeatedly tested negative for the virus— and has not engaged in any risky behavior.

People should either abstain from having sex or use latex condoms, which may offer partial protection, during oral, anal, or vaginal sex. Only condoms made of latex should be used, and water-based lubricants should be used with latex condoms.

Although some laboratory evidence shows that spermicides can kill HIV, researchers have not found that these products can prevent a person from getting HIV.

The risk of HIV transmission from a pregnant woman to her baby is significantly reduced if she takes AZT during pregnancy, labor and delivery, and her baby takes it for the first six weeks of life.

HIV Infection in Adolescents

Overview

The human immunodeficiency virus (HIV), which causes AIDS, ranks seventh among the leading causes of death for US children 5 to 14 years of age and sixth for young people 15 to 24 years of age. Because the average period of time from HIV infection to the development of AIDS is 10 years, most young adults with AIDS were likely infected with HIV as adolescents. Almost 18 percent of all reported cases of AIDS in the United States have occurred in people between the ages of 20 and 29.

In the United States, through June 1999, 3,564 cases of AIDS in people aged 13 through 19 had been reported to the Centers for Diseases Control and Prevention (CDC). Many other adolescents are currently infected with HIV but have not yet developed AIDS. Data from the 31 states that conduct HIV case surveillance indicate that among adolescents aged 13 through 19:

- 46 percent were male
- 54 percent were female
- 28 percent were non-Hispanic white
- 66 percent were non-Hispanic black
- 5 percent were Hispanic
- less than 1 percent were Asian/Pacific Islander or American Indian/Alaskan Native

Transmission

Most adolescents recently infected with HIV are exposed to the virus through sexual intercourse or injection drug use. Through June 1999, HIV surveillance data suggest that nearly half of all HIV-infected adolescent males are infected through sex with men. A small percentage of males appear to be exposed by injection drug use and/or heterosexual contact. The same data suggest that almost half of all adolescent females who are infected with HIV were exposed through heterosexual contact and a very small percentage through injection drug use.

CDC studies conducted every two years in high schools (grades nine through 12) consistently indicate that approximately 60 percent of the students have had sexual intercourse by grade 12; half report use of a latex condom during last sexual intercourse, and about one-fifth have had more than four lifetime sex partners.

Approximately two-thirds of the 12 million cases of sexually transmitted diseases (STDs) that are reported in the United States each year are in individuals under the age of 25 and one-quarter are among teenagers. This is particularly significant because if either partner is infected with another STD, the risk of HIV transmission increases substantially. If one of the partners is infected with an STD that causes the discharge of pus and mucus, such as gonorrhea or chlamydia, the risk of HIV transmission is three to five times greater. If one of the partners is infected with an STD that causes ulcers, such as syphilis or genital herpes, the risk of HIV transmission is nine times greater.

Treatment

Adolescents tend to think they are invincible, and therefore they tend to deny any risk. This belief may cause them to engage in risky behavior, to delay HIV-testing, and if they test positive, to delay or refuse treatment. Doctors report that many young people, when they learn they are HIV-positive, take several months to accept their diagnosis and return for treatment. Health care professionals may be able to help these adolescents by explaining the information slowly and carefully, eliciting questions from them, and emphasizing the success of newly available treatments.

According to the "Guidelines for the Use of Antiretroviral Agents in HIV-Infected Adults and Adolescents" (produced by theDepartment of Health and Human Services), adolescents who were exposed to HIV sexually or via injection drug use appear to follow a clinical course that is more similar to HIV disease in adults than in children. At this time, most adolescents with sexually acquired HIV are in a relatively early stage of infection and are ideal candidates for early intervention. Adolescents who were infected at birth or via blood products as young children follow a unique clinical course that may differ from other adolescents and long-term surviving adults. Physicians should refer to the treatment guidelines for detailed information about the treatment of HIV-infected adolescents.

Clinical Trials

The National Institute of Allergy and Infectious Diseases (NIAID) supports clinical trials at many clinics and medical centers throughout the United States. These studies help evaluate promising therapies to fight HIV infections, prevent and treat the opportunistic infections and cancers associated with AIDS, and reconstitute HIV-damaged immune systems.

Recruiting adolescents into clinical trials is important to ensure that research results will be applicable to therapy for that age group. Most clinical trials are open to adolescents, but in reality very few enroll. Of the 53,000 participants in studies conducted in the NIAID-supported AIDS Clinical Trials Groups, for pediatric and adult HIV-infected people, 812 (1.5 percent) were adolescents. To encourage participation by more adolescents, the Pediatric AIDS Clinical Trials Group (also funded by the National Institute of Child Health and Human Development [NICHD]) has developed an Adolescent Initiative to fund a research agenda on clinical studies relevant to HIV-infected youth.

The Adolescent Medicine HIV/AIDS Research Network was formed in 1994 to plan and conduct research on the medical, biobehavioral and psychosocial aspects of HIV and AIDS in young people. Funded by the National Institute of Allergy and Infectious Diseases (NIAID), the National Institute of Child Health and Human Development (NICHD), the National Institute on Drug Abuse (NIDA), the National Institute of Mental Health (NIMH), the network is currently recruiting participants for a study called REACH (Reaching for Excellence in Adolescent Care and Health). Researchers will learn about disease progression in adolescents by examining a number of immunological and virological factors. The goal is to enroll at least 360 high-risk, HIV-infected and HIV-uninfected adolescents. The results of this study are expected to assist researchers and policy makers in developing the agenda for future adolescent clinical trials. REACH is a national, observational study that is being conducted in 16 sites in 13 cities. Participants must be between the ages of 12 and 18, have a health care provider, and have been infected through sexual contact or injection drug use. To enroll a patient or obtain more information, physicians may contact the National Institute of Child Health and Human Development at (301) 496-7339.

Section 38.7

Syphilis

Excerpted from "Some Facts about Syphilis," National Center for HIV,
STD, and TB Prevention, Centers for Disease Control and Prevention (CDC),
http://www.cdc.gov/nchstp/dstd/Fact_Sheets/Syphilis_Facts.htm, October 1999.

What Is Syphilis?

Syphilis is a complex sexually transmitted disease (STD) caused
by the bacterium *Treponema pallidum*. It has often been called the
great imitator because so many of the signs and symptoms are indis-
tinguishable from those of other diseases.

How Is Syphilis Spread?

The syphilis bacterium is passed from person to person through
direct contact with a syphilis sore. Sores mainly occur on the external genitals, vagina, anus, or in the rectum. Sores also can occur on
the lips and in the mouth. Transmission of the organism occurs during vaginal, anal, or oral sex. Pregnant women with the disease can
pass it to the babies they are carrying. Syphilis cannot be spread by
toilet seats, door knobs, swimming pools, hot tubs, bath tubs, shared
clothing, or eating utensils.

What Are the Signs and Symptoms in Adults?

The time between picking up the bacterium and the start of the
first symptom can range from 10–90 days (average 21 days). The primary stage of syphilis is marked by the appearance of a single sore (called
a chancre). The chancre is usually firm, round, small, and painless. It
appears at the spot where the bacterium entered the body. The chancre
lasts 1–5 weeks and will heal on its own. If adequate treatment is not
administered, the infection progresses to the secondary stage.

The second stage starts when one or more areas of the skin break
into a rash that usually does not itch. Rashes can appear as the chancre
is fading or can be delayed for weeks. The rash often appears as rough,

"copper penny" spots on both the palms of the hands and the bottoms of the feet. The rash also may appear as a prickly heat rash, as small blotches or scales all over the body, as a bad case of old acne, as moist warts in the groin area, as slimy white patches in the mouth, as sunken dark circles the size of a nickel or dime, or as pus-filled bumps like chicken pox. Some of these signs on the skin look like symptoms of other diseases. Sometimes the rashes are so faint they are not noticed. Rashes typically last 2–6 weeks and clear up on their own. In addition to rashes, second stage symptoms can include fever, swollen lymph glands, sore throat, patchy hair loss, headaches, weight loss, muscle aches, and tiredness. A person can easily pass the disease to sex partners when first or second stage signs or symptoms are present.

The latent (hidden) stage of syphilis begins when the secondary symptoms disappear. If the infected person has not received treatment, he/she still has syphilis even though there are no signs or symptoms. The bacterium remains in the body and begins to damage the internal organs, including the brain, nerves, eyes, heart, blood vessels, liver, bones, and joints. In about one-third of untreated persons, this internal damage shows up many years later in the late or tertiary stage of syphilis. Late stage signs and symptoms include not being able to coordinate muscle movements, paralysis, no longer feeling pain, gradual blindness, dementia (madness) or other personality changes, impotency, shooting pains, blockage or ballooning of the heart vessels, tumors or "gummas" on the skin, bones, liver, or other organs, severe pain in the belly, repeated vomiting, damage to knee joints, and deep sores on the soles of the feet or toes. This damage may be serious enough to cause death.

Can a Newborn Get Syphilis?

An infected pregnant woman has about a 40% chance of having a stillbirth (syphilitic stillbirth) or giving birth to a baby who dies shortly after birth. A baby born to a mother with either untreated syphilis or syphilis treated after the 34th week of pregnancy has a 40%–70% chance of being infected with syphilis (congenital syphilis). An infected baby may be born without symptoms but may develop them within a few weeks, if not treated immediately. These signs and symptoms can be very serious and include skin sores, a very runny nose, which is sometimes bloody (and infectious), slimy patches in the mouth, inflamed arm and leg bones, a swollen liver, anemia, jaundice, or a small head. Untreated babies may become retarded or may have seizures. About 12% of infected newborns will die because of the disease.

How Is Syphilis Diagnosed?

The syphilis bacterium can be detected by a health care provider who examines material from infectious sores under a microscope. Shortly after infection occurs, the body produces syphilis antibodies that are detected with a blood test. A syphilis blood test is accurate, safe, and inexpensive. A low level of antibodies will stay in the blood for months or years after the disease has been successfully treated, and antibodies can be found by subsequent blood tests. Because untreated syphilis in a pregnant woman can infect and possibly kill her developing baby, every pregnant woman should have a blood test for syphilis.

How Common Is Syphilis?

In the United States, nearly 38,000 cases of syphilis were detected by health officials in 1998, including 7,000 cases of primary and secondary syphilis and 800 cases of congenital syphilis in newborns. More cases occur each year than come to the attention of health officials. The eight states with the highest 1998 syphilis rates were located in the southern region of the US. These states had rates 2–5 times higher than the national rate. In 1998, 28 counties accounted for 50% of all primary and secondary syphilis cases. Three hundred twelve counties had syphilis rates greater than the Year 2000 objective of 4 cases per 100,000. Ninety-one percent of these were in the South.

In 1998, syphilis occurred primarily in persons aged 20 to 39 and slightly more frequently in males than females. Syphilis rates in females were higher in the 20–24 age group, while male rates were higher in the 30 to 39 age group. Some fundamental societal problems, such as poverty, inadequate access to health care, and lack of education are associated with disproportionately high levels of syphilis in certain populations. Cases in 1998 had the following race or ethnicity distribution: African-Americans 80%, whites 13%, Hispanics 6%, and others 1%. Syphilis is one of the most glaring examples of racial disparity in health status, with the rate for African-Americans nearly 34 times the rate for whites.

What Is the Link between Syphilis and Human Immunodeficiency Virus (HIV)?

While the health problems caused by the syphilis bacterium for adults and newborns are serious in their own right, it is now known that the genital sores caused by syphilis in adults also make it easier to transmit and acquire HIV infection sexually. There is a 2- to 5-fold increased risk of acquiring HIV infection when syphilis is present. Areas of the US that have the highest rates of syphilis also have the fastest-growing HIV infection rates in women of childbearing age.

Is There a Cure for Syphilis?

One dose of the antibiotic penicillin will cure a person who has had syphilis for less than a year. More doses are needed to cure someone who has had it for longer than a year. A baby born with the disease needs daily penicillin treatment for 10 days. There are no home remedies or over-the-counter drugs that cure syphilis. Penicillin treatment will kill the syphilis bacterium and prevent further damage, but it will not repair any damage already done. Persons who receive syphilis treatment must abstain from sexual contact with new partners until the syphilis sores are completely healed. Persons with syphilis must notify their sex partners so that they also can receive treatment.

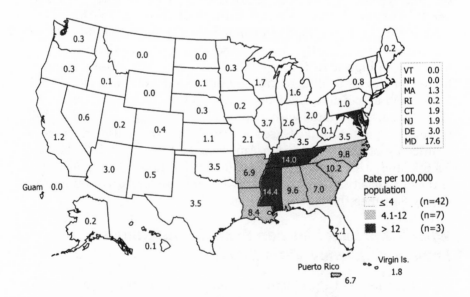

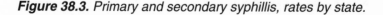

Figure 38.3. *Primary and secondary syphillis, rates by state.*

Will Syphilis Recur?

Having had syphilis does not protect a person from getting it again. Antibodies are produced as a person reacts to the disease, and, after treatment, these antibodies may offer partial protection from getting infected again, if exposed right away. Even though there may be a short period of protection, the antibody levels naturally decrease in the blood, and people become susceptible to syphilis infection again if they are sexually exposed to syphilis sores.

How Can People Protect Themselves against Infection?

Two people who know they are not infected and who have sex with no one but each other cannot contract syphilis. When a person has sex with a person whose syphilis status is unknown, a latex condom put on before beginning sex and worn until the penis is withdrawn is a good defense against infection. Only lab tests can confirm whether someone has syphilis. Because syphilis sores can be hidden in the vagina, rectum, or mouth, it may not be obvious that a sex partner has syphilis. Washing the genitals, urinating, or douching after sex does not prevent sexually transmitted diseases (STDs), including syphilis. Any unusual discharge, sore, or rash, especially in the groin area, should be a signal to stop having sex and to see a doctor at once.

Section 38.8

Trichomoniasis

Excerpted from "Trichomoniasis," National Center for HIV, STD, and TB Prevention, Centers for Disease Control and Prevention (CDC), http://www.cdc.gov/nchstp/dstd/Fact_Sheets/FactsTrichomoniasis.htm, September 2000.

What Is Trichomoniasis?

Trichomoniasis is a common sexually transmitted disease (STD) that affects both women and men, although symptoms are more common in women.

What Causes Trichomoniasis?

Trichomoniasis is caused by the single-celled protozoan parasite Trichomonas vaginalis. The vagina is the most common site of infection in women, and the urethra is the most common site of infection in men.

How Do People Get Trichomoniasis?

Trichomoniasis is a sexually transmitted disease that is spread through penis-to-vagina intercourse or vulva-to-vulva contact with an infected partner. Women can acquire the disease from infected men or women, whereas men usually contract it only from infected women.

How Common Is Trichomoniasis?

Trichomoniasis is the most common curable STD in young, sexually active women. An estimated 5 million new cases occur each year in women and men.

What Are the Signs and Symptoms of Trichomoniasis?

Most men with trichomoniasis do not have signs or symptoms. Men with symptoms may have an irritation inside the penis, mild discharge, or slight burning after urination or ejaculation.

Many women do have signs or symptoms of infection. In these women, trichomoniasis causes a frothy, yellow-green vaginal discharge with a strong odor. The infection may also cause discomfort during intercourse and urination. Irritation and itching of the female genital area and, in rare cases, lower abdominal pain can also occur.

When Do Symptoms Appear?

Symptoms usually appear within 5 to 28 days of exposure in women.

What Are the Complications of Trichomoniasis?

Trichomoniasis in pregnant women may cause premature rupture of the membranes and preterm delivery. The genital inflammation caused by trichomoniasis might also increase a woman's risk of acquiring human immunodeficiency virus (HIV) infection if she is exposed to HIV. Trichomoniasis in a woman who is also infected with HIV can increase the chances of transmitting HIV infection to a sex partner.

How Is Trichomoniasis Diagnosed?

To diagnose trichomoniasis, a health care provider must perform a physical examination and laboratory test. In women, a pelvic examination can reveal small red ulcerations on the vaginal wall or cervix. Laboratory tests are performed on a sample of vaginal fluid or urethral fluid to look for the disease-causing parasite. The parasite is harder to detect in men than in women.

Who Is at Risk for Trichomoniasis?

Any sexually active person can be infected with trichomoniasis.

What Is the Treatment for Trichomoniasis?

Trichomoniasis can usually be cured with the prescription drug metronidazole given by mouth in a single dose. The symptoms of trichomoniasis in infected men may disappear within a few weeks without treatment. However, an infected man, even a man who has never had symptoms or whose symptoms have stopped, can continue to infect a female partner until he has been treated. Therefore, both partners should be treated at the same time to eliminate the parasite. Persons being treated for trichomoniasis should avoid sex until they and their sex partners complete treatment and have no symptoms. Metronidazole can be used by pregnant women.

How Can Trichomoniasis Be Prevented?

Practice sexual abstinence, or limit sexual contact to one uninfected partner.

Use condoms correctly every time you have sex. The use of latex or polymethane condoms during vaginal intercourse can prevent the transmission of trichomoniasis. However, condoms do not provide complete protection from all STDs. Sores and lesions of other STDs on infected men and women may be present in areas not covered by the condom, resulting in transmission of infection to another person.

Limit the number of sex partners, and do not go back and forth between partners.

If you think you are infected, avoid sexual contact and see a health care provider. Any genital symptoms such as discharge or burning during urination or an unusual sore or rash should be a signal to stop having sex and to consult a health care provider immediately. If you are told you have trichomoniasis or any other STD and receive treatment, you should notify all of your recent sex partners so that they can see a health care provider and be treated.

References

American Social Health Association. *Sexually transmitted diseases in America: How many cases and at what cost?* Research Triangle Park, NC, 1998.

CDC. "1998 guidelines for treatment of sexually transmitted diseases." *Morbidity and Mortality Weekly Report* 1998;47(RR-1).

Krieger JN and Alderete JF. "Trichomonas vaginalis and trichomoniasis." In: K. Holmes, P. Markh, P. Sparling et al (eds). *Sexually Transmitted Diseases, 3rd Edition.* New York: McGraw-Hill, 1999, 587–604.

Chapter 39

Dating Violence Fact Sheet

Dating violence may be defined as the perpetration or threat of an act of violence by at least one member of an unmarried couple on the other member within the context of dating or courtship. This violence encompasses any form of sexual assault, physical violence, and verbal or emotional abuse.

Scope of the Problem

Violent behavior that takes place in a context of dating or courtship is not a rare event. Estimates vary because studies and surveys use different methods and definitions of the problem.

- A review of dating violence research found that prevalence rates of nonsexual, courtship violence range from 9% to 65%, depending on whether threats and emotional or verbal aggression were included in the definition.

- Data from a study of 8th and 9th grade male and female students indicated that 25% had been victims of nonsexual dating violence and 8% had been victims of sexual dating violence.

- Summarizing many studies, the average prevalence rate for nonsexual dating violence is 22% among male and female high

"Dating Violence," National Center for Injury Prevention and Control, Centers for Disease Control and Prevention (CDC), http://www.cdc.gov/ncipc/factsheets/datviol.htm, reviewed January 27, 2000.

school students and 32% among college students. Females are somewhat more likely than males to report being victims of violence.

- In a national study of college students, 27.5% of the women surveyed said that they had suffered rape or attempted rape at least once since age 14. Only 5% of those experiences were reported to the police. The term "hidden rape" has emerged because this survey and many other studies found that sexual assaults are seldom reported to the police.

- Over half of a representative sample of more than 1,000 female students at a large urban university had experienced some form of unwanted sex. Twelve percent of these acts were perpetrated by casual dates and 43% by steady dating partners.

- Studies of college students and high school students suggest that both males and females inflict and receive dating violence in equal proportion, but the motivation for violence by women is more often for defensive purposes. Other studies have found that women and girls were victims of dating violence twice as often as men and boys, and that females suffer significantly more injuries than males.

- A recent National Crime Victimization survey found that women were 6 times more likely than men to experience violence at the hands of an intimate partner. Intimate partners include current or former spouses, boyfriends, girlfriends, dating partners, regardless of whether they are cohabiting or not.

- Nearly half of the 500,000 rapes and sexual assaults reported to the police by women of all ages were committed by friends or acquaintances. From 80% to 95% of the rapes that occur on college campuses are committed by someone known to the victim.

Risk Factors

Characteristics of Victims

- Young women aged 12–18 who are victims of violence are more likely than older women to report that their offenders were acquaintances, friends, or intimate partners.

- The likelihood of becoming a victim of dating violence is associated with having female peers who have been sexually victimized, lower church attendance, greater number of past dating partners, acceptance of dating violence, and personally having experienced a previous sexual assault.

Characteristics of Perpetrators

* Studies have found the following to be associated with sexual assault perpetration: the male having sexually aggressive peers; heavy alcohol or drug use; the man's acceptance of dating violence; the male's assumption of key roles in dating such as initiating the date, being the driver, and paying dating expenses; miscommunication about sex; previous sexual intimacy with the victim; interpersonal violence; traditional sex roles; adversarial attitudes about relationships; and rape myths.

* Men who have a family history of observing or experiencing abuse are more likely to inflict abuse, violence, and sexual aggression.

* As the consumption of alcohol by either the victim or perpetrator increases, the rate of serious injuries associated with dating violence also increases.

Selected References

[Editors note: Original, complete document, found at http://www. cdc.gov/ncipc/factsheets/datviol.htm contains all the references.]

Abbey, A.; Ross, L. T.; Mcduffie, D.; Mcauslan, P. Alcohol and dating risk factors for sexual assault among college women. *Psychology of Women Quarterly* 1996; 20(1)147–169.

Bachman, R; Saltzman, L.E. Violence Against Women: Estimates from the redesigned survey, Bureau of Justice Statistics, Special Report, U.S. Department of Justice, August 1995.

Foshee, V.A.; Linder, G.F.; Bauman, K.E.; Langwick, S.A.; Arriaga, X.B.; Heath, J.L.; McMahon, P.M.; Bangdiwala, S. The Safe Dates Project: Theoretical Basis, Evaluation Design, and Selected Baseline Findings. Youth Violence Prevention: Description and baseline data from 13 evaluation projects (K. Powell; D. Hawkins, Eds.). *American Journal of Preventive Medicine*, Supplement, 1996; 12 (5):39–47.

Gray, H.M.; Foshee, V. Adolescent Dating Violence: Differences between one-sided and mutually violent profiles. *Journal of Interpersonal Violence* 1997;12(1)126–141.

Koss, M. P. Defending Date Rape. *Journal of Interpersonal Violence* 1992;7(1) 121–126.

Chapter 40

Rape Fact Sheet

Prevalence and Incidence

- The revised National Crime Victimization Survey for 1992–1993 estimates that annually 172,400 women were victims of rape.

- There were 71 forcible rapes per 100,000 females reported to United States law enforcement agencies in 1996.

- Data from the National Women's Study, a longitudinal telephone survey of a national household probability sample of women at least 18 years of age, show 683,000 women forcibly raped each year and that 84% of rape victims did not report the offense to the police.

- Using Uniform Crime Report data for 1994 and 1995, the Bureau of Justice Statistics found that of rape victims who reported the offense to law enforcement, about 40% were under the age of 18, and 15% were younger than 12.

- In a national survey 27.7% of college women reported a sexual experience since the age of fourteen that met the legal definition of rape or attempted rape, and 7.7% of college men reported perpetrating aggressive behavior which met the legal definition of rape.

Excerpted from "Rape Fact Sheet, Family and Intimate Violence Prevention Team," Centers for Disease Control and Prevention (CDC), http://www.cdc.gov/ncipc/dvp/fivpt/spotlite/rape.htm, September, 1998.

Risk Factors

- The National Crime Victimization Survey indicates that for 1992–1993, 92% of rapes were committed by known assailants. About half of all rapes and sexual assaults against women are committed by friends and acquaintances, and 26% are by intimate partners.

- Risk factors for perpetrating sexual violence include: early sexual experience (both forced and voluntary), adherence by men to sex role stereotyping, negative attitudes of men towards women, alcohol consumption, acceptance of rape myths by men.

- Non-forceful verbal resistance and lack of resistance are associated with rape completion.

Consequences

- The adult pregnancy rate associated with rape is estimated to be 4.7%. This information, in conjunction with estimates based on the U.S. Census, suggest that there may be 32,101 annual rape-related pregnancies among American women over the age of 18.

- Non-genital physical injuries occur in approximately 40% of completed rape cases. As many as 3% of all rape cases have non-genital injuries requiring overnight hospitalization.

- Victims of rape often manifest long-term symptoms of chronic headaches, fatigue, sleep disturbance, recurrent nausea, decreased appetite, eating disorders, menstrual pain, sexual dysfunction, and suicide attempts. In a longitudinal study, sexual assault was found to increase the odds of substance abuse by a factor of 2.5.

- Estimates of the occurrence of sexually transmitted diseases resulting from rape range from 3.6% to 30%. HIV (human immunodeficiency virus) transmission risk rate from rape is estimated at 1 in 500, although a few probable cases have been documented in Sweden and Great Britain.

- Victims of marital or date rape are 11 times more likely to be clinically depressed, and 6 times more likely to experience social phobia than are non-victims. Psychological problems are still evident in cases as long as 15 years after the assault.

- Fatalities occur in about 0.1% of all rape cases.

- A study examining the use of health services over a five year period by female members of a health maintenance program found that the number of visits to physicians by rape victims increased 56% in the year following the crime, compared to a 2% utilization increase by non-victims.

Promising Primary Prevention Programs

Although few prevention initiatives in this area have been evaluated, the following programs represent strategies which have promise for rape prevention.

- A program of peer facilitated groups among men help men recognize their role in sexual assault prevention.

- The STOP IT NOW Program, currently operating in Vermont, provides a number of preventive services including an anonymous help-line number which provides information to abusers before they act on thoughts of child sexual abuse.

- A home-based program utilizing visiting nurses to instruct parents on child development and care with a focus on preventing child abuse and other forms of family violence which may act as a primary prevention for the children as they mature since early sexual experience is a risk factor for perpetration.

- The Safe Dates Program is a school-based curriculum that targets gender-role stereotyping dating violence norms, conflict management skills, help-seeking, and cognitive factors associated with help-seeking. Preliminary evaluation suggests the program reduces the perpetration of dating sexual violence.

Chapter 41

Parenting the Sexually Abused Child

What Is Child or Adolescent Sexual Abuse?

Child or adolescent sexual abuse is any forced or tricked sexual contact by an adult or older child with a child. Usually the adult or older child is in a position of power or authority over the child. Physical force is generally not used, since there is usually a trusting relationship between the adult or older child and the child who is abused.

There are various types of sexual activity which may take place. It can include open mouth kissing, touching, fondling, manipulation of the genitals, anus or breasts with fingers, lips, tongue or with an object. It may include intercourse. Children or adolescents may not have been touched themselves but may have been forced to perform sexual acts on an adult or older child. Sometimes children are forced or tricked into disrobing for photography or are made to have sexual contact with other children while adults watch.

Sexual abuse does not always involve physical touching. It can include any experience or attitude imposed on a child that gets in the way of the development of healthy sexual responses or behaviors. For example, a child may be a victim of "emotional incest." If a mother tells her son, in great detail, about her sexual exploits, or if a father promises his daughter that she will be his life partner when she turns 18, these would be scenarios in which the child could be considered

Excerpted from Rosemary Narimanian and Julie Marks, "Parenting the Sexually Abused Child," National Adoption Information Clearinghouse, http://www.calib.com/naic/pubs/f_abused.htm, 1990. Updated August 2, 2000.

sexually abused. Siblings who are aware of a brother or sister's victimization, but are not actually abused themselves, may also suffer many of the same effects as an abused child.

In addition, some children experience ritualistic and/or satanic abuse. Ken Wooden, founder of the National Coalition for Children's Justice, defines ritualistic abuse as a bizarre, systematic, continuing abuse which is mentally, physically, and sexually abusive of children, and for the purpose of implanting evil.

How Often Does Child and Adolescent Sexual Abuse Occur?

Estimates are that approximately 1 in 4 girls and 1 in 8 boys experience sexual abuse in some way before they are 18. Data on how many of these children live in foster or adoptive homes are not available. Foster care and adoption social workers are now saying they believe the percentages of boys and girls in foster care who have been sexually abused are much higher than in the general population, perhaps as high as 75%. Many came into foster care initially because of sexual abuse and others are children who were re-victimized while in foster care, either by an older foster child or by an adult.

What Behaviors or Signs Might You See in a Child or Adolescent Who Has Been Sexually Abused?

While no one sign or behavior can be considered absolute proof that sexual abuse has occurred, you should consider the possibility of sexual abuse when one or several of these signs or behaviors are present.

Physical Signs

- scratches, bruises, itching, rashes, cuts or injuries, especially in the genital area
- venereal disease
- pregnancy in (young) adolescents
- blood or discharge in bedding or clothes, especially underwear

Behavioral Signs

- aggressive behavior towards younger children
- advanced sexual knowledge for the child's age

- seductive or "sexy" behavior towards adults or peers

- pseudo-mature behavior (for instance, a girl who is eight and dresses like a 16 year-old, wears makeup and generally acts "too old for her age," or a young boy who attempts to be his mother's "man" in every sense of the word)

- regressed behavior (for example, the child who has been toilet trained starts wetting the bed)

- excessive masturbation, masturbation in public places, difficulty with being re-focused to another behavior

- poor relationships with peers

- fear of a particular person, place or thing (for example, if the abuse occurred in the bathroom, the child may show fear in that room)

- sudden or extreme changes in behavior (for instance, a previously good student starts having trouble with school work, a child who was not sad before starts crying frequently or acting sad, or a formerly cooperative child acts defiantly or is uncooperative or unusually overly cooperative)

- eating disorders (overeats, undereats)

Additional Behavioral Signs in Pre-teens and Adolescents

- self-mutilation (the child may repeatedly pick at scabs, cut him/herself with a razor blade, bite his/her finger or arm, burn him/herself with a cigarette)

- threatening or attempting suicide

- using drugs or alcohol

- becoming promiscuous (a child is sexually active without discrimination, or just has that reputation)

- being prudish (the child avoids any sexuality, does not see him/herself as a sexual being in any way)

- prostitution

- fire-setting

- lying, stealing

- running away

- isolating self or dropping friends

- pre-occupation with death (the child may write poems about death, may ask a lot of questions about death, such as "What does it feel like and where do people go?")

Some Additional Behavioral Signs in Children Who Have Been Ritualistically/Satanically Abused

- bizarre nightmares

- sadistic play (for example, mutilation of dolls or small animals)

- self-mutilation

- pre-occupation with death

- increased agitation on certain dates which represent satanic high holy days

- a constant fear of harm and extreme fear of being alone

Do Boys Who Are Abused Have Special Issues?

Boys who are sexually abused face some additional problems because of persistent myths in our society. Males are rarely viewed as fitting the victim role. When boys get hurt, they are often told "act like a man," "don't be a sissy," "control your emotions." The message to boys is to stand on their own two feet and to take care of themselves. Under these circumstances, a male victim is less likely to tell and therefore cannot begin a healing process. This increases the chances that he may take on the role of the victimizer in an attempt to master his own experience.

A further complication for boys is that the media portray boys who have sexual experiences with older women as going through a "rite of passage" rather than as victims of sexual exploitation. Movies such as "Summer of '42" and "Get Out Your Handkerchiefs" are prime examples of this.

What about Juvenile Sex Offenders?

Some children who have been sexually abused go on to abuse other children. While this is a serious problem, the exact percentage of sexual abuse victims who become abusers is not known.

It is important to realize that these children are victims as well as offenders and need to receive counseling from qualified therapists who understand both aspects of the problem. The therapist must be able to be empathic and understanding of the "victim" but confrontational with the "victimizer."

Victimizers have triggers that precede their behavior. For example, a child may abuse another child when he or she finds him or herself in a vulnerable or stressful situation. Sometimes this is because he or she lacks control or power. This may be when the child gets called a name at school or believes he or she is being punished unfairly. The therapist must help the child to not only recognize his/her own individual triggers but also, to understand the consequences of acting out these impulses.

In other instances, past experiences have left the child overly sexually stimulated. The child needs education and suggestions of alternative positive behaviors to replace the sexually victimizing behavior.

What Do Parents Need to Be Aware of about Themselves?

It is very important for you to be honest with yourselves and with others about a number of things:

Is there a history of sexual abuse in either the mother or father's past? If there is, how were those experiences resolved? Did you decide to "just forget about it" and chalk it up as one of those things that just happened? Or did you get help, from your parents, a teacher, a minister, a therapist, or someone who could help you work through your feelings about having been abused? Parents with unresolved abuse experiences in their history may be at greater risk for either abusing the child again, or for keeping too much physical and emotional distance, for fear of abusing the child. Both parents and survivors in local support groups regularly address these phenomena.

How comfortable are you as parents with your own sexuality and with your sexual relationship(s)? Can you talk comfortably about sex? Do you give yourselves permission to acknowledge your own sexual feelings, thoughts, fantasies and fears? Do you have a well-established relationship which allows for direct and open communication? A child who has been sexually abused may need to talk about what happened to him or her. The child's behavior may be seductive or blatantly sexual at times. A parent must be able to deal with this.

What Do Parents Need to Be Aware of about Their Child Who Has Been Sexually Abused?

Children who have experienced sexual abuse will probably need help in learning new behaviors and ways of relating. Some of the behaviors and emotions you may see expressed by your child are:

Withdrawal. Overwhelmed by the feelings she or he has experienced, the child may retreat physically or emotionally. As a parent, you may feel confused or resentful. It can be very isolating to have someone close to you tune you out. Unless you think there is danger of physical harm to the child or others, the best course of action is to reassure the child that you care and that you will provide the limits and boundaries that your child needs.

Mood swings. A moment's tenderness can quickly explode into anger. The child may be full of confidence one day, only to sink into despair the next. It is difficult to see someone you care about in pain, but you cannot control the feelings of someone else. Point out that these mood swings are occurring. Do not allow yourself to be unfairly blamed. Try to stay calm and accepting that sometimes the child does not even know when or why his/her mood swings are occurring. Crying jags can be part of these mood swings. Accept that it is beyond your power to make it all better. Sometimes when a parent tries to rescue a child from his or her pain, he or she ends up feeling guilty, resentful and frustrated when it does not work. When a caterpillar is emerging from the cocoon, it must have a period of time to build strength in its wings. If the butterfly is released from its cocoon before its time, its strength will be diminished and it will not be able to survive on its own.

Anger. The first target for the child's angry feelings may be the person he or she has come to feel the safest with— you. When a person's angry feelings are completely out of proportion to what is going on, it probably has nothing to do with the present situation. Something in the present is triggering and re-stimulating old memories and feelings. The safety of the current situation allows these feelings to be expressed. Recognize that this is actually a sign of health, but do not accept unacceptable behavior; and never expose yourself to physical violence.

You can assure your child that you are willing to work out the problem at hand, but in a safe and supportive manner. For example, a child may be offered a pillow to beat on in order to vent his or her anger.

Unreasonable demands. Some children learn the survival skills of manipulation and control. They may feel entitled to make unreasonable demands for time, money or material goods. It is important not to play into or get trapped by these demands. You need to maintain a healthy relationship with your child. This will help the child reduce these demands.

Sexual behaviors. Since the abuse was acted out sexually, the child needs help in sorting out the meaning of abuse, sex, love, caring and intimacy. Some children may try to demand sexual activity, while others may lose interest in any form of closeness. Think of all the needs that are met through sex: intimacy, touch, validation, companionship, affection, love, release, nurturing. Children need to be re-taught ways that these needs can be met that are not sexual.

A child who has been sexually abused may feel:

- I am worthless and bad.

- No person could care for me without a sexual relationship.

- I am "damaged goods" (no one will want me again).

- I must have been responsible for the sexual abuse because

    - it sometimes felt good physically.

    - it went on so long.

    - I never said "no."

    - I really wasn't forced into it.

    - I never told anyone.

- I hate my body.

- I am uncomfortable with being touched because it reminds me of the abuse.

- I think I was abused but sometimes I think I must have imagined it.

- I blame my (biological) mother or father for not protecting me but I can't talk about it; I don't want to hurt him/her.

A child who has been sexually abused will benefit from clear guidelines that set the rules both in the home and outside. These kinds of rules will help provide the structure, comfort and security which all children need to grow into healthy adults. The following guidelines address topics with specific reference to children who have been sexually abused.

Privacy. Everyone has a right to privacy. Children should be taught to knock when a door is closed and adults need to role model the same behavior.

Bedrooms and bathrooms. These two locations are often prime stimuli for children who have been sexually abused, since abuse commonly occurs in these rooms.

By the time children enter first grade, caution should be used about children of the opposite sex sharing bedrooms or bath times.

It is not advisable to bring a child who has been sexually abused into your bed. Cuddling may be overstimulating and misinterpreted. A safer place to cuddle may be the living room couch.

Touching. No one should touch another person without permission. A person's private parts (the area covered by a bathing suit) should not be touched except during a medical examination or, in the case of young children, if they need help with bathing or toileting.

Clothing. It is a good idea for family members to be conscious of what they wear outside of the bedroom. Seeing others in their underclothes or pajmas may be overstimulating to a child who has been sexually abused.

Saying "no." Children need to learn that it is their right to assertively say "no" when someone touches them in a way they do not like. Help them to practice this.

Sex education. All children, including the child who has been sexually abused, need basic information about how they develop sexually. They also will benefit from an atmosphere in which it is OK to talk about sex. Appropriate words for body parts, such as penis, vagina, breasts and buttocks, will give the child the words to describe what happened to him or her. Suggestive or obscene language is sometimes a trigger for old feelings for a child who was sexually abused, and should not be allowed.

No "secrets." Make it clear that no secret games, particularly with adults, are allowed. Tell children if an adult suggests such a game, they should tell you immediately.

Being alone with one other person. If your child is behaving seductively, aggressively or in a sexually acting out manner, these are high risk situations. During those times, it is advisable not to put yourself in the vulnerable position of being accused of abuse. In addition, other children may be in jeopardy of being abused. Therefore, whenever possible during these high risk situations, try not to be alone with your child or allow him/her to be alone with only one other child.

Wrestling and tickling. As common and normal as these childhood behaviors are, they are often tinged with sexual overtones. They can put the weaker child in an overpowered and uncomfortable or humiliating position. Keep tickling and wrestling to a minimum.

Behaviors and feelings. Help children differentiate between feelings and behaviors. It is normal to have all kinds of feelings, including sexual feelings. However, everyone does not always act on all the feelings he or she has. Everyone has choices about which feelings he or she acts on, and everyone (except very young children) must take responsibility for his or her own behavior.

Will Our Child and Family Need Professional Help?

It is very likely that at some time or other parents of a child who was sexually abused will need professional help and support for themselves and their child. The type of therapy that will be the most helpful, that is, individual, couple or family therapy, will depend on a family's particular situation. When a child is being seen in individual therapy, it is important that the parents, who have the primary responsibility for the child, be in close contact with the therapist, or included in the therapy. Try to choose a therapist who is knowledgeable about sexual abuse and with whom you feel comfortable. If parents are not familiar with the therapy resources in their area, they may want to ask their local mental health center for a referral. There are also some resources listed at the end of this *Sourcebook* which may be helpful with referrals to therapists who are knowledgeable about sexual abuse.

Support groups for parents or sexually abused children and support groups for victims/survivors are another helpful resource. Parents who have had a chance to talk with others who understand the experience of parenting a sexually abused child say that this kind of sharing is very useful. Dr. Nicholas Groth, a leading psychologist in the field of sexual abuse, along with many children and adult victims/

survivors, say that groups for children can be most effective in the healing process. The opportunity to talk and share with other children who have also experienced sexual abuse reduces a child's sense of isolation and belief that he/she is the only one to whom this has ever happened.

Is the Healing Ever Completed?

Recovery from child sexual abuse is an on-going process. As this process unfolds, the child will ideally move from victim to survivor to thriver. Developmental stages, particularly adolescence and young adulthood, may trigger old feelings about the abuse. For example, the time when an adolescent's body begins to develop physically, or when he or she marries, or becomes a parent may restimulate old feelings and memories.

As discussed earlier, so many factors can influence the extent of the damage to the abused child. While parents cannot erase what happened to their child earlier in his/her life, you have a wonderful opportunity to provide your child with new, healthier experiences. Those who have made the commitment to parenting a sexually abused child say that the rewards of helping a child grow into a healthy, vibrant adult are very satisfying indeed.

Part Four

Drug Abuse in Adolescents

Chapter 42

Alcohol and Young Teens

How Does Alcohol Affect the World of a Child?

Ask Yourself

As Parents

- Do you know how to discuss alcohol use with your child and where to get information to help you?

- Do you know your child's friends, and do you feel that they provide positive influences on your child's activities?

- Do you know the extent of drinking by children in your neighborhood and how to find local organizations that are working on the issue?

- Do you know the legal consequences if your child is caught drinking alcohol?

The Child

- Almost 42% of ninth grade students reported having consumed alcohol before they were 13.

This chapter contains text from "How Does Alcohol Affect the World of a Child?" National Institute on Alcohol Abuse and Alcoholism (NIAAA), National Institutes of Health (NIH), http://www.niaaa.nih.gov/publications/childcontent-text.htm, 1999, and "Make a Difference, Talk to Your Child about Alcohol," NIAAA, NIH Pub. No. 00-4314, http://www.niaaa.nih.gov/publications/children.pdf, 2000.

- About 44% of ninth grade students reported drinking in the past month. In contrast, only 33% of ninth graders reported smoking in the past month.

- One fourth (25%) of ninth grade students reported binge drinking (having had five or more drinks on one occasion) in the past month.

- Rates of drinking differ among racial and ethnic minority groups. Among ninth graders, binge drinking was reported by 27% of non-Hispanic white students and 30% of Hispanic students, but only 15% of African American students and 5% of Asian-Pacific Islander students.

- The gap between alcohol use by boys and girls has closed. Girls consume alcohol and binge drink at rates equal to boys.

- Forty percent of children who start drinking before the age of 15 will become alcoholics at some point in their lives. If the onset of drinking is delayed by 5 years, a child's risk of serious alcohol problems is decreased by 50%.

Family

- Current research suggests children are less likely to drink when their parents are involved with them and when they and their parents report feeling close to each other.

- Adolescents drink less and have fewer alcohol-related problems when their parents discipline them consistently and set clear expectations.

- Nearly 17% of children under 14 and 20% of children under 18 live with a parent (or responsible adult) who drinks heavily or has an alcohol problem.

- Parents' drinking behaviors and favorable attitudes about drinking have been associated with adolescents' initiating and continuing drinking.

- The immediate family members of alcoholics are 2 to 7 times more likely than the general population to develop problems with alcohol during their lifetime.

- Drinking during pregnancy has been associated not only with fetal alcohol syndrome but with offspring learning and behavioral problems into adolescence.

- Elevated rates of alcoholism are consistently found in parents of youth with Attention Deficit/Hyperactivity Disorder (ADHD).

School

- Evidence suggests that alcohol use by peers is a strong predictor of adolescent use and misuse of alcohol.

- According to a 1995 national survey of fourth through sixth graders who read the *Weekly Reader*, 30% of students reported that they received "a lot" of pressure from their classmates to drink beer.

- Three-quarters of eighth graders reported having friends who use alcohol. In fact, one-fourth of eighth graders said that most or all of their friends drink.

- Among eighth graders, students with higher grade point averages reported less alcohol use in the past month.

- Among eighth graders, higher truancy rates were associated with greater rates of alcohol use in the past month.

- One national study found that students are less likely to use alcohol if they are close to people at school, are a part of their school, and if they feel that teachers treat students fairly.

- According to the 1995 *Weekly Reader* survey, over half (54%) of fourth through sixth graders reported learning about the dangers of illicit drugs at school, but less than a third (30%) learned about the dangers of drinking and smoking at school.

- In 1995, 76% of seventh through twelfth grade teachers polled felt that underage student drinking was a serious or somewhat serious problem.

Impact on Children's Health and Safety

- In 1997, nearly 10% of ninth graders reported driving one or more times while drinking. Thirty-three percent of ninth graders reported having ridden in a car driven by someone who had been drinking alcohol.

- Of all children under age 15 killed in vehicle crashes in 1998, 20% were killed in alcohol-related crashes.

- Among 12-to 17-year-old current drinkers, 31% had extreme levels of psychological distress, and 39% exhibited serious behavioral problems.

- In 1994, suicides or homicides accounted for 18% of the estimated number of alcohol-related deaths of children aged 9–15.

- Current drinkers among a nationally representative sample of youth aged 12–16 had higher levels of diastolic blood pressure than did their non-drinking counterparts.

- Adolescent females who drink exhibit higher levels of estradiol (an estrogen) and testosterone than non-drinking girls. High levels of estrogen may contribute to increased risk for specific diseases, including breast cancer, and high levels of testosterone are associated with an increased risk of substance use.

- Girls, aged 12–16, who were current drinkers were four times more likely than their non-drinking counterparts to suffer depression.

Make a Difference, Talk to Your Child about Alcohol

Introduction

Kids who drink are more likely to be victims of violent crime, to be involved in alcohol-related traffic accidents, and to have serious school-related problems. You have more influence on your child's values and decisions about drinking before he or she begins to use alcohol. Parents can have a major impact on their children's drinking, especially during the preteen and early teen years.

With so many drugs available to young people these days, you may wonder, "Why develop a chapter about helping kids avoid alcohol?" Alcohol is a drug, as surely as cocaine and marijuana are. It's also illegal to drink under the age of 21. And it's dangerous. Kids who drink are more likely to:

- be victims of violent crime.

- have serious problems in school.

- be involved in drinking-related traffic accidents.

Keep in mind that the suggestions on the following pages are just that—suggestions. Trust your instincts. Choose ideas you are comfortable with, and use your own style in carrying out the approaches you find useful. Your child looks to you for guidance and support in making life decisions—including the decision not to use alcohol.

"But my child isn't drinking yet," you may think. "Isn't it a little early to be concerned about drinking?" Not at all. This is the age at which some children begin experimenting with alcohol. Even if your child is not yet drinking, he or she may be receiving pressure to drink. Act now. Keeping quiet about how you feel about your child's alcohol use may give him or her the impression that alcohol use is OK for kids.

It's not easy. As children approach adolescence, friends exert a lot of influence. Fitting in is a chief priority for youth, and parents often feel shoved aside. Kids will listen, however. Study after study shows that even during the teen years, parents have enormous influence on their children's behavior. The bottom line is that most young youth don't yet drink. And parents' disapproval of youthful alcohol use is the key reason children choose not to drink. So make no mistake: You can make a difference.

Kids and Alcohol: The Risks

For young people, alcohol is the number one drug of choice. In fact, youth use alcohol more frequently and heavily than all other illicit drugs combined. Although most children ages 10 to 14 have not yet begun to drink, early adolescence is a time of special risk for beginning to experiment with alcohol.

While some parents and guardians may feel relieved that their youth is "only" drinking, it is important to remember that alcohol is a powerful, mood-altering drug. Not only does alcohol affect the mind and body in often unpredictable ways, but kids lack the judgment and coping skills to handle alcohol wisely. As a result:

- Alcohol-related traffic accidents are a major cause of death and disability among youth. Alcohol use also is linked with youthful deaths by drowning, fire, suicide, and homicide.

- Youth who use alcohol are more likely to become sexually active at earlier ages, to have sexual intercourse more often, and to have unprotected sex than youth who do not drink.

- Young people who drink are more likely than others to be victims of violent crime, including rape, aggravated assault, and robbery.

- Youth who drink are more likely to have problems with school work and school conduct.

- An individual who begins drinking as a young teen is four times more likely to develop alcohol dependence than someone who waits until adulthood to use alcohol.

The message is clear: Alcohol use is very risky business for young people. And the longer children delay alcohol use, the less likely they are to develop any problems associated with it. That's why it is so important to help your child avoid any alcohol use.

A Young Person's World

Early adolescence is a time of enormous and often confusing changes for your child, which makes it a challenging time for both your youngster and you. Being tuned in to what it's like to be a youth can help you stay closer to your child and have more influence on the choices he or she makes including decisions about using alcohol.

Thinking skills. Most youth are still very "now" oriented and are just beginning to understand that their actions such as drinking have consequences. They also tend to believe that bad things won't happen to them, which helps to explain why they often take risks. Therefore, it is very important for adults to invest time in helping kids understand how and why alcohol-related risks do apply to them.

Social and emotional changes. As children approach adolescence, friends and "fitting in" become extremely important. Youth increasingly look to friends and the media for clues on how to behave and begin to question adults' values and rules. Given these normal developments, it is perhaps not surprising that parents often experience conflict with their kids as they go through early adolescence. During this sometimes stormy time, perhaps your toughest challenge is to try to respect your child's growing drive for independence while still providing support and appropriate limits.

The Bottom Line: A Strong Parent-Child Relationship

You may wonder why a guide to preventing youth alcohol use is putting so much emphasis on parents' need to understand and support their children. But the fact is, the best way to influence your child to avoid drinking is to have a strong, trusting relationship with him or her. Research shows that youth are much more likely to delay drinking when they feel they have a close, supportive tie with a parent or guardian. Moreover, if your son or daughter eventually does begin to drink, a good relationship with you will help protect him or her from developing alcohol-related problems.

The opposite is also true: When the relationship between a parent and youth is full of conflict or is very distant, the youth is more likely to use alcohol and to develop drinking-related problems. This connection between the parent-child relationship and a child's drinking habits makes a lot of sense when you think about it. First, when children have a strong bond with a parent, they are apt to feel good about themselves and therefore be less likely to cave in to peer pressure to use alcohol. Second, a good relationship with you is likely to influence your children to try to live up to your expectations, because they want to maintain their close tie with you. Here are some ways to build a strong, supportive bond with your child:

- Establish open communication. Make it easy for your youth to talk honestly with you.

- Show you care. Even though youth may not always show it, they still need to know they are important to their parents. Make it a point to regularly spend one-on-one time with your child—time when you can give him or her your loving, undivided attention. Some activities to share: a walk, a bike ride, a quiet dinner out, or a cookie-baking session.

- Draw the line. Set clear, realistic expectations for your child's behavior. Establish appropriate consequences for breaking rules and consistently enforce them.

- Offer acceptance. Make sure your youth knows that you appreciate his or her efforts as well as accomplishments. Avoid hurtful teasing or criticism.

- Understand that your child is growing up. This doesn't mean a hands-off attitude. But as you guide your child's behavior, also make an effort to respect his or her growing need for independence and privacy.

Tips for Communicating with Your Youth

Developing open, trusting communication between you and your child is essential to helping your child avoid alcohol use. If your child feels comfortable talking openly with you, you'll have a greater chance of guiding him or her toward healthy decision making. Some ways to begin:

Encourage conversation. Encourage your child to talk about whatever interests him or her. Listen without interruption and give your child a chance to teach you something new. Your active listening to your child's enthusiasms paves the way for conversations about topics that concern you.

Ask open-ended questions. Encourage your youth to tell you how he or she thinks and feels about the issue you're discussing. Avoid questions that have a simple "yes" or "no" answer.

Control your emotions. If you hear something you don't like, try not to respond with anger. Instead, take a few deep breaths and acknowledge your feelings in a constructive way.

Make every conversation a "win-win" experience. Don't lecture or try to "score points" on your youth by showing how he or she is wrong. If you show respect for your child's viewpoint, he or she will be more likely to listen to and respect yours.

Talking to Your Teen about Alcohol

For many parents, bringing up the subject of alcohol is no easy matter. Your young teen may try to dodge the discussion, and you yourself may feel unsure about how to proceed. To boost your chances for a productive conversation, take some time to think through the issues you want to discuss before you talk with your child. Also, think about how your child might react and ways you might respond to your youngster's questions and feelings. Then choose a time to talk when both you and your child have some "down time" and are feeling relaxed.

Keep in mind, too, that you don't need to cover everything at once. In fact, you're likely to have a greater impact on your child's drinking by having a number of talks about alcohol use throughout his or her adolescence. Think of this discussion with your child as the first part of an ongoing conversation.

And remember, do make it a conversation, not a lecture! Following are some topics for discussion:

Your child's views about alcohol. Ask your young teen what he or she knows about alcohol and what he or she thinks about youth drinking. Ask your child why he or she thinks kids drink. Listen carefully without interrupting. Not only will this approach help your child to feel heard and respected, but it can serve as a natural "lead-in" to discussing alcohol topics.

Important facts about alcohol. Although many kids believe they already know everything about alcohol, myths and misinformation abound. Here are some important facts to share:

- Alcohol is a powerful drug that slows down the body and mind. It impairs coordination; slows reaction time; and impairs vision, clear thinking, and judgment.

- Beer and wine are not "safer" than hard liquor. A 12-ounce can of beer, a 5-ounce glass of wine, and 1 ounce of hard liquor all contain the same amount of alcohol and have the same effects on the body and mind.

- On average, it takes 2 to 3 hours for a single drink to leave the body's system. Nothing can speed up this process, including drinking coffee, taking a cold shower, or "walking it off."

- People tend to be very bad at judging how seriously alcohol has affected them. That means many individuals who drive after drinking think they can control a car but actually cannot.

- Anyone can develop a serious alcohol problem, including a youth.

The magic potion myth. The media's glamorous portrayal of alcohol encourages many youth to believe that drinking will make them popular, attractive, happy, and "cool." Research shows that youth who expect such positive effects are more likely to drink at early ages. However, you can help to combat these dangerous myths by watching TV shows and movie videos with your child and discussing how alcohol is portrayed in them. For example, television advertisements for beer often show young people having an uproariously good time, as though drinking always puts people in a terrific mood. Watching such a commercial with your child can be an opportunity to discuss the many ways that alcohol can affect people—in some cases bringing on feelings of sadness or anger rather than carefree high spirits.

Good reasons not to drink. In talking with your child about reasons to avoid alcohol, stay away from scare tactics. Most youth are aware that many people drink without problems, so it is important to discuss the consequences of alcohol use without overstating the case. For example, you can talk about the dangers of riding in a car with a driver who has been drinking without insisting that "all kids who ride with drinkers get into accidents." Some good reasons that youth shouldn't drink:

- You want your child to avoid alcohol. Be sure to clearly state your own expectations regarding your child's drinking and to establish consequences for breaking rules. Your values and attitudes count with your child, even though he or she may not always show it.

- To maintain self-respect. In a series of focus groups, youth reported that the best way to persuade them to avoid alcohol is to appeal to their self-respect—letting them know that they are too smart and have too much going for them to need the crutch of alcohol.

- Drinking is illegal. Because alcohol use under the age of 21 is illegal, getting caught may mean trouble with the authorities. Even if getting caught doesn't lead to police action, the parents of your child's friends may no longer permit them to associate with your child. If drinking occurs on school grounds, your child could be suspended.

- Drinking can be dangerous. One of the leading causes of teen injuries and death is drunk driving. Alcohol is also a major factor in other types of fatal accidents among youth, such as drownings, burns, falls, and alcohol poisoning from drinking too much, too fast. Drinking also makes a young person more vulnerable to sexual assault and unprotected sex. And while your youth may believe he or she wouldn't engage in hazardous activities after drinking, point out that because alcohol impairs judgment, a drinker is very likely to think such activities won't be dangerous.

- You have a family history of alcoholism. If one or more members of your immediate or extended family has suffered from alcoholism, your child may be somewhat more vulnerable to developing a drinking problem. Your child needs to know that for him or her, drinking may carry special risks.

How to handle peer pressure. It's not enough to tell your youth that he or she should avoid alcohol you also need to help your child figure out how. What can your daughter say when she goes to a party and a friend offers her a beer? Or what should your son do if he finds himself in a home where kids are passing around a bottle of wine and parents are nowhere in sight? What should their response be if they are offered a ride home with an older friend who has been drinking? Brainstorm with your youth for ways that he or she might handle these and other difficult situations, and make clear how you are willing to support your child. An example: "If you find yourself at a home where kids are drinking, call me and I'll pick you up and there will be no scolding or punishment." The more prepared your child is, the better able he or she will be to handle high-pressure situations that involve drinking.

Mom, Dad, did you drink when you were a kid? This is the question many parents dread yet it is highly likely to come up in any family discussion of alcohol. The reality is that many parents did drink before they were old enough to legally do so. So how can one be honest with a child without sounding like a hypocrite who advises, "Do as I say, not as I did"?

This is a judgment call. If you believe that your drinking or drug use history should not be part of the discussion, you can simply tell your child that you choose not to share it. Another approach is to admit that you did do some drinking as a teenager, but that it was a mistake and give your youth an example of an embarrassing or painful moment that occurred because of your drinking. This approach may help your child better understand that youthful alcohol use does have negative consequences.

How to Host a Teen Party

- Agree on a guest list and don't admit party crashers.

- Discuss ground rules with your child before the party.

- Encourage your youth to plan the party with a responsible friend so that he or she will have support if problems arise.

- Brainstorm fun activities for the party.

- If a guest brings alcohol into your house, ask him or her to leave.

- Serve plenty of snacks and non-alcoholic drinks.

- Be visible and available but don't join the party!

Six Ways to Say No to a Drink

At some point, your child will be offered alcohol. To resist such pressure, youth say they prefer quick "one-liners" that allow them to dodge a drink without making a big scene. It will probably work best for your youth to take the lead in thinking up comebacks to drink offers so that he or she will feel comfortable saying them. But to get the brainstorming started, here are some simple pressure-busters from the mildest to the most assertive.

- No thanks.
- I don't feel like it—do you have any soda?
- Alcohol's NOT my thing.
- Are you talking to me? FORGET it.
- Why do you KEEP pressuring me when I've said NO?
- Back off!

Taking Action! Prevention Strategies for Parents

While parent-child conversations about drinking are essential, talking isn't enough—you also need to take concrete action to help your child resist alcohol. Research strongly shows that active, supportive involvement by parents and guardians can help youth avoid underage drinking and prevent later alcohol misuse.

In a survey of sixth graders, over half said it would be easy for a kid their age to get alcohol at a party. And in a recent national survey, 75 percent of eighth graders said alcohol was "fairly easy" or "very easy" to get. The message is clear: Youth still need plenty of adult supervision. Some ways to provide it:

Monitor alcohol use in your home. If you keep alcohol in your home, keep track of the supply. Make clear to your child that you don't allow unchaperoned parties or other youth gatherings in your home. If possible, however, encourage him or her to invite friends over when you are at home. The more entertaining your child does in your home, the more you will know about your child's friends and activities.

Connect with other parents. Getting to know other parents and guardians can help you keep closer tabs on your child. Friendly relations can make it easier for you to call the parent of a youth who is having a party to be sure that a responsible adult will be present and that alcohol will not be available. You're likely to find out that you're not the only adult who wants to prevent youthful alcohol use—many other parents share your concern.

Keep track of your child's activities. Be aware of your youth's plans and whereabouts. Generally, your child will be more open to your supervision if he or she feels you are keeping tabs because you care, not because you distrust him or her.

Develop family rules about youth drinking. When parents establish clear "no alcohol" rules and expectations, their children are less likely to begin drinking. While each family should develop agreements about youth alcohol use that reflect their own beliefs and values, some possible family rules about drinking are:

- Kids will not drink alcohol until they are 21.

- Older siblings will not encourage younger brothers or sisters to drink and will not give them alcohol.

- Kids will not stay at youth parties where alcohol is served.

- Kids will not ride in a car with a driver who has been drinking.

Once you have chosen rules for your family, you will need to establish appropriate consequences for breaking those rules. Be sure to choose a penalty that you are willing to carry out. Also, don't make the consequences so harsh that they become a barrier to open communication between you and your youth. The idea is to make the penalty "sting" just enough to make your child think twice about breaking the rule. A possible consequence might be temporary restrictions on your child's socializing.

Finally, you must be prepared to consistently enforce the consequences you have established. If your children know that they will lose certain privileges each and every time an alcohol use rule is broken, they will be more likely to keep their agreements.

Set a good example. Parents and guardians are important role models for their children—even children who are fast becoming teenagers. Studies indicate that if a parent uses alcohol, his or her children are more likely to drink themselves. But even if you use alcohol, there may be ways to lessen the likelihood that your child will drink. Some suggestions:

401

- Use alcohol moderately.

- Don't communicate to your child that alcohol is a good way to handle problems. For example, don't come home from work and say, "I had a rotten day. I need a drink."

- Instead, let your child see that you have other, healthier ways to cope with stress, such as exercise; listening to music; or talking things over with your spouse, partner, or friend.

- Don't tell your kids stories about your own drinking in a way that conveys the message that alcohol use is funny or glamorous.

- Never drink and drive or ride in a car with a driver who has been drinking.

- When you entertain other adults, make available alcohol-free beverages and plenty of food. If anyone drinks too much at your party, make arrangements for them to get home safely.

Don't support youth drinking. Your attitudes and behavior toward youth drinking also influence your child. Avoid making jokes about underage drinking or drunkenness, or otherwise showing acceptance of youth alcohol use. In addition, never serve alcohol to your child's underage friends. Research shows that kids whose parents or friends' parents provide alcohol for youth get-togethers are more likely to engage in heavier drinking, to drink more often, and to get into traffic accidents. Remember, too, that it is illegal in most states to provide alcohol to minors who are not family members. You can also join school and community efforts to discourage alcohol use by youth. By working with school officials and other members of your community, you can help to develop policies to reduce alcohol availability to youth and to enforce consequences for underage drinking.

Help your child build healthy friendships. If your child's friends use alcohol, your child is more likely to drink too. So it makes sense to try to encourage your youth to develop friendships with kids who do not drink and who are otherwise healthy influences on your child. A good first step is to simply get to know your child's friends better. You can then invite the kids you feel good about to family get-togethers and outings and find other ways to encourage your child to spend time with those youth. Also, talk directly with your youngster about the qualities in a friend that really count, such as trustworthiness and kindness, rather than popularity or a "cool" style. When you disapprove of one of your child's friends, the situation can be tougher to handle. While it may be tempting to simply forbid your child to see that friend, such a move may make your child even more determined to hang out with him or her. Instead, you might try pointing out your reservations about the friend in a caring, supportive way. You can also limit your child's time with that friend through your family rules, such as how after-school time can be spent or how late your child can stay out in the evening.

Encourage healthy alternatives to alcohol. One reason kids drink is to beat boredom. Therefore, it makes sense to encourage your child to participate in supervised after-school and weekend activities that are challenging and fun. According to a recent survey of youth, the availability of enjoyable, alcohol-free activities is a big reason for deciding not to use alcohol.

If your community doesn't offer many supervised activities, consider getting together with other parents and youth to help create some. Start by asking your child and other kids what they want to do, since they will be most likely to participate in activities that truly interest them. Find out whether your church, school, or community organization can help you sponsor a project.

Could My Child Develop a Drinking Problem?

While this text is mainly concerned with preventing youth alcohol use, we also need to pay attention to the possibility of youthful alcohol abuse. Certain children are more likely than others to drink heavily and encounter alcohol-related difficulties, including health, school, legal, family, and emotional problems. Kids at highest risk for alcohol-related problems are those who:

- Begin using alcohol or other drugs before the age of 15.

- Have a parent who is a problem drinker or an alcoholic.

- Have close friends who use alcohol and/ or other drugs.

- Have been aggressive, antisocial, or hard to control from an early age.

- Have experienced childhood abuse and/ or other major traumas.

- Have current behavioral problems and/ or are failing at school.

- Have parents who do not support them, do not communicate openly with them, and do not keep track of their behavior or whereabouts.

- Experience ongoing hostility or rejection from parents and/or harsh, inconsistent discipline.

The more of these experiences a child has had, the greater the chances that he or she will develop problems with alcohol. Having one or more risk factors does not mean that your child definitely will develop a drinking problem. It does suggest, however, that you may need to act now to help protect your youngster from later problems. For example, if you have not been openly communicating with your child, it will be important to develop new ways of talking and listening to each other. Or, if your child has serious behavioral difficulties, you may want to seek help from your child's school counselor, physician, and/or a mental health professional. Some parents may suspect that their child already has a drinking problem. While it can be hard to know for sure, certain behaviors can alert you to the possibility of an alcohol problem. If you think your child may be in trouble with drinking, consider getting advice from a health care professional specializing in alcohol problems before talking with your youth. To find a professional, contact your family doctor or a local hospital. Other sources of information and guidance may be found in your local Yellow Pages under "Alcoholism" or through one of the resources listed at the end of this book.

Warning Signs of a Drinking Problem

While the following behaviors may indicate an alcohol or other drug problem, some also reflect normal teenage growing pains. Experts believe that a drinking problem is more likely if you notice several of these signs at the same time, if they occur suddenly, and if some of them are extreme in nature.

- Mood changes: flare-ups of temper, irritability, and defensiveness.

- School problems: poor attendance, low grades, and/or recent disciplinary action.

- Rebelling against family rules.

- Switching friends, along with a reluctance to have you get to know the new friends.

- A "nothing matters" attitude: sloppy appearance, a lack of involvement in former interests, and general low energy.

- Finding alcohol in your child's room or backpack, or smelling alcohol on his or her breath.

- Physical or mental problems: memory lapses, poor concentration, bloodshot eyes, lack of coordination, or slurred speech.

Action Checklist

- Establish a loving, trusting relationship with your child.

- Make it easy for your youth to talk honestly with you.

- Talk with your child about alcohol facts, reasons not to drink, and ways to avoid drinking in difficult situations.

- Keep tabs on your young teen's activities, and join with other parents in making common policies about youth alcohol use.

- Develop family rules about youth drinking and establish consequences.

- Set a good example regarding your own alcohol use and your response to youth drinking.

- Encourage your child to develop healthy friendships and fun alternatives to drinking.

- Know whether your child is at high risk for a drinking problem; if so, take steps to lessen that risk.

- Know the warning signs of a youth drinking problem and act promptly to get help for your child.

- Believe in your own power to help your child avoid alcohol use.

Chapter 43

Tobacco

Chapter Contents

Section 43.1

Health Effects of Smoking among Young People

Centers for Disease Control and Prevention (CDC), National Center for Chronic Disease Prevention and Health Promotion, Office on Smoking and Health, http://www.cdc.gov/tobacco/research_data/youth/stspta5.htm, August 1996, last reviewed November 02, 2000.

Among young people, the short-term health consequences of smoking include respiratory and nonrespiratory effects, addiction to nicotine, and the associated risk of other drug use. Long-term health consequences of youth smoking are reinforced by the fact that most young people who smoke regularly continue to smoke throughout adulthood.

- Cigarette smokers have a lower level of lung function than those persons who have never smoked.

- Smoking reduces the rate of lung growth.

- In adults, cigarette smoking causes heart disease and stroke. Studies have shown that early signs of these diseases can be found in adolescents who smoke.

- Smoking hurts young people's physical fitness in terms of both performance and endurance—even among young people trained in competitive running.

- On average, someone who smokes a pack or more of cigarettes each day lives 7 years less than someone who never smoked.

- The resting heart rates of young adult smokers are two to three beats per minute faster than nonsmokers.

- Smoking at an early age increases the risk of lung cancer. For most smoking-related cancers, the risk rises as the individual continues to smoke.

- Teenage smokers suffer from shortness of breath almost three times as often as teens who don't smoke, and produce phlegm more than twice as often as teens who don't smoke.

- Teenage smokers are more likely to have seen a doctor or other health professionals for an emotional or psychological complaint.

- Teens who smoke are three times more likely than nonsmokers to use alcohol, eight times more likely to use marijuana, and 22 times more likely to use cocaine. Smoking is associated with a host of other risky behaviors, such as fighting and engaging in unprotected sex.

Section 43.2

What to Do If Your Kid Smokes or Chews Tobacco

This section contains text from Russell G. Robertson, MD, "Smoking Teens: Some Good News and Some Bad," http://healthlink.mcw.edu/article/ 972578004.html, October 2000, and "What You Can Do to Prevent Teen Smoking," http://healthlink.mcw.edu/article/916868831.html, January 1999, copyright 2000, Medical College of Wisconsin. Reprinted with permission.

Smoking Teens: Some Good News and Some Bad

First the good news. A recent study by the Centers for Disease Prevention and Control (CDC) has for the first time documented a slight decrease in smoking among high-schoolers questioned in 1999. The decline was attributed to teen smoking prevention programs and the higher cost of cigarettes. The CDC said that 34.8% of high school students reported that they had smoked a cigarette in the past 30 days—down from 36.4 % in 1997 and the first overall decline since the government's first study in 1991. Smoking dropped 17% in freshman, which was seen as a particularly good sign.

Despite the positive tone of this new information, the number of high school seniors smoking rose from 39.6% to 42.8%. And the number of frequent smokers, defined as those having smoked at least 20 of the past 30 days, rose to 16.8%—about one third higher than it was in 1991. The government's goals are to cut teen smoking in half—to 16% by 2010. Surgeon General David Satcher said the study offers hope that the figures have peaked, but notes that only 5% of American schools have adopted the CDC's guidelines for discouraging smoking.

The bad news is that a study of 12 and 13 years olds found that after only a few cigarettes, tobacco addition occurred. This was surprising result as the authors of the study expected to find that prolonged exposure to smoking would lead to addiction. The study also demonstrates the vulnerability of adolescents to tobacco's grip and the easy availability of cigarettes. It also supports previous findings that show that nicotine is more addictive than heroin.

What this means to parents is twofold. First, it is every parent's obligation to mimimize their children's exposure to tobacco. This last study puts the kibosh on the idea that it is normal for kids to "experiment" with smoking. Tragically, such "experimentation" can lead to lifelong addiction.

Remember that teens are no more successful at smoking cessation than are adults. There is also evidence that teens who smoke are more likely to use alcohol and participate in premarital sex. This means that tobacco use may not be an isolated phenomenon.

Second, parents must adopt a zero-tolerance policy if they discover their teens smoking. This policy also must begin with mom and dad. If either of you is a smoker, your credibility is zero if you expect to be able to stop your kids from doing so. Do everything you can to stop smoking because of what it means to your children, if not for yourself.

Confront your son or daughter regularly if you know they are smoking. Comments like, "I know you are smoking and I am so sad at that choice you are making," or "I love you so much and it hurts me to know what you are doing to your body by doing this" are loving but direct statements that let them know you are not going to ignore the behavior. Offer to pay for smoking cessation classes, nicotine patches or Zyban. Don't be a nag, but don't let up.

Look carefully at their peer group. If the habit stems from friends, try to steer your kids towards activities and friends who are less likely to smoke. Be alert to the fact that some young women use tobacco as an appetite suppressant.

This is a winnable battle but not for the faint of heart. Prevention is the best strategy and requires relentless dedication due to the ubiquity of tobacco use in our society. The most solid foundation is set by the behavior of responsible adults. Actively discourage experimentation and definitely don't normalize it. Be lovingly relentless if you learn that your kids have started to smoke. If they know you love them, you'll have more impact than they may lead you to believe.

What You Can Do to Prevent Teen Smoking

The sheer numbers of our children who have taken up the habit of tobacco is beyond belief.

How can it be that with the known dangerous effects of smoking so clearly defined, record numbers of young people are choosing this addiction?

Popular targets for culpability include the tobacco industry and its alleged manipulation of nicotine content, print advertising, and lack of government regulation. Although the aforementioned play a role in decision making, in reality children smoke for two reasons.

The first reason children smoke is because the people they admire smoke. In many American homes, they are simply modeling themselves after one or both parents, grandparents, or other key people in the household.

One also need look no farther than Hollywood, where there has been a significant increase in instances of onscreen smoking that is also amplified by the current cigar craze. Adolescents, by definition, grasp at the trappings of adulthood and as smoking is an adult activity that is forbidden, its allure is further intensified.

The second reason ties in teen cravings for affirmation and acceptance. They will associate with the individuals or group that is the most powerfully affirming and accepting. They will adopt the standards and behaviors of that group, no matter how dangerous or unhealthy, as failure to do so could mean rejection, expulsion, ridicule, or worst of all, loneliness.

Adolescents have an acute need for expressed, felt love. Paradoxically they appear to be uncomfortable responding to that love, highlighting a mistake that many parents make as they begin an apparent retreat from their children once they reach adolescence.

The reasons having been delineated, a preventive response is mandatory. This is essential because the addictive nature of tobacco use, once begun, is so profound. Surveys of teens have clearly indicated that they experimented with cigarettes because they assume they could easily stop at some time in the future, yet sadly they are no more successful in quitting than most adults.

Beyond prevention of smoking's dangers we also know that tobacco is clearly a gateway drug to other drugs and unhealthy activities. Kids who smoke cigarettes are more likely to use marijuana and other drugs as well as engage in sexual intercourse.

There are two steps that you can take as the parent of an adolescent to prevent your son or daughter from becoming a smoker. The ideal time to begin these interventions is when your children are between the ages of 8 and 10, although it is never too late to start.

No. 1, if you are a smoker, QUIT. I cannot imagine a more powerful message than sitting down with your son or daughter and telling them that you realize what an unhealthy and dangerous habit your smoking has become and that your love for them is so deep that you are willing to take whatever steps necessary to stop. You already know that they are worried about you and the unhealthy effects of your smoking. Besides setting a good example for your kids, you will also relieve them of some of the concerns they already have for you and your health.

The second step requires more effort and consideration. If parental support and love for one's children is perceived to be more important than that of friends, they will seek parental favor over that of their peers. In effect you can by the power of parental love, transcend the negative influences of their peer groups.

This can only be successful if you are prepared to make large investments of time and to set a higher priority for the emotional needs of your children than for yourself. Following a few of these suggestions is a start:

- Have one meal each day together as a family.

- Set aside one night per week for family-only activities.

- Adjust your play with your children as they age.

- Be there, wherever "there" is—at a school play, a sporting event, a musical performance, etc.

- If you are married, honor your commitment to your spouse. If you are a single parent or noncustodial parent, work out a plan that allows for regular and loving participation in the life of your child.

- Resist the temptation to reduce your involvement in your child's life during adolescence.

412

- Do not leave teens in groups in unsupervised settings. As a parent, call ahead to see if there is anything you can do to help with a gathering and ask if there will be an adult present.

Be encouraged that adolescence means that you're almost finished with the active role of being a parent. Taking an involved role at this time will not only keep your child from the clutches of tobacco, but set the stage for a wonderful transition to adulthood and lifelong friendship with your children.

—by Russell G. Robertson, MD

Dr. Robertson is Associate Professor of Family and Community Medicine at the Medical College of Wisconsin. His biweekly column of medical advice, "The Doctor Is In," appears in the CNI Community Newspapers throughout metropolitan Milwaukee.

Chapter 44

Marijuana

What Is Marijuana? Are There Different Kinds?

Marijuana is a green, brown, or gray mixture of dried, shredded leaves, stems, seeds, and flowers of the hemp plant (*Cannabis sativa*). Before the 1960s, many Americans had never heard of marijuana, but today it is the most often used illegal drug in this country.

Cannabis is a term that refers to marijuana and other drugs made from the same plant. Strong forms of cannabis include sinsemilla (sin-seh-me-yah), hashish ("hash" for short), and hash oil.

All forms of cannabis are mind-altering (psychoactive) drugs; they all contain THC (delta-9-tetrahydrocannabinol), the main active chemical in marijuana. They also contain more than 400 other chemicals.

Marijuana's effect on the user depends on the strength or potency of the THC it contains. THC potency has increased since the 1970s but has been about the same since the mid-1980s. The strength of the drug is measured by the average amount of THC in test samples confiscated by law enforcement agencies.

What Are the Current Slang Terms for Marijuana?

There are many different names for marijuana. Slang terms for

Excerpted from "Marijuana: Facts Parents Need to Know," National Institute on Drug Abuse (NIDA), National Institutes of Health (NIH), http://www.nida.nih.gov/MarijBroch/MarijParentstxt.html, revised November, 1998, page last updated April 20, 2000.

drugs change quickly, and they vary from one part of the country to another. They may even differ across sections of a large city.

Terms from years ago, such as pot, herb, grass, weed, Mary Jane, and reefer, are still used. You might also hear the names Aunt Mary, skunk, boom, gangster, kif, or ganja.

There are also street names for different strains or "brands" of marijuana, such as "Texas tea," "Maui wowie," and "Chronic." A recent book of American slang lists more than 200 terms for various kinds of marijuana.

How Is Marijuana Used?

Most users roll loose marijuana into a cigarette (called a joint or a nail) or smoke it in a pipe. One well-known type of water pipe is the bong. Some users mix marijuana into foods or use it to brew a tea. Another method is to slice open a cigar and replace the tobacco with marijuana, making what's called a blunt. When the blunt is smoked with a 40 ounce bottle of malt liquor, it is called a "B-40."

Lately, marijuana cigarettes or blunts often include crack cocaine, a combination known by various street names, such as "primos" or "woolies." Joints and blunts often are dipped in PCP and are called "happy sticks," "wicky sticks," "love boat," or "tical."

How Many People Smoke Marijuana?
At What Age Do Children Generally Start?

A recent government survey tells us:

- Marijuana is the most frequently used illegal drug in the United States. Nearly 69 million Americans over the age of 12 have tried marijuana at least once.

- About 10 million had used the drug in the month before the survey.

- Among teens 12 to 17, the average age of first trying marijuana was 14 years.

A yearly survey of students in grades 8 through 12 shows that 23 percent of 8th-graders have tried marijuana at least once, and by 10th grade, 21 percent are "current" users (that is, used within the past month). Among 12th-graders, nearly 50 percent have tried marijuana/hash at least once, and about 24 percent were current users.

Other researchers have found that use of marijuana and other drugs usually peaks in the late teens and early twenties, then declines in later years.

How Can I Tell If My Child Has Been Using Marijuana?

There are some signs you might be able to see. If someone is high on marijuana, he or she might

- seem dizzy and have trouble walking

- seem silly and giggly for no reason

- have very red, bloodshot eyes

- have a hard time remembering things that just happened

When the early effects fade, over a few hours, the user can become very sleepy.

Parents should be aware of changes in their child's behavior, although this may be difficult with teenagers. Parents should look for withdrawal, depression, fatigue, carelessness with grooming, hostility, and deteriorating relationships with family members and friends. In addition, changes in academic performance, increased absenteeism or truancy, lost interest in sports or other favorite activities, and changes in eating or sleeping habits could be related to drug use. However, these signs may also indicate problems other than use of drugs.

In addition, parents should be aware of:

- signs of drugs and drug paraphernalia, including pipes and rolling papers

- odor on clothes and in the bedroom

- use of incense and other deodorizers

- use of eye drops

- clothing, posters, jewelry, etc., promoting drug use

Why Do Young People Use Marijuana?

Children and young teens start using marijuana for many reasons. Curiosity and the desire to fit into a social group are common reasons. Certainly, youngsters who have already begun to smoke cigarettes and/or use alcohol are at high risk for marijuana use.

417

Also, our research suggests that the use of alcohol and drugs by other family members plays a strong role in whether children start using drugs. Parents, grandparents, and older brothers and sisters in the home are models for children to follow.

Some young people who take drugs do not get along with their parents. Some have a network of friends who use drugs and urge them to do the same (peer pressure). All aspects of a child's environment—home, school, neighborhood—help to determine whether the child will try drugs.

Children who become more heavily involved with marijuana can become dependent, and that is their prime reason for using the drug. Others mention psychological coping as a reason for their use—to deal with anxiety, anger, depression, boredom, and so forth. But marijuana use is not an effective method for coping with life's problems, and staying high can be a way of simply not dealing with the problems and challenges of growing up.

Researchers have found that children and teens (both male and female) who are physically and sexually abused are at greater risk than other young people of using marijuana and other drugs and of beginning drug use at an early age.

Does Using Marijuana Lead to Other Drugs?

Long-term studies of high school students and their patterns of drug use show that very few young people use other drugs without first trying marijuana. The risk of using cocaine has been estimated to be more than 104 times greater for those who have tried marijuana than for those who have never tried it. Although there are no definitive studies on the factors associated with the movement from marijuana use to use of other drugs, growing evidence shows that a combination of biological, social, and psychological factors are involved.

Marijuana affects the brain in some of the same ways that other drugs do. Researchers are examining the possibility that long-term marijuana use may create changes in the brain that make a person more at risk of becoming addicted to other drugs, such as alcohol or cocaine. While not all young people who use marijuana go on to use other drugs, further research is needed to determine who will be at greatest risk.

What Are the Effects of Marijuana?

The effects of marijuana on each person depend on the:

- type of cannabis and how much THC it contains
- way the drug is taken (by smoking or eating)
- experience and expectations of the user
- setting where the drug is used
- whether drinking or other drug use is also going on

Some people feel nothing at all when they first try marijuana. Others may feel high (intoxicated and/or euphoric).

It's common for marijuana users to become engrossed with ordinary sights, sounds, or tastes, and trivial events may seem extremely interesting or funny. Time seems to pass very slowly, so minutes feel like hours. Sometimes the drug causes users to feel thirsty and very hungry—an effect called "the munchies."

How Is Marijuana Harmful?

Marijuana can be harmful in a number of ways, through both immediate effects and damage to health over time.

Marijuana hinders the user's short-term memory (memory for recent events), and he or she may have trouble handling complex tasks. With the use of more potent varieties of marijuana, even simple tasks can be difficult.

Because of the drug's effects on perceptions and reaction time, users could be involved in auto crashes. Drug users also may become involved in risky sexual behavior. There is a strong link between drug use and unsafe sex and the spread of HIV (Human Immunodeficiency Virus), the virus that causes AIDS (Acquired Immunodeficiency Syndrome).

Under the influence of marijuana, students may find it hard to study and learn. Young athletes could find their performance is off; timing, movements, and coordination are all affected by THC.

What Are the Long-Term Effects of Marijuana?

While all of the long-term effects of marijuana use are not yet known, there are studies showing serious health concerns. For example, a group of scientists in California examined the health status of 450 daily smokers of marijuana but not tobacco. They found that the marijuana smokers had more sick days and more doctor visits for respiratory problems and other types of illness than did a similar group who did not smoke either substance.

Findings so far show that the regular use of marijuana or THC may play a role in cancer and problems in the respiratory, immune, and reproductive systems.

Cancer

It is hard to find out whether marijuana alone causes cancer because many people who smoke marijuana also smoke cigarettes and use other drugs. Marijuana smoke contains some of the same cancer-causing compounds as tobacco, sometimes in higher concentrations. Studies show that someone who smokes five joints per week may be taking in as many cancer-causing chemicals as someone who smokes a full pack of cigarettes every day.

Tobacco smoke and marijuana smoke may work together to change the tissues lining the respiratory tract. Marijuana smoking could contribute to early development of head and neck cancer in some people.

Immune System

Our immune system protects the body from many agents that cause disease. It is not certain whether marijuana damages the immune system of people. But both animal and human studies have shown that marijuana impairs the ability of T-cells in the lungs' immune defense system to fight off some infections. People with HIV and others whose immune system is impaired should avoid marijuana use.

Lungs and Airways

People who smoke marijuana often develop the same kinds of breathing problems that cigarette smokers have. They have symptoms of daily cough and phlegm (chronic bronchitis) and more frequent chest colds. They are also at greater risk of getting lung infections such as pneumonia. Continued marijuana smoking can lead to abnormal function of the lungs and airways. Scientists have found signs of lung tissue injured or destroyed by marijuana smoke.

Can a Person Become Addicted to Marijuana?

Yes. While not everyone who uses marijuana becomes addicted, when a user begins to seek out and take the drug compulsively, that person is said to be dependent on the drug or addicted to it. In 1995, 165,000 people entering drug treatment programs reported marijuana as their primary drug of abuse, showing they needed help to stop using.

Some heavy users of marijuana show signs of dependence because when they do not use the drug, they develop withdrawal symptoms. Some subjects in an experiment on marijuana withdrawal had symptoms, such as restlessness, loss of appetite, trouble with sleeping, weight loss, and shaky hands.

According to one study, marijuana use by teenagers who have prior serious antisocial problems can quickly lead to dependence on the drug. That study also found that, for troubled teenagers using tobacco, alcohol, and marijuana, progression from their first use of marijuana to regular use was about as rapid as their progression to regular tobacco use, and more rapid than the progression to regular use of alcohol.

What Is "Tolerance" for Marijuana?

"Tolerance" means that the user needs increasingly larger doses of the drug to get the same desired results that he or she previously got from smaller amounts. Some frequent, heavy users of marijuana may develop tolerance for it.

Are There Treatments to Help Marijuana Users?

Up until a few years ago, it was hard to find treatment programs specifically for marijuana users. Treatments for marijuana dependence were much the same as therapies for other drug abuse problems. These include detoxification, behavioral therapies, and regular attendance at meetings of support groups, such as Narcotics Anonymous.

Recently, researchers have been testing different ways to attract marijuana users to treatment and help them abstain from drug use. There are currently no medications for treating marijuana dependence. Treatment programs focus on counseling and group support systems. From these studies, drug treatment professionals are learning what characteristics of users are predictors of success in treatment and which approaches to treatment can be most helpful.

Further progress in treatment to help marijuana users includes a number of programs set up to help adolescents in particular. Some of these programs are in university research centers, where most of the young clients report marijuana as their drug of choice. Others are in independent adolescent treatment facilities. Family physicians are also a good source for information and help in dealing with adolescents' marijuana problems.

How Can I Prevent My Child from Getting Involved with Marijuana?

There is no magic bullet for preventing teenage drug use. But parents can be influential by talking to their children about the dangers of using marijuana and other drugs, and remain actively engaged in their children's lives. Even after teenage children enter high school, parents can stay involved in schoolwork, recreation, and social activities with their children's friends. Research shows that appropriate parental monitoring can reduce future drug use, even among those adolescents who may be prone to marijuana use, such as those who are rebellious, cannot control their emotions, and experience internal distress. To address the issue of drug abuse in your area, it is important to get involved in drug abuse prevention programs in your community or your child's school. Find out what prevention programs you and your children can participate in together.

Chapter 45

Inhalants

What Are Inhalants?

Inhalants are volatile substances that produce chemical vapors that can be inhaled to induce a psychoactive, or mind-altering, effect. Although other abused substances can be inhaled, the term "inhalants" is used to describe a variety of substances whose main common characteristic is that they are rarely, if ever, taken by any route other than inhalation. This definition encompasses a broad range of chemicals found in hundreds of different products that may have different pharmacological effects. As a result, precise categorization of inhalants is difficult. One classification system lists four general categories of inhalants—volatile solvents, aerosol, gases, and nitrites—based on the form in which they are often found in household, industrial, and medical products.

Volatile solvents are liquids that vaporize at room temperatures. They are found in a multitude of inexpensive, easily available products used for common household and industrial purposes. These include paint thinners and removers, dry-cleaning fluids, degreasers, gasoline, glues, correction fluids, and felt-tip marker fluids.

Aerosols are sprays that contain propellants and solvents. They include spray paints, deodorant and hair sprays, vegetable oil sprays for cooking, and fabric protector sprays.

"Inhalant Abuse," National Institute on Drug Abuse (NIDA), National Institutes of Health (NIH), http://www.nida.nih.gov/ResearchReports/Inhalants/Inhalants2.html, last updated January 24, 2001.

Gases include medical anesthetics as well as gases used in household or commercial products. Medical anesthetic gases include ether, chloroform, halothane, and nitrous oxide, commonly called "laughing gas." Nitrous oxide is the most abused of these gases and can be found in whipped cream dispensers and products that boost octane levels in racing cars. Household or commercial products containing gases include butane lighters, propane tanks, whipped cream dispensers, and refrigerants.

Nitrites often are considered a special class of inhalants. Unlike most other inhalants, which act directly on the central nervous system (CNS), nitrites act primarily to dilate blood vessels and relax the muscles. And while other inhalants are used to alter mood, nitrites are used primarily as sexual enhancers. Nitrites include cyclohexyl nitrite, isoamyl (amyl) nitrite, and isobutyl (butyl) nitrite. Cyclohexyl nitrite is found in room odorizers. Amyl nitrite is used in certain diagnostic procedures and is prescribed to some patients for heart pain. Illegally diverted ampules of amyl nitrite are called "poppers" or "snappers" on the street. Butyl nitrite is an illegal substance that is often packaged and sold in small bottles also referred to as "poppers."

What Are the Patterns of Inhalant Abuse?

Inhalants—particularly volatile solvents, gases, and aerosols—are often among the first drugs that young children use. One national survey indicates about 6 percent of US children have tried inhalants by the time they reach fourth grade. Inhalants also are one of the few substances abused more by younger children than by older ones. Nevertheless, inhalant abuse can become chronic and extend into adulthood.

Generally, inhalant abusers will abuse any available substance. However, effects produced by individual inhalants vary, and some individuals will go out of their way to obtain their favorite inhalant. For example, in certain parts of the country, "Texas shoe-shine," a shoe-shining spray containing the chemical toluene, is a local favorite. Silver and gold spray paints, which contain more toluene than other spray colors, also are popular inhalants.

Data from national and State surveys suggest inhalant abuse reaches its peak at some point during the seventh through ninth grades. For example, the American Drug and Alcohol Survey of children in the 4th through 12th grades indicates that the percentage of children who have ever used inhalants peaks in the 8th grade. In the

Monitoring the Future (MTF) study, an annual NIDA-supported survey of the Nation's secondary school students, 8th-graders also regularly report the highest rate of current, past year, and lifetime inhalant abuse; 10th- and 12th-graders report less abuse.

Gender differences in inhalant abuse have been identified at different points in childhood. One study indicates inhalant abuse is higher for boys than girls in grades 4 through 6, occurs at similar rates in grades 7 through 9—when overall use is highest—and becomes more prevalent again among boys in grades 10 through 12. The National Household Survey on Drug Abuse (NHSDA), an annual survey of drug use among the Nation's noninstitutionalized civilians, reports that similar percentages of 12- to 17-year-old boys and girls abused inhalants in 1998. However, the percentage of 18- to 25-year-old males who abused inhalants was more than twice that of females in that age group, suggesting that sustained abuse of inhalants is more common among males.

People who abuse inhalants are found in both urban and rural settings. Research on factors contributing to inhalant abuse suggests that adverse socioeconomic conditions, rather than racial or cultural factors per se, may account for most reported racial and ethnic differences in rates of inhalant abuse. Poverty, a history of childhood abuse, poor grades, and dropping out of school all are associated with inhalant abuse. Native American youths who live on reservations, where socioeconomic distress and school dropout rates are high, typically have higher rates of inhalant abuse than both the general population of young people and those Native American youths who do not live on reservations.

What Is the Scope of Inhalant Abuse?

Inhalant abuse among the Nation's 8th-, 10th-, and 12th-graders declined in 1999, continuing an apparent gradual decline that began in 1996, according to the latest MTF data. For example:

- The percentage of high school seniors who abused any inhalants declined to 5.6 percent in 1999 from a peak of 8 percent in 1995. Abuse of nitrites, specifically, also declined to less than 1 percent (0.9) among seniors in 1999.

- Abuse of all inhalants by 10th-graders declined to 7.2 percent in 1999, from 9.6 percent in 1995.

- Among eighth-graders, abuse declined to 10.3 percent in 1999 from 12.8 percent in 1995.

Despite the declines in abuse among schoolchildren in recent years, inhalants are still being abused at higher rates than they were a decade ago, according to the NHSDA. The 1998 survey indicates that the rate of first use among 12- to 17-year-olds rose significantly from 8.4 to 18.8 per 1,000 potential new users from 1989 to 1995 and remained at those levels through 1997. The rate of first use of inhalants for young adults aged 18 to 25 also rose, from 3.7 to 10.7 per 1,000 potential new users between 1989 and 1996, before leveling off in 1997.

MTF's lifetime prevalence figures also indicate that the percentages of students who have tried inhalants remain at high levels. In 1999, 19.7 percent of 8th-graders, 17.0 percent of 10th-graders, and 15.4 percent of 12th-graders said they had abused inhalants at least once in their lives. These data raise a question: How can fewer 12th-graders than 8th-graders consistently report they have ever abused inhalants? Possibly, many 12th-graders fail to recall their much earlier use of inhalants or, more troubling, many 8th-grade inhalant abusers may have dropped out of school by the 12th grade and are no longer included in the survey population. The latter explanation is supported by research that shows higher rates of inhalant abuse among children who have poor grades or have dropped out of school than among their classmates who remain in good standing in school.

Chapter 46

Stimulants

Unlike the narcotics and other depressants, stimulants increase activity in the central nervous system, speeding up metabolism and unleashing feelings of energy and confidence while curbing appetite and fatigue.

The stimulants group (commonly and collectively known as speed) is an extremely diverse chemical mixed bag, and one that young people have been sampling from in a big way in recent years. Just the legal side of the bag deserves special consideration: It includes a variety of readily available, over-the-counter products marketed to, and increasingly used by, young people:

- *Caffeine.* The old standby, caffeine is dispensed in liquid form by espresso machines and in even more concentrated form as stay-awake tablets (No-Doz, Vivarin) and "performance boosters" (UpTime) at the local mini-mart.

- *PPA.* The appetite suppressant and stimulant drug phenylpropanolamine (PPA) is the active ingredient in such over-the-counter diet aids as Accutrim and Dexatrim, commonly used by teen (and pre-teen) girls for weight control. [See updated information about PPA at the end of this chapter.]

Erica Wittenberg and Jim Parker, "Drug Proofing the Family: How to Raise 'I'm Okay' Kids in a 'No You're Not' World (Chapter 6)," http://doitnow.org/pages/204/204ch6s.html, April 1998, copyright 2000 by D.I.N Publications/Do It Now Foundation; reprinted with permission.

- *Ephedra.* A variety of commercial teas, nutritional supplements, and bodybuilding aids contain the Chinese herb ma huang (ephedra). In addition to curbing appetite and increasing fat metabolism, ephedra is a potent central nervous system (CNS) stimulant.

- *Herbal "Ecstasy."* Sold at head shops, concerts, and dance clubs, a number of herbal drug blends are promoted as substitutes for controlled substances, particularly the popular psychedelic stimulant MDMA.

On the other, controlled side of the stimulant equation are drugs commonly prescribed for kids with hyperactivity or attention-deficit disorder—including methylphenidate (Ritalin), Dexedrine, and Cylert —and such illicit drugs as methamphetamine ("crystal meth") and MDMA ("Ecstasy"). Rounding out the list is cocaine, which is still around, still expensive, and still causing serious problems.

Like alcohol and downers, stimulants are all much more alike than they are different, both in their effects and the risks they pose. That's why we'll discuss the various chemicals as a group—and to underscore the simple, often-ignored point that, in spite of significant differences in both cost and legal status, stimulants are stimulants. Speed is speed.

It's not that illegal ones are "bad" and legal ones are "good" or "safe"—they're not, at least not all the time. Speed is speed; and just like the other form we're all familiar with, it doesn't matter that much whether you're in a car or on a plane: the faster you go, the more likely you are to crash.

One reason that users tend to crash so often is because speed causes a rapid buildup of tolerance, which means that the drugs' effects fade after a few weeks, unless dosage is increased. For some reason, this doesn't generally apply to stimulants prescribed for attention-deficit disorder, but it does apply to the ones prescribed for weight control. And it especially applies to crystal meth, which causes such powerful feelings of euphoria that users want to increase dosage.

What they don't want, but get anyway, are other risks that go with the territory:

- *Emotional problems.* Heavy use can unleash profound psychological changes. In its most severe form, a toxic psychosis can emerge, characterized by hallucinations, paranoia, a feeling of bugs crawling on the skin, and bizarre behavior.

- *Physical hazards.* Since stimulants enable the body to go for long periods without food or sleep, a number of physical problems and nutritional deficiencies have been linked to use of the drugs.

- *Overdose.* High doses can trigger heart attack, respiratory collapse, seizures, stroke, and death.

Note about PPA

On November 6, 2000 the U.S. Food and Drug Administration (FDA) issued a Public Health Advisory concerning the safety of phenylpropanolamine (PPA). The following text is excerpted from the advisory. The full text can be found in the internet at www.fda.gov/cder/drug/infopage/ppa/advisory.htm:

The Food and Drug Administration (FDA) is issuing a public health advisory concerning phenylpropanolamine hydrochloride. This drug is widely used as a nasal decongestant (in over-the-counter and prescription drug products) and for weight control (in over-the-counter drug products). FDA is taking steps to remove phenylpropanolamine from all drug products and has requested that all drug companies discontinue marketing products containing phenylpropanolamine.

Phenylpropanolamine has been marketed for many years. A recent study reported that taking phenylpropanolamine increases the risk of hemorrhagic stroke (bleeding into the brain or into tissue surrounding the brain) in women. Men may also be at risk. Although the risk of hemorrhagic stroke is very low, FDA recommends that consumers not use any products that contain phenylpropanolamine.

Chapter 47

Steroids and Sports Are a Losing Combination

Ben Johnson, the Canadian sprinter, expected the 1988 Summer Olympics in Seoul, South Korea, to be the zenith of his track and field career. He would compete against his arch-rival, American sprinter Carl Lewis, in the event that was his specialty: the 100-meter dash. When the starting pistol sounded, Johnson was off like a man possessed. He crossed the finish line victorious and became the toast of the athletic world, as well as a hero to his fellow Canadians. The next morning, however, events took a 180-degree turn. Johnson became the shame of his country and his cherished gold medal was stripped. Tests revealed that he used steroids.

A 23-year old bodybuilder, complaining of severe groin pains, was taken to the hospital. Doctors found his liver and kidneys had stopped working. He immediately rushed to the intensive-care unit. Four days later he died when his heart stopped. His autopsy revealed that he was a steroid abuser.

While preparing for his prom night, a high school senior drank a "health formula," which he had been taking for some time to increase muscle and reduce fat. His evening of romance was never to be. Twenty minutes after drinking the formula, which contained GHB (an illegal drug promoted as an anabolic steroid alternative), he lapsed into a coma. His parents found him sprawled on the floor and rushed

Raja Mishra, *FDA Consumer*, September 1991, http://www.fda.gov/bbs/topics/CONSUMER/CON00107.html, updated in January, 2001 by Dr. David A. Cooke, MD, Diplomate, American Board of Internal Medicine.

him to the hospital. Doctors said if he had been found half an hour later, he probably would have died.

These three cases, though different, all involve the illegal use of anabolic steroids or similar "performance-enhancing" drugs.

What Exactly Are These Drugs That Have Damaged So Many Lives?

Steroids are a synthetic version of the human hormone called testosterone. Testosterone stimulates and maintains the male sexual organs. It also stimulates development of bones and muscle, promotes skin and hair growth, and can influence emotions. In males, testosterone is produced by the testes and the adrenal gland. Women have only the amount of testosterone produced by the adrenal gland—much less than men have. This is why testosterone is often called a "male" hormone.

The average adult male naturally produces 2.5 to 11 milligrams of testosterone daily. The average steroid abuser often takes more than 100 mg a day, through "stacking" or combining several different brands of steroids. Researchers first developed steroids in the 1930s to rebuild and prevent the breakdown of body tissues from disease.

The controversy surrounding steroids began in the 1950s during the Olympic Games when the athletic community discovered that athletes from Russia and some East European nations, which had dominated the games, had taken large doses of steroids. Many of the male athletes developed such large prostate glands (a gland located near the bladder and urethra that aids in semen production) that they needed a tube inserted in order to urinate. Some of the female athletes developed so many male characteristics, chromosome tests were necessary to prove that they were still women.

Even though the side effects of steroid abuse had become known, the demand for them increased in the athletic community. Since then, the sale of steroids has ballooned into a $100-million-a-year black market.

Dangers Abound

Steroids fool the body into thinking that testosterone is being produced. The body, sensing an excess of testosterone, shuts down bodily functions involving testosterone, such as bone growth. The ends of long bones fuse together and stop growing, resulting in stunted growth. Steroid abuse has many dangerous side effects.

Adding to the danger is the way some steroids are manufactured and distributed. The drugs are often made in motel rooms and warehouses in Mexico, Europe, and other countries and then smuggled into the United States. The potency, purity and strength of the steroids produced this way are not regulated and therefore it is almost impossible for users to know how much they are taking. Counterfeit steroids are also sold as the real thing. So it's often impossible to tell exactly what some products contain. Contamination of steroids with other substances have caused illnesses in some users.

In addition to the myriad physical side effects seen with anabolic steroid use, concerning psychological changes have also been seen. Psychological addiction has been widely reported, with users developing an emotional need to continue taking the drugs. Additionally, violent mood changes, uncontrollable rage, and impaired judgement have occurred in many steroid users.

New Trends

A new, alarming trend, is the use of other drugs to achieve the "performance-enhancing" effects of steroids. These steroid "alternatives" are sought in order to avoid the stiff penalties now in effect against those who possess anabolic steroids without a valid prescription. The two most common are gamma hydroxybutyrate (GHB) and clenbuterol.

GHB is a deadly, illegal drug that is a primary ingredient in many of these "performance-enhancing" formulas. The GHB that caused the prom night tragedy was marketed under the name "Somatomax PM." Rumors among teens that it caused a "high" increased the public health problems with GHB. In fact, the drug does not produce a high. It does, however, cause headaches, nausea, vomiting, diarrhea, seizures, and other central nervous system disorders, and, possibly, death. GHB has been implicated in a number of deaths of young people in recent years, and has been criminalized in most areas.

Clenbuterol, another steroid "alternative," has become an extremely popular item on the black market. The drug is used in some countries for certain veterinary treatments, but is not approved for any use—in animals or humans—in the United States. In Spain, 135 people became ill with muscle tremors, fast heart rates, headaches, dizziness, nausea, fever, and chills after eating beef liver that contained residues of the drug.

"The lack of information about clenbuterol is its greatest hazard. Most of the research we do have is from humans who ingested the drug by eating meat from animals who had been administered it, but as far as ingestion straight into humans, much work needs to be done," says Donald Legget, a compliance officer with FDA's (Food and Drug Administration) Center for Drug Evaluation and Research who deals with enforcement of laws against steroid distribution.

Why Does Anyone Use Them?

With so many harmful effects from steroids and similar illegal drugs, why do so many young people continue to use them?

One answer is social pressures. Many young men feel they need to look "masculine," that is, strong and muscular. Bodybuilding stresses such muscularity, and some men—and women—abuse anabolic steroids to increase muscle mass and definition.

And then there's the "winning isn't everything, it's the only thing" philosophy common in so many school athletic programs. Some student athletes feel so pressured to succeed in their respective sports that they resort to steroids for help.

Another reason, say many experts, lies in the basic nature of young people not to concern themselves with long-term effects. The desire to make the football team or to impress peers is much more immediate than the future prospect of possible damage to the liver, heart, and other vital organs.

In its effort to alert teenagers to the dangers of steroid abuse, FDA has developed a series of pamphlets, posters, and public service announcements. Recently, anabolic steroids were placed in the same regulatory category as cocaine, heroin, LSD, and other habit-forming drugs. This means that, in addition to FDA, the Drug Enforcement Agency helps to enforce laws relating to their abuse.

Celebrities like bodybuilding champs Arnold Schwarzenegger and Lee Haney and professional wrestler Jesse Ventura have spoken out against steroid use. Major magazines, ranging from *Newsweek* to *Muscle and Fitness*, have published articles warning of the dangers of steroid abuse.

The courts are handing down stiff sentences for people dealing in illegal steroids and similar drugs. Distributors have been sentenced to three to six years in jail and fined up to six figures. FDA, working with other law enforcement agencies, has made hundreds of arrests and broken up several large distribution and manufacturing rings.

Athletic organizations have joined the fight. The Olympic Games are now closely monitored to prevent athletes who use steroids from participating, as Ben Johnson found out. The National Football

League has a strict testing policy in its training camps and hands down fines and suspensions for those who test positive, and bans for repeat offenders. The National Collegiate Athletic Association, too, has established stricter measures for testing and disciplining steroid users.

Although it may be true that in combination with intensive weight training and a high-calorie, high-protein diet, steroids can augment short-term muscle gain, teens need to ask themselves: Is it worth all the short-term health effects and the possibility of long-term, permanent damage? Is it worth the disgrace of being eliminated from competition, or even of being arrested?

After taking a long, hard look at the facts, most teens will realize that using drugs to boost athletic performance is a no-win situation.

Steroids May Give You More Than You Bargained For

Established side effects and adverse reactions:

- acne
- genital changes
- water retention in tissue
- yellowing of eyes and skin
- oily skin
- stunted growth
- fetal damage
- coronary artery disease
- sterility
- liver tumors and disease
- death

In women:

- male pattern baldness
- hairiness
- voice deepening
- decreased breast size
- increased body hair
- and menstrual irregularities

Other possible side effects and adverse reactions:

- abdominal pains
- hives
- chills
- euphoria
- diarrhea
- fatigue
- fever
- muscle cramps
- headache
- unexplained weight loss/gain
- nausea and vomiting
- vomiting blood
- bone pains
- depression
- impotence
- breast development in men
- aggressive behavior
- urination problems
- sexual problems
- gallstones
- high blood pressure
- kidney disease

Part Five

Social Issues and Other Parenting Concerns Affecting Adolescent Health and Safety

Chapter 48

Adolescents and Peer Pressure

As children grow, develop, and move into early adolescence, involvement with one's peers and the attraction of peer identification increases. As pre-adolescents begin rapid physical, emotional and social changes, they begin to question adult standards and the need for parental guidance. They find it reassuring to turn for advice to friends who understand and sympathize—friends who are in the same position themselves. By "trying on" new values and testing their ideas with their peers, there is less fear of being ridiculed or "shot down." Yet, mention the word "peer pressure" and many adults cringe because the words are laden with negative connotations. The idea that someone, or something, lures our children into learning dangerous and destructive behavior by discarding all parental behaviors and values, scares adults.

The fact is, peer pressure can be positive. It keeps youth participating in religious activities, going to 4-H meetings and playing on sports teams, even when they are not leaders. It keeps adults going to religious services, serving on community committees, and supporting worthwhile causes. The peer group is a source of affection, sympathy,

This chapter contains text from "Adolescence and Peer Pressure," Nebraska Cooperative Extension NF95-211, December 1995, and Rey A. Carr, "Positive Peer Pressure, a Transition Perspective," Family Service Canada, http://www.cfc-efc.ca/docs/00000410.htm, 1996, and Herbert G. Lingren. Documents reprinted with permission of copyright holders. Despite the age of these documents, readers seeking an understanding of peer pressure will find this information useful.

439

and understanding; a place for experimentation; and a supportive setting for achieving the two primary developmental tasks of adolescence. These are: (1) identity—finding the answer to the question "Who Am I?" and (2) autonomy—discovering that self as separate and independent from parents. It is no wonder, then, that adolescents like to spend time with their peers.

Peers and Adolescence

At adolescence, peer relations expand to occupy a particularly central role in young people's lives. New types (e.g., opposite sex, romantic ties) and levels (e.g., "crowds") of peer relationships emerge. Peers typically replace the family as the center of a young person's socializing and leisure activities. Teenagers have multiple peer relationships, and they confront multiple "peer" cultures that have remarkably different norms and value systems.

The adult perception of peers as having one culture or a unified front of dangerous influence, is inaccurate. More often than not, peers reinforce family values, but they have the potential to encourage problem behaviors as well. Although the negative peer influence is overemphasized, more can be done to help teenagers experience the family and the peer group as mutually constructive environments. Here are some facts about parent, adolescent, and peer relations:

- During adolescence, parents and adolescents become more physically and psychologically distant from each other. This normal distancing is seen in decreases in emotional closeness and warmth, increases in parent-adolescent conflict and disagreement, and an increase in time adolescents spend with peers. Unfortunately, this sometimes is caused because parents are emotionally unavailable to their teenaged children.

- Increases in family strains (economic pressures, divorce, etc.) have prompted teenagers to depend more on peers for emotional support. By the high school years, most teenagers report feeling closer to friends than parents. Stress caused by work, marital dissatisfaction, family break-up caused by divorce, entering a step-family relationship, lower family income, or increasing expenses, all produce increased individual and family stress.

- Parent-adolescent conflict increases between childhood and early adolescence, although in most families, its frequency and intensity remain low. Typically, conflicts are the result of relationship negotiation and continuing attempts by parents to socialize their adolescents and do not signal the breakdown of parent-adolescent relations. Parents need to include adolescents in decision-making and rule-setting that affects their lives.

- In 10 to 20 percent of families, parents and adolescents are in distressed relationships characterized by emotional coldness and frequent outbursts of anger and conflict. Unresolved conflicts produce discouragement and withdrawal from family life. Adolescents in these families are at high risk for various psychological and behavioral problems.

- Youth gangs, commonly associated with inner-city neighborhoods, are becoming a recognizable peer group among youth in smaller cities, suburbs, and even rural areas. Gangs are particularly visible in communities with a significant portion of economically disadvantaged families and when the parent is conflictual, distant, or unavailable.

- Formal dating patterns of two generations ago have been replaced with informal socializing patterns in mixed-sex groups. This may encourage casual sexual relationships that heighten the risk of exposure to AIDS and other sexually transmitted diseases.

- As high schools become more culturally diverse environments, ethnicity is replacing individual abilities or interests as the basis for defining peer "crowds." Crowds can be an important source of ethnic identity, but also the center of racial and ethnic tension in schools.

- There has been an increase in part-time employment among youth, but it has had little impact on peer relations. To find time for work, teenagers drop extracurricular activities, reduce time spent on homework, and withdraw from family interactions, but they "protect" time spent with friends.

Adolescents and the Community

All of these factors may or may not fit a particular community, school or family. However, there is a tendency to deny some of these changes that are taking place. Sometimes communities think it is the family's total responsibility to monitor the negative effects of peer relationships over which they have little control. It is critically important that communities provide a safe, supportive, nurturing environment for adolescents as they grow up. At the same time, families must provide limits and expectations for all members to live by.

The community an adolescent lives in has a major impact on whether she or he will pay more attention to adults or to other young people. Findings from a study of several hundred teenagers in several communities—a rural area, a poor inner-city neighborhood with many minority residents, and an upper-middle class suburb—tell us that we cannot draw sweeping conclusions about teenagers as if they were all alike.

Urban teenagers faced with conflicting standards of family, school, and social agencies were apt to reject all these values and create their own, often among peers. Suburban and rural teens, however, were more likely to have values very close to those held by the important adults in their lives—they might question adult values, but they wanted consistent rules and standards they could evaluate.

Effective Strategies for Coping with Peer Pressure

If the negative effect of peer pressure is to be minimized, youth, parents, school, and community leaders must come together to establish workable and effective strategies to guide teen behavior and to support their transition from children to mature, responsible adults. Here are several strategies to consider:

- Relinquish the stereotype of peers as a uniformly negative influence on youth. Although some teenage peer groups encourage drug use, delinquent activities, and poor school performance, others discourage deviant activity in favor of school achievement and involvement in sports or other extra-curricular activities (e.g., 4-H, music, religious activities).

- Nurture teenagers' abilities and self-esteem so they can forge positive peer relationships. The parent, schools, and other agencies can be taught how to help develop the adolescent's self-concept and self-worth so he or she is a valued person.

- Empower parents and educators to help teenagers pursue and maintain positive peer relationships. They can provide adolescents with the opportunity to succeed in constructive ways which are valued by the teen, the parent, and the community alike.

- Encourage cross-ethnic and "cross-class" peer interactions and guide teenagers in dealing positively with cultural diversity and individual differences. Parents, teachers, community leaders, and clergy can model appreciation for ethnic differences and support cross-class and cross-ethnic friendships. Schools and youth organizations can assist by encouraging youth from diverse backgrounds to work and play together.

- Place sensible restraints on part-time teen employment. This could ease adolescents' compliance with peer pressures to "buy" acceptance into a peer group (i.e., to have enough money for the "right" clothes, the "right" shoes, the "right" CDs, etc.). Increases in part-time employment among youth have had little impact on the time they spend with peers.

- Support parent education programs for families with teenagers. Parents need to be better informed about the dynamics of adolescent peer groups and the demands and expectations teenagers face in peer relationships.

- Establish intervention programs for pre-adolescents with low social skills or aggressive tendencies. Addressing these problems before adolescence will decrease the chances of these youth joining anti-social peer groups that will reinforce their problem behaviors.

Summary

During adolescence, peers play a large part in a young person's life and typically replace family as the center of a teen's social and leisure activities. But teenagers have various peer relationships, and they interact with many peer groups. Often "peer cultures" have very different values and norms. Thus, the adult perception of peers as a "united front of dangerous influence" is inaccurate.

More often than not, peers reinforce family values, but they have the potential to encourage problem behaviors as well. Although the negative influence of peers is over-emphasized, more can be done to help teenagers experience the family and the peer group as mutually constructive environments. To accomplish this, families, communities, churches, schools, 4-H, and other youth groups must work together because it "takes a whole village to raise a child."

Positive Peer Pressure, a Transition Perspective

By the time I made it to the last year of my elementary school, I had collected whatever badges, brownie points, and extracurricular awards that were available. I had become one of the mighty, one of the elite, and one of the kids who controlled the school. As far as I was concerned, I and my other 11 year-old peers were pretty much the rulers of our domain.

However, each day as I walked to my kingdom, I had to pass the cavernous junior high school into which most of history's previous grade sixers had disappeared. My movement past this monolithic building with its massive chain-link fences, and playground filled with big kids wearing strange clothes was often interrupted by monstrous-size kids lunging towards me, yelling at me, and threatening to tear something off me that I didn't even know I had yet. I learned to navigate this terror zone pretty quickly.

Just a few days following the awards, recognition, and graduation ceremony at my elementary school where I spent most of the time giving out or receiving some accolade, I started at ground zero. On my first day at junior high I had nothing, I was nothing, and I was scared. Instead of self-esteem, I brought the echoes of dozens of stories I had been told about kids being crushed in lockers, books being burned on the playground, and seventh grade students being "punched out" by powerful grade nine sluggers.

Although this experience of being full of esteem one day and being reduced to unworthiness on another day happened to me many years ago, the vivid recollection of this period of time has led me, in part, to focus on the role of "transition" in the life-span. There are many kinds of transitions in our lives: leaving home and entering school for the first time; changing schools; going through puberty; getting a job; losing a job; losing a parent by death or divorce; getting married; playing on a team; becoming a parent; parenting a teenager; overcoming an addiction; and so on.

While transitions may be similar for most adolescents, and transitions may be unique to particular adolescents, all adolescents share one common occurrence—the experience of transition. These experiences may be successful and lead to happiness, or they may be troublesome and lead to failure. Parents and peers play a crucial role in assisting adolescents with the outcomes of transitions, and this article will focus on how peers can assist each other with transitions and the role parents can play in helping their children make successful transitions.

Although there is a common perception that "peer pressure" is the reason for many negative behaviors of adolescents, in reality, peers are necessary and crucial in helping adolescents make successful transitions. Peers can and do act as positive role models. Peers can and do demonstrate appropriate social behaviors. Peers often listen to, accept, and understand the frustrations, challenges, and concerns associated with being a teenager.

Peers provide an opportunity for teens to meet their needs, to feel capable, to belong, to be respected, and to have fun. While young people often experience these needs being met within the family, the peer group provides unique and different opportunities to meet these needs. The peer group encourages autonomy, mutuality, and experimentation with self guided roles. While many families assist teens to find out who they really are and to help teens feel proud and confident of their unique traits, backgrounds, and abilities, the peer group may often be more accepting of the feelings, thoughts, and actions associated with this search for self-identity.

In families where children do not have these needs met, young people will likely turn to the peer group for attention, affection, and support as a replacement for family. This transition often occurs too early in a child's development and consequently the peer group can only partially fulfil these needs. Young people in this circumstance often spend much time with peers, but they rarely have someone within the group that they experience as a close or intimate friend. The ability to make and keep friends is one of the most powerful indications of successful, positive peer group interactions.

Parents may be particularly concerned about the kinds of "friends" their teenagers are "hanging" with. We all want our children to be with persons who will have a positive influence, and stay away from persons who will encourage our children to engage in harmful, destructive, immoral, or illegal activities. However, being a teenager means finding out how to manage these influences, and as parents, we cannot protect or shield our teens from the existence of these influences. We can, however, help teens develop an ability to resist or reduce the impact of these negative influences. One way to accomplish the harm-reduction goal is to provide your teen with the opportunity to discuss and describe their transition experiences. When adolescents have an opportunity to 1) consider and describe their experience, 2) discuss their feeling and reactions, 3) determine the meaning(s) the experience has for them, and 4) decide on actions to build on such meaning(s), then it is more likely that adolescents will be able to recover and benefit from troubling or adverse transitions between life events as well as learn from successful life event transitions.

This focus on discussing experiences is the basis for peer helper training as designed by Carr and Saunders, and deRosenroll, Saunders, and Carr. The deRosenroll, Saunders, and Carr model concentrates on helping adolescents learn from their experiences, and does not impose any particular value or lesson, but instead follows the lead of the adolescent in examining any particular experience. By providing certain types of prompts or questions called "anchors" at various points in the processing of the experience, the learning model both supports adolescent learning and challenges adolescents to deeper reflection, understanding, search for personal and communal meaning, and action planning.

Helping other adolescents talk about their experience in a way that preserves self-esteem, contributes to interpersonal relations, builds on cognitive abilities to abstract and reflect, and places concerns in manageable portions through a sense of control and goal setting, allows adolescents to take a more active role in their ability to benefit from the myriad of transitions they experience within their lives.

Schools throughout the country have recognized the valuable roles peers play in helping each other and have established a variety of peer programs across the province. Peer programs exist in elementary schools, junior highs, secondary schools and even in colleges and universities. Peer programs are even available for senior citizens! If you would like more information about peer programs in your community, contact your local school counselor.

Transition Anchors for Parents

Instead of issuing a command such as : "I don't want you hanging out with that person. He is a bad influence." Try opening a door by saying, "I want to learn about your friendships. Tell me how being with (person's name) is valuable to you."

Then try to gain a description by asking: "What is it like to hang out with (person's name)?"

Then gain a deeper perspective by asking: "What do you get out of being with (person's name)?"

If you gain information that indicates dangers are present, then help with action planning by asking: "What risks might there be in hanging out with (person's name)?"

The create some concrete plans by asking: "What are your plans to deal with the risks?"

Finally, to provide support and alliance: "What role do you want me to play in helping you with your plan?"

Chapter 49

You and Your Teen: Discipline That Works

A world without limits or rules would be a nightmare for every person living in it. Just imagine the complete chaos that would happen if everyone "did his own thing," no matter what!

Teenagers may think they don't want or need discipline, but the truth is without limits a person is insecure, may feel unloved, and will have a very hard time becoming a responsible, happy member of society.

For most parents, setting and reinforcing family rules without cramping the teen's style or taking away his or her independence is difficult. Many parents recognize the need to change the methods their own parents used to discipline but aren't sure what will work in today's fast-paced world. Parents sometimes struggle from one problem to the next hoping that somehow the teen will change his behavior. This is unlikely! Instead, parents can become involved by giving guidance through discipline. Remember that discipline is a tool used to teach, never to punish.

As parents, we don't have to solve or act upon all our teen's problems. We must be careful to recognize that some problems belong to the teen alone and should be solved by the teen, with our strong encouragement and support, but not interference. On the other hand, problems affecting us have to be solved using good discipline methods.

Excerpted from "You and Your Teen: Discipline That Works," an undated document published by Grey Bruce Health Unit, available on the Internet at http://www.publichealthgreybruce.on.ca/FamilyTeens/FamilyYourteendiscipline thatworksFS.html, accessed in November 2001.

Is it sometimes hard to tell which problems are ours and which are theirs....? You bet! It might help to look at each problem and consider:

1. Who is complaining or concerned about the problem?

2. Who is affected by the problem?

3. Who is prevented from doing what he/she wants because of the problem?

If the answer to each question is "your teen," help him or her become a good problem solver. On the other hand if the answer is "yourself," it is your problem to solve.

If the problem belongs to you, wouldn't it be wonderful if hassles could be avoided? They can. Suppose for example, your daughter decides to get her driver's license. Think about what problems could happen.....ahead of time. Sit down with your teen and set clear limits that avoid unpleasant surprises and resentment later on. Discuss what's expected and what will happen if she violates the limits. Don't be a dictator! Listen to your teen's point of view and negotiate rules you can both live with. Whose fault is it if your teen messes up and breaks rules she doesn't understand or know existed!

Unfortunately, some problems can't be predicted ahead of time and must be managed as they happen. If your teen's behavior must change, try a polite request first. She will be more likely to listen if you talk respectfully to her as you would to a friend. Shout and demand and you've turned off the teen and lost your cool.

If polite requests don't work, then try "I" messages. "I messages" are friendly but firm statements that are very clear. Describe the behavior and how it makes you feel and why; ask for a change. Frustrated complaints like "look at this mess" may be ignored.

Try instead: "When you leave the bathroom in a mess, I feel taken advantage of. It means I have to spend time cleaning up. I want you to clean the tub and put the towels in the hamper."

If you then say....."Will you do that?" and "When," your message becomes stronger. Never leave "I" messages unchecked. If they work, thank your teen.

If these techniques haven't worked; what do you do next? Do you give up, get angry or do you keep calm and take the next step.

Natural Consequences

Reinforce that all behavior results in consequences. There are two types of consequences: natural and logical. As parents, we're always hearing about letting our children learn from their mistakes. Natural consequences give us that chance because they follow naturally after the teen's action or lack of action (with no interference from the parent.) For instance, a young person who oversleeps will be late for school or work. Let him be late, but give him encouragement and support to solve his problem so it won't happen again. Hopefully, he has learned a valuable lesson. As parents we must always be very careful not to use natural consequences if the result will harm the teen or someone else.

Logical Consequences

If the teen's behavior still isn't changing, it is time to try logical consequences. Remember, logical consequences should be logically connected to the behavior. If your teen is always late for supper and you take away his stereo, you probably won't be successful. However, if he's late for supper and he has to make his own supper and clean up the kitchen, he is less likely to be late again. Remember, discipline is teaching. It is not punishment; never give the logical consequences in anger. Anger breeds anger, and before you know it you'll be in the middle of a "battle royal." Calm down and give the teen a choice: "Either put your clothes in the hamper or wash them yourself. You decide." Or.... "When you have finished your homework, then you may go out."

When developing logical consequences, remember to keep the following in mind:

- Be careful to set consequences that are reasonable and you can live with.

- Be firm but calm.

- Ask your teen for input regarding the consequences.

- Give the choice once and then follow up.

- Expect challenges. Your teen is testing to see if you really mean it.

- Allow the young person to try again after experiencing the consequences.

If misbehavior continues the consequences may need to be revised. Be patient.

You'll be more successful if you include the teen in discussing the expectations and the consequences. Parents who listen respectfully and who negotiate curfews and other issues have fewer problems. Parents who rule with an iron fist usually have major problems.

If your teenager does not respond to any of your efforts and appears to be "out of control" you may need to seek professional help. Help is available through your family doctor, the guidance department of your school, and local mental health counseling services.

Chapter 50

Adolescents and the Internet

The newest street corners, arcades, and malls that serve as teen hangouts can be found right within the walls of the homestead. They are electronic mockups of the real thing—accessed easily by the family's modem-equipped computer. For many adolescents these cyberspace hangouts are no less treasured or real than the "real" thing.

What draws adolescents to the world of the Internet? What are the benefits and dangers of their exploring this new realm that may very well become a cornerstone of the new millennium into which they will grow as adults?

Where Adolescents Hang Out

In case there are readers who aren't familiar with the Internet, let me briefly explain some of the places where adolescents might hang out. I'll break the rather complex world of cyberspace into five basic categories:

- Web pages—By this I mean documents or collections of documents that adolescents can read. It might be a short one-page description of a rock star, other teens' home pages in which they describe themselves, an article about the French revolution, or

Excerpted from "Adolescents in Cyberspace" by John Suler, Ph.D,, from http://www.rider.edu/users/suler/psycyber/adoles.html, June 1998. Reprinted with permission of the author.

an entire online book. Web pages may also include pictures, video clips, sounds, and music. Web pages are, essentially, a vast multimedia online library covering almost any topic you can imagine.

• Email dyads and groups—Email is one of the most easy to use, flexible, and powerful means to communicate. It's more than just an electronic letter launched through the Internet. Rapid email exchanges are more like a conversation. Subtle and complex relationships can form through frequent email interactions. The email itself becomes a psychological "space" in which the adolescents live together. Email within a couple can create a very intimate, emotional relationship. Groups of people also can communicate with each other through email lists, also known as "listservs." For some people, the attractive feature of email communication is that you can't see or hear the other person. This may make the relationship feel somewhat ambiguous and anonymous.

• Chat rooms, Instant Messaging (IM), and MUDs (Multiple User Dimension)—These also are a favorite for many teens. In chat rooms and instant messaging, the adolescents communicate with each other in "real time." In other words, everyone in the group is sitting at their computer at the same time, typing messages to each other that scroll down the screen. Everyone can see the messages as people "talk" to their friend or to a group of friends. It's also possible to send a private message to another person that the group can't see. In the multimedia chat environments such as Palace, the text conversations occur in a visual room and the participants use tiny visual icons called "avatars" to represent themselves. Some adolescents like to present themselves in an imaginative way, by changing their name, age, identity, or even their gender. Some chat environments (e.g., MUDs) become a very intricate fantasy world where adolescents create all sorts of imaginative roles and scenarios. It's like a living novel complete with characters and plots, or a very elaborate Halloween party with its own idiosyncratic rules and culture. As with email, not being able to see or hear the other person makes chat a rather ambiguous and anonymous mode of communication—especially since other people may not even know your real name, but just your username, which can be any imaginative name you choose.

- Message Boards—Sometimes called by a variety of other names ("forums," "discussion groups," "newsgroups"), a message board is like an electronic bulletin board. People connect to a specific site on the Internet and post messages to each other. Unlike chat, this is not a real-time conversation. Whenever you want, you can go to the site and read the messages that others have written. Each newsgroup usually is devoted to a specific topic of discussion. Usenet, the original home of the newsgroup, contains tens of thousands of groups devoted to almost any topic you can imagine. Some of these groups are the homes-away-from-home for many teens. Some web sites also use this "bulletin board" format. Once again, as with email and chat, newsgroup posts can be a very anonymous style of communicating.

- Video-conferencing is another newer feature of cyberspace. Using a video camera and microphone, people can see and hear each other as they talk. However, the expense and variety of technical problems associated with high quality video-conferencing makes it a much less common form of communication for adolescents. Usually, only more hardcore computer techies are up to the challenge. My guess, too, is that it's not as much fun for the adolescent as the more anonymous and/or fantasy-based modes of hanging out in cyberspace.

Now that we are all familiar with the places where adolescents might hang out, let's focus on the pros and cons of what they are doing there. The important thing to remember about cyberspace is that its strengths are its weaknesses. Like many things in life, the bad comes with the good.

In the Know: Finding Information

One way adolescents establish their own individual identity is by acquiring new facts and philosophies, which includes the skills that may develop from that information. Maybe one attractive feature of the Internet for teens is that there are no holds barred on the information out there. It's not controlled by the government, school, parents, or even just by adults. Other kids are publishing on the web too. Cyberspace is a new frontier of information just waiting to be pioneered. Exploring that information can satisfy that need to feel separate and unique from one's parents.

The Internet is a vast library covering any topic imaginable. In some respects, it's better than most libraries—at least it is from the perspective of the adolescent. How much information can you find at the public library about rock groups or your favorite TV stars? My daughter spent hours online looking for information about the Titanic. She pulled up information that amazed me. Some people might claim that much of the information on the web is junk. Of course, one person's garbage is another's jewel. Perhaps the positive aspect of this dilemma is that adolescents are placed in the position of deciding for themselves what is good information, and what isn't. They will have to become savvy consumers of information in this Information Age of ours.

Now for the bad news. Some of the information and skills that adolescents might seek is better left alone. Pornography, drugs, methods of inflicting violence. It's all there on the Internet. No parent wants their child to learn how to concoct a sex drug or build a bomb. But other scenarios may be more ambiguous. What if, for personal reasons, an adolescent wants information about abortion or being gay? Should they have access to it? Freedom of information, the quality control of information, and the values that influence our attitudes about information are all issues that everyone must confront.

Where Everyone Knows Your Name

More so than anything else, adolescents are drawn to cyberspace because they make friends there. They find new groups to join—a place where they feel like they belong, where everyone knows their name. Just being an onliner automatically makes you part of the in-crowd, and from there you can pick, choose, and create almost any other specific type of group you want. Cyberspace technology excels in all sorts of methods for forming groups—and adolescents take advantage of it because joining and shaping a new group is so important to their evolving identity. What do they do once they're in the group? They joke and play games, complain about their parents and teachers, talk about their lives, support and give advice to each other... the same things they do in "real" life.

Once again, there's a down side. Teens may join online groups that are not in their best interests. Radical political groups, Satanic cults, online "orgies." Of course, these groups exist in the real world too. It's just a lot easier to participate in them when you're sitting at the computer in your bedroom.

The more common pitfall of online friendships and cliques is that they can be somewhat artificial, shallow, and transient. Cyberspace may seem so surreal, so much like a fantasy inside your head, that some people don't take it seriously even though emotions and commitment seem to run high. It's like a great interactive TV program that really gets you emotionally involved, but it's just a TV program. To the adolescent craving for a group of good friends, it can be heartbreaking when those pals unexpectedly and unexplainably change their "tune," withdraw, or disappear completely. With just a mouse click, you're gone, almost without leaving any traces behind. It's too easy to say good bye, especially when you can easily exit without even having to say "good bye."

This sometimes shallow and transient quality of online relationships doesn't apply in all cases. People do find and keep good friends in cyberspace. But artificial best buddies do appear often enough to be a very problematic disappointment, especially to adolescents who are so sensitized to issues about intimacy, trust, and loyalty.

Cybersex

Since we're on the topic of intimacy, let's delve into that other magnet that lures some teens into cyberspace—cybersex. It certainly isn't shocking news that adolescents are keenly interested in sex. It's an adventure, it calls out to their rising hormone levels, it's a way to separate from—as well as worry, aggravate, and outrage—their parents. It means, to them, that they're developing an adult identity.

What exactly is cybersex? Mostly, just talking dirty to each other via typed text—describing in detail who is doing what to whom, and how they feel doing it. People may masturbate while they type. Sometimes pictures are exchanged, but that can become an unnecessary technical complication that may ruin the free play of imagination.

Whether or not parents consider this a bad thing for adolescents is largely determined by their values. Some may think that the anonymity of cybersex is wrong—that it is superficial, artificial, unnatural—or that sex in any form is inappropriate for adolescents. Others may think that adolescents are going to experiment with sex no matter what adults do, so why not permit them to satisfy their sexual interests and learn about sex via cyberspace encounters?

Adult Predators

One dilemma of online life is that you can never be sure that other people indeed are who they say they are. That 17 year old flirtatious girl could be a 47 year old man. Some chat rooms are supervised in order to protect children from predatory adults, but many are not. Even in those communities that are well supervised, there is little that can be done to prevent predatory adults from pretending to be teens in order to win the favors of young people. If a predator doesn't use an adolescent disguise, he (and usually they are males) may present himself as a supportive, sympathetic confidant who encourages the adolescent to discuss personal problems and become emotionally attached to him. Troubled adolescents who feel alienated from their parents are especially vulnerable. These are the same types of strategies used by predators in the in-person world. The Internet is just another avenue they use to launch their abuse against children. Children need to be taught the same sorts of rules that apply to real world encounters with questionable adults:

- Don't divulge personal information to strangers. Don't give out your phone number or address.

- Log off if someone makes you uncomfortable or asks you to do something that is wrong. Write down the username of that person, and inform your parents about it so they can contact the people who operate the chat room.

- Don't accept gifts from strangers or call someone, even if they invite you to call collect.

- Never meet anyone offline without adult family supervision.

Caught in the Net: Addiction

Because cyberspace can satisfy so many of the adolescent's needs, there is the possibility of becoming "addicted" to it. Are all teens susceptible to this danger?... No. Some will always be casual users, some may just go through phases of intense Internet use. The ones who do fall prey to the net most likely are experiencing problems in their real lives. Cyberspace becomes an escape, a place to vent, a place to act out or even cry out for help.

What are some of the danger signals of excessive Internet use? In her book, Dr. Young identifies several warning signs:

- Denial and lying about the amount of time spent on the computer or about what they are doing on the computer.

- Excessive fatigue and changes in sleeping habits, such as getting up early or staying up late (in order to spend more time online).

- Academic problems, usually grades slipping. Sometimes parents might overlook the fact that the computer is the culprit since they assume their children are doing school work at the keyboard.

- Withdrawal from friends and declining interest in hobbies (online friends and activities are taking the place of the "real" world).

- Loss of appetite; irritability when cut-off from computer use; a decline in their appearance or hygiene.

- Disobedience and acting out. Teens may become very hostile when parents confront them. They may deliberately break the computer-use rules that are set. Their reactions may be so intense because they feel that they are being cut off from their attachments to cyberfriends.

How Should Parents Be Involved?

Although the Internet may be one way adolescents attempt to establish themselves as separate, unique individuals who have a social world of their own, that doesn't mean parents shouldn't be involved. Exactly the opposite is true. As is true of all adolescent activities, they need at least some supervision to stay on track and avoid trouble.

But getting involved doesn't just mean supervising in order to avert trouble. The computer and cyberspace also can become an excellent way for parents and adolescents to have fun together, to get to know each other better. There will be a part of the adolescent—maybe even a part that they try to hide—that will love this.

- Get knowledgeable and join in: To be most effective in supervising the adolescent's cyberspace activities, the parent needs to know something about the topic. You don't have to become a hacker yourself, but read up on the topic. Discuss it with other parents. Better yet, explore cyberspace yourself. Better still, talk to your kids about cyberspace and join them in some of their online activities. Cruise web sites together. Use a search engine to find people with your same last name. Build a web page for your family. Even hang out with your child and their friends in a chat room (for a short period of time, if they can tolerate your presence!). There are numerous possibilities.

- Talk to them: The old warning "Do you know where your children are?" applies to cyberspace as well as to the real world.

Ask them about their Internet use. What web sites are they visiting? To avoid an accusatory tone, ask them what web sites they like and why. Sit down with them at the computer and let them take you to their Internet hangouts. Be curious, in a parental but congenial sort of way. Ask them about their cyberfriends, what they talk about, what they do on the Internet. Avoid interrogation. Instead, show them that you are interested in knowing more about their cyberfriends.

- Acknowledge the good and the bad: Don't vilify cyberspace— that will only alienate the adolescent. Talk about both the pros and cons. Show an acceptance of their cyberlife, but discuss some of the dangers and what steps they should take if they encounter unsavory situations or people.

- Make the computer visible: Privacy is a tricky balancing act with the adolescent. They want and need some, but the parent must weigh that demand against the necessity of supervising their activities. Generally speaking, it's probably a good idea to avoid placing the modem-equipped computer in the adolescent's bedroom. Put it in a family area. That makes supervision a lot easier, and it also encourages computering as a family activity. If they suddenly quit the program as you walk in, you know something is up. It may not be anything serious, but it's worth talking about.

- Set reasonable rules: Parents don't let their kids stay out all night, watch any movie they want, or drive anywhere they want. Adolescents need rules. In fact, believe it or not, they secretly want rules so they don't feel out of control and unprotected by a seemingly uncaring parent. Set limits on when (e.g., after homework) and how much time they can spend socializing and entertaining themselves in cyberspace. Create rules about what exactly they can and can't do on the Internet.

- Encourage a balance: Cyberspace is great, but there's more to life than that. Encourage the adolescent to stay involved in "real world" activities too.

- Software controls: There are a variety of commercial programs that can be used to monitor and control the adolescents activities in cyberspace. These programs can keep a record of web sites they visit, block access to particular web sites or programs, prevent files from being downloaded, and set limits on when and for how much time the Internet is being used. Of course, if parents want to install such programs they have to be fairly knowledgeable about computers. The programs aren't perfect either. There are loopholes, and a technically sophisticated adolescent will be able to defeat them. Probably the last thing a parent wants is an ongoing technical battle of wits with their child. If that happens, something has gone awry. Software controls are a tool in the supervision of the adolescent. They are not a substitute for talking and being more personally involved. In other words, they are not a substitute for a relationship.

- Intervening with addiction: In her book, Dr. Kimberly Young describes some strategies for parents who need to help their children who have fallen into excessive Internet use. Don't try to take the computer away or ban them from using it. This strategy can backfire. Show your caring for the teenager's predicament.

- Discipline misbehavior/encourage humaneness: Most parents apply punishment when a child misbehaves in the real world. The same should be true of their cyberspace misconduct. If a parent discovers that an adolescent is harassing others online or attempting to hack online systems (a phone call from the administrators of the system or online community can be an eye-opener!), discipline is in order.

Chapter 51

What You Need to Know about Teen Safety on the Job

Teen Safety

Is Your Job Safe?

Every year, more than 4 million teens under 18 will work at jobs. For the majority of teens, work will be a rewarding experience. However, a sizable number of teens will risk being injured or killed on the job. Statistics show that each year 70 teens are killed on the job, about one every 5 days. 210,000 working teens are injured; 70,000 teens are injured seriously enough to require hospital emergency room treatment.

Where Teens Work/How They Are Hurt

Most teens (51 percent) work in the retail industry, which includes fast-food outlets and food stores. An additional 34 percent work in the service industry, including health, education, and entertainment or recreation.

This chapter includes text from "Teen Safety," http://www.dol.gov/dol/esa/public/youth/tshome.htm, and "Work Safe This Summer 'Teen' Tips for Parents," US Department of Labor, 1996. Despite the age of this document, information on teen job safety will be useful to the reader. Statistics in this chapter were taken from the Occupational Safety and Health Administration's (OSHA) 1995 report, however, the figures are still quite accurate. OSHA's current report (updated November 2000) can be found at http://www.bls.gov/opub/rylf/rylfhome.htm.

Fifty-four percent of teen occupational injuries occur in the retail industry, followed by the service industry (20 percent), agriculture (7 percent), and manufacturing (4 percent). Some tasks and tools associated with a large number of injuries include:

- driving a car
- driving heavy equipment, especially tractors
- using power tools, especially meat slicers

Teens are killed at work, most often, while driving or traveling as passengers in motor vehicles. Machine-related accidents, electrocution, homicide, and falls also account for many deaths. A National Institute for Occupational Safety and Health (NIOSH) study has determined that the risk of injury death for workers age 16 and 17 was 5.1 per 100,000 full-time equivalent workers, compared with 6.0 for adult workers over age 18. This is of particular concern when you take into consideration the fact that as a whole teens work fewer hours than adult employees.

Safety Protections for Working Teens

Child labor laws and regulations govern the ages and types of jobs children under 18 may work and the hours they may work. In June 1994, the Labor Department increased penalties for death or serious injury of minors employed in violation of child labor laws as a deterrent to employers. The new penalties allow a fine of up to $10,000 for each violation that leads to the serious injury or death of a child. The former penalty was a fine of up to $10,000 for each minor seriously injured or killed.

From October 1, 1995, through September 30, 1996, Department of Labor investigators found more than 7,000 young people working in violation of child labor laws and regulations, and assessed $6.8 million in civil money penalties for violations involving 1,341 establishments.

Virtually all workers, including teenagers, are protected by safety and health standards set by the Occupational Safety and Health Administration. These standards cover fire and electrical safety, chemical hazards, machine guarding, and many other on-the-job risks. Employers with 10 or more employees in more hazardous industries must keep records of injuries and illnesses that occur at their sites. All employers must report to the Occupational Safety and Health Administration (OSHA) incidents in which one or more workers are killed or three are more are hospitalized.

Prohibited Jobs and Hours Limitations

Prohibited Jobs

Seventeen hazardous non-farm jobs, as determined by the Secretary of Labor, are out of bounds for teens below the age of 18. Jobs marked with "*" indicate that limited exemptions are provided for apprentices and student-learners under specified standards. Generally, teens may not work at jobs that involve:

1. manufacturing or storing explosives

2. driving a motor vehicle and being an outside helper on a motor vehicle

3. coal mining

4. logging and sawmilling

5. power-driven wood-working machines*

6. exposure to radioactive substances and to ionizing radiations

7. power-driven hoisting equipment

8. power-driven metal-forming, punching, and shearing machines*

9. mining, other than coal mining

10. meat packing or processing (including power-driven meat slicing machines)

11. power-driven bakery machines

12. power-driven paper-products machines*

13. manufacturing brick, tile, and related products

14. power-driven circular saws, band saws, and guillotine shears*

15. wrecking, demolition, and ship-breaking operations

16. roofing operations*

17. excavation operations*

Hours Limitations

1. Youths 18 or older may perform any job, whether hazardous or not, for unlimited hours, in accordance with minimum wage and overtime requirements.

2. Youths 16 and 17 years old may perform any nonhazardous job, for unlimited hours.

3. Youths 14 and 15 years old may work outside school hours in various nonmanufacturing, nonmining, nonhazardous jobs up to:

   - 3 hours on a school day.
   - 18 hours in a school week.
   - 8 hours on a non-school day.
   - 40 hours in a non-school week.

Also, work must be performed between the hours of 7 a.m. and 7 p.m., except from June 1 through Labor Day, when evening hours are extended to 9 p.m.

Frequently Asked Questions about Teen Safety

What Happens If I Don't Feel Safe on the Job?

You should know that you have the right to work in a safe and healthful place. Injuries are not "cool" and we must stay alert to prevent them. Let the person in charge know when you are doing a task for the first time, especially if it looks tricky or dangerous. Ask how to do it in a safe manner. Then, learn to do it the right way. Always do it the same way—safely—don't take any dangerous shortcuts.

Can I Work on Machines?

If you are under 16 years of age, you are prohibited from working on most machines. No supervisor should ask you, and you should refuse to operate any power-driven machines (except office machines). Ask your parents to help you discuss this with the person in charge if you are unsure.

Why Do Some Machines Have Guards and Shields?

These help protect workers and reduce injuries. Make sure that all guards and safety devices are kept on machines, even if they slow you down a little.

What Happens If I Get Injured on the Job?

Be sure to report all injuries, and seek treatment for all injuries from the first aid station, nurse, doctor or hospital. Don't ignore injuries. Make sure that the supervisor and the medical person that treats you know that the incident that caused the injury happened on the job.

Work Safe This Summer "Teen" Tips for Parents

Kids are often encouraged to visit their parents' workplace to learn about what they do. During the summer—when more than 3 million teens go to work—is a good time to do the reverse. Parents should pay a visit to their teen's place of employment to make sure that their children are working in a safe and healthful environment.

Parents have a special role in preventing on-the-job injuries suffered by 200,000 teen workers every year. The Labor Secretary offers the following "Teen Tips" to parents:

Talk to your kids. Make sure you know all the tasks your child will be performing at work, their hours and pay rate, and who their supervisors and coworkers are.

Engage their employer. Meet with your teen's employer. Let them know you're concerned about safety.

Educate yourself. There are some jobs and work tasks that teens are not allowed to do, and there are certain laws that apply to the hours teens are allowed to work. Find out more by visiting our web site at http://www.dol.gov/dol/teensafety.htm or call your local Department of Labor Wage and Hour office (listed under Department of Labor in the blue pages of your local telephone book).

Know to say NO! Both parents and teens should know that no worker under age 18 is allowed to perform hazardous jobs. "No" is a good answer if a teen worker is asked to drive a car or ride in the back of an open truck, use a power-driven meat slicer or bakery machine, operate a power-driven woodworking machine or circular saw, or do any type of roofing or excavation work.

Chapter 52

Safe Driving for Teenagers

Chapter Contents

Section 52.1

Teens Behind the Wheel: What Parents Need to Know

Excerpted from Jennifer Nelson "Teens Behind the Wheel: What Parents Need to Know" Teenagers Today/iParenting, http://teenagerstoday.com/resources/articles/teendriving.htm, 2001.

With the advent of my son's 16th birthday came some new and challenging experiences—especially driving. While many teens look forward to this milestone birthday, parents riding shotgun know the often scary and startling statistics that come with teen driving. If you have a teen driver in your home or soon will have—listen up. There are some things that both parents and teens need to know.

The Facts

The Insurance Institute for Highway Safety reports that 16-year-old drivers get in wrecks nearly nine times more often than those ages 20 and over. For 17-year-olds the rate is six times higher than the adult rate. According to the American Automobile Association, teens account for only 7 percent of all drivers, yet they are involved in 14 percent of all fatal auto accidents and 20 percent of all accidents.

The statistics are scary and seem to reflect poorly on teen drivers. However, facts and figures are not a personal reflection of every teen's judgement. But sweet 16 or not, teens and their parents need to be aware of the numbers and understand how to decrease the chances of harm and increase chances for safe, crash-free driving.

What You Can Do

Only you can decide when your teen is ready to drive without adult supervision, and riding with your teen while he practices on a learner's permit is a great way to judge his skills. If your teen is not logging 30 minutes to an hour of practice each week, you're wasting precious learning experiences. All those errands, shopping and after-school activities around town are perfect trips for driving practice. "I just can't stress enough about getting experience behind the wheel," Cooper says.

When a teen gets a license, she's still gaining the experience she'll need to be a safe driver. Rather than simply handing over the keys, it's up to parents to set rules and guidelines regarding when, where, how and with whom teens may drive. Here's a list of some important guidelines:

- Limit the number of passengers in the car. Teens are likely to have trouble concentrating on the road with laughter, music, food, and other distractions, which increase with the number of passengers.

- Insist on seatbelts. Teens tend to use their safety belts less frequently than other drivers do. Insist that your teen and all passengers wear safety belts at all times.

- Limit driving during high-risk times. Statistics show that the highest numbers of driving crashes occur on Friday and Saturday nights and early Saturday and Sunday mornings. Limit teen driving during these peak times.

- Take a "no tolerance" stance on drugs and alcohol. Aside from any legal punishment, a violation of driving under the influence should be cause for the revocation of driving privileges by parents.

- Have your teen sign a safe driving contract. Explain how seriously you take the contract.

What about Driver's Ed?

For decades, driver education classes were believed to help prevent accidents. While there's no proof that the high school courses reduce crash numbers in the long term, it's still not a bad idea for teens to take the course—and is still required in many areas. The AAA (American Automobile Association) and the NHTSA (National Highway Traffic Safety Administration) are currently designing a state-of-the-art driver education curriculum that they hope will become part of the GDL program. Driver education focuses on defensive driving. The skills taught, such as anticipating problems and knowing how to correct them, are crucial abilities for teen drivers to master.

Winter Driving

Another obstacle for teens is winter driving. Parents should work with teens to help them gain the experience they need to safely drive in ice, wind, and snow. "Young drivers may not have any frame of reference for what it's like to be on an icy highway or overpass," Cooper says. Under close supervision, teens need practice with slow-speed maneuvers on an open snow- or ice-covered parking lot. Have your teen practice hard breaking and steering in skidding situations. Make sure tires and brakes are in top condition. Always make sure the vehicle is equipped with the proper emergency gear for winter, including a flashlight, blankets, jumper cables, sand, and a small shovel or ice scraper. And finally, teach teens to use far more caution during hazardous winter conditions.

Preventing teen drivers from becoming statistics and helping them master the skills needed for good driving is the goal of both parents and organizations such as the AAA and NHTSA. Through strict parental rules, continued practice and education, state programs like GDL (Graduated Drivers License) and driver education classes, parents and teens can work together to put teens on the road to safe driving.

Section 52.2

Fact and Fiction of Seat Belt Use

This section contains text from "Fact or Fiction of Seat Belt Use," http://safeprogram.com/pub_factfiction.html, and "Occupant Protection," http://safeprogram.com/pub_instructor.html, copyright 2000 Stay Alive from Education. Reprinted with permission.
See http://www.safeprogram.com for additional materials.

Seat belts are your best protection against other drivers. They keep you in the safest place during a crash—in your seat and in your car. Safety belts keep drivers in place so they can retain control of the car. They also keep passengers from becoming human projectiles in the event of a crash. Unbelted occupants colliding with each other cause many serious injuries. Seat belts are designed to absorb most of the force of the impact and distribute it to the strongest parts of the body, the shoulders and pelvis. Lap/shoulder belts reduce the risk of fatal injury to front-seat occupants by 45% and the risk of moderate-to-critical injury by 50%. The bottom line is safety belts can be the difference between life and death!

Here are some excuses that you will hear why people won't wear seat belts:

I Won't Ever Be in a Crash. It Can't Happen to Me

Motor vehicle crashes are the leading cause of death for all persons between the ages of 6 and 27, out distancing deaths from homicide, suicide, other accidental injuries, drug dependency, or AIDS (acquired immune deficiency syndrome). Over 41,000 people were killed and 3,511,000 were injured in traffic crashes in 1996. Still think it can't happen to you?

I'm Not Going Far

According to the National Highway Traffic Safety Administration (NHTSA), three out of four crashes occur within 25 miles of home. Distance has nothing to do with safety.

I'm a Very Good Driver

That may be true, but not everyone that you have to share the road with is a good driver. Alcohol, drugs, or lack of sleep can affect driving and judgment abilities. A blown tire, failed brakes, bad weather, or poor road conditions can cause crashes even for good drivers.

I Don't Need One—I Sit in the Back Seat

In a motor vehicle crash, there are three collisions: the car's collision, the human collision, and the human body's internal collision. Sitting in the back can protect you from a frontal car collision, but unbelted occupants are still traveling at the vehicle's original speed when they slam into some part of the vehicle's interior during the human collision after the vehicle stops. Unbelted occupants colliding with each other, sometimes with fatal force, also cause many serious injuries.

I Don't Have to Wear My Safety Belt, My Car's Equipped with Air Bags

Air bags were designed to supplement safety belts, not replace them. They provide little protection in side, rear, and rollover crashes since frontal impacts activate them. Not wearing your seat belt can put you in the wrong place at the wrong time when your air bag deploys, possibly causing serious injury or even death.

If I'm Thrown Clear of the Crash, My Chances of Survival Increase

Wrong! You are much more likely to be killed or injured if you are thrown from the car. In fatal crashes, 73% of passenger car occupants who were ejected from the car were killed. The forces in a collision can be great enough to throw a person as far as 150 feet (about 15 car lengths).

I'm Pregnant. The Seat Belt Will Hurt My Baby

By protecting the mother, the baby has the best chance of surviving a crash. Pregnant women should always wear the lap and shoulder belt with the lap belt firmly placed under the belly and across the hips.

Other Facts You Should Know about Seat Belts

- Not buckling up contributes to more fatalities than any other behavior.

- Every 14 seconds someone in America is injured in a traffic crash. Every 12 minutes, someone is killed.

- Seat belts and child safety seats work. Yet, fewer than 40 percent of both adults and children who died in traffic crashes were properly restrained.

- The average age of death from all causes was 71 years. The average age of death for people killed in motor vehicle crashes was 40.

- Research shows that 70 percent of the time if the driver is unbuckled, children riding in that vehicle won't be restrained either.

- In a 30 mile per hour crash, an unbuckled child is hit with a force equivalent to falling from a third-story window.

- On-the-job crashes cost employers almost $22,000 per crash and $110,000 per injury.

- Increasing the national seat belt use rate to 90 percent would prevent an estimated 5,536 fatalities, 132,670 injuries, and save the nation $8.8 billion annually including $356 million in Medicare and Medicaid.

- The lap belt should be adjusted so it is low across the hips and pelvis, never across the stomach. Adjust the belt so it is snug. The shoulder belt should cross the chest and collarbone and be snug. The belt should never cross the front of the neck or face. Do not add excessive slack (more than one inch) into the shoulder belt.

- Your seat belts cannot work properly if you have the seat back in a reclined position or if you are slouched in your seat. The shoulder belt will not be against your chest and the lap belt could ride up over your stomach. For the best protection, keep the seat upright and sit back in the seat. Do not put the shoulder belt behind your back or under your arms. Your head and chest could strike the steering wheel, the dashboard, or the back of the front seat. You could break ribs and be seriously hurt.

- Restrain infants and children in age- and size-appropriate child safety seats. Safety belts do not provide the best protection.

- The best place for a child is in the back seat whether or not the car has air bags. Children who cannot be properly secured by the adult belt system should be restrained in a booster seat to help the adult belt fit.

Occupant Protection

Injuries from motor vehicles crashes are the number one cause of death for young people, the number one cause of on-the-job fatalities, and the third largest cause of all deaths in America. In the next ten years of normal driving, most of us will almost certainly be involved in a serious motor vehicle crash. By taking advantage of occupant protection systems, we can greatly improve our chances of surviving a crash without severe or critical injury. Remember we are not saying that seat belts and air bags will save your life and prevent all injuries all of the time, but rather seat belts will greatly increase the odds in your favor of preventing serious injuries or death.

It is important that we can relay to youth what actually happens in a crash while trying to be descriptive as possible. If we can effectively relay this information to youth they will understand the significance of occupant protection.

473

The Three Collisions of a Crash

Crash # 1, the car's collision. The first collision causes the car to buckle and bend as it hits something and comes to an abrupt stop. The crushing of the front absorbs some of the force of the crash and cushions the rest of the car. As a result, the passenger compartment comes to a more gradual stop than the front of the car and is relatively undamaged by the crash. The important thing to relay is that the passenger compartment most always remains intact and can potentially allow a crash to be a survivable crash.

Crash #2, the human collision. The human collision is when the car's occupants hit some part of the vehicle. This is where the law of physics comes into play once again. If the car was traveling 50 miles per hour, how fast is the person in the vehicle traveling? At the moment of impact, unbelted occupants are traveling at the vehicle's original speed. Just after the vehicle comes to a complete stop, these unbelted occupants will slam into the steering wheel or the windshield or some other part of the interior of the car. This is the human collision.

Another form of human collision is the person-to-person impact. Unbelted occupants colliding with each other cause many serious injuries. In a crash, occupants tend to move toward the point of impact, not away from it. Rear seat passengers who have become high-speed projectiles often strike people in the front seat. Occupants smash heads, sometimes with fatal force. Children held in an adult's lap are crushed against the dashboard. In a side collision, a person can crash into nearby passengers and force them out a window or door. In a 30-mile-per-hour crash, an occupant strikes the interior of the car with a force of several thousand pounds.

Crash # 3, the internal collision. Even after the occupant's body comes to a complete stop, the internal organs are still moving forward. Suddenly, these organs hit other organs or the skeletal system. This third collision, the internal collision, often causes considerable and potentially fatal injury. When the head collides with the windshield or the dashboard, the brain hits the inside of the skull. The result may only be a mild concussion, but, in many cases, blood vessels are broken or the brain is bruised and torn. These injuries to the brain can cause permanent brain damage. Motor vehicle crashes account for about 45.2 percent of all spinal cord injuries reported. Almost one-third of these cases result in partial paralysis. Of the known causes of epilepsy, head trauma such as that received in an automobile crash is one of the most frequently identified.

Section 52.3

Helping Your Child Avoid Prom Night Drunk Driving

Excerpted from Julia Rosien "A Prom Night Plan: Working with Your Child to Avoid the Perils of Drunk Driving," Teenagers Today/iParenting, http:// teenagerstoday.com/resources/articles/promplan.htm, 2001.

Alcohol related crashes kill more people ages 16 to 20 than any other age group. Nearly half of all fatal car accidents involve alcohol, according to the National Highway Traffic Safety Act (NHTSA). Parents and school officials are looking for a way to drive home the idea that alcohol and cars don't mix.

Teenagers, parents, and teachers know the enemy. Whether they call it "Prom Safe Ride Home," "Prom Promise," or "Lock-In," it all adds up to the same thing: banding together to eliminate drunk driving. And the numbers show that it may be working. The NHTSA says that fatalities are dropping slowly—but they still have a long way to fall.

What's Turning the Tide?

Prom Safe Ride Home

At Lake Washington High School in Seattle, parents and community volunteers meet at Overlake Hospital and wait for the calls to come in on prom night. Calling before 2 a.m. ensures a safe, free, nonjudgmental ride home for teenagers in at-risk situations. This program is so successful for the community that organizers now provide it for all major school functions.

Not every kid reaches for the phone when a friend has the keys and is too intoxicated to drive. Groups like M.A.D.D. (Mothers Against Drunk Driving), and S.A.D.D. (Students Against Drunk Driving), go to schools to teach kids how to stay out of situations over which they have no control. Members give kids information and support to make the right choices when it comes to drinking and driving.

Lock-in

By far the most popular program across the country is the post-prom party that lasts all night. At North Little Rock High School (NLRHS) students pay $5 each for the post-prom party, which includes a T-shirt, all the food and drinks (non-alcoholic) they want and "play" money to buy prizes until dawn.

Linda Harper, guidance secretary at NLRHS, estimates that three quarters of the seniors go to the post-prom party. "No one may leave and come back in," Harper says. "It's a firm rule." The prizes at the end of the evening encourage everyone to stay for the whole party. The big prize is $500 cash, and one year they offered 20 cash prizes of $100 each. Organizers also draw names for microwaves, dorm re-frigerators, televisions and stereo "boxes"—things kids heading off to university or college always need. "Every year it gets bigger and better," Harper says. "The students love it!"

After the all-night bash, parents invite the kids at NLRHS into their homes for a big breakfast. Because so many students partici-pate, they influence each other and more get involved each year.

Paramount Canada's Wonderland

Heather Bushwald graduated from Burford District High school in Ontario with great memories of an entire night spent at an amuse-ment park. "We [student council] wanted to do something really dif-ferent and when Canada's Wonderland started this program, we knew it was the one for us."

Bushwald's high school is one of many that choose an alternative to the glitz and glamour of a formal prom. The night is open to all schools in Ontario. All kids must arrive and leave the park by bus. Check in time is 6 p.m., departure time is 5 a.m., and the park gates are locked at night.

The park is closed to the public and many companies set up booths giving freebies to the kids. Karaoke, a live band and all-night rides add to the fun and excitement. The flat-rate entry fee supplies kids with food coupons to last the night.

The fact that organizers searched bags before entry didn't bother most kids. "It made us feel safe knowing that no one could smuggle drugs or alcohol into the park," Bushwald says. One classmate had prescription sleeping pills in her purse and they were confiscated. "It's no different than going to a concert," she says. "You just don't bring that kind of stuff."

Staging a Mock Crash

Students at Glen Rock High School in Glen Rock, NJ, feel their mock demonstrations are successful with their peers. It's real education before the big night.

A week before the prom, the staged accident involves a smashed car and students looking hurt or dead. Paramedics arrive and start cleaning up the bodies, as students look on. Rescue workers bring out the body bags, and the reality of drinking and driving is instantly realized. Some kids scoff, believing it could never happen to them. But many take it seriously.

Catherine Nauccme's kids thought the whole thing was hokey at first. "They heard the words of the drink and drive campaign, sloughed it off as 'corny' but the visual, thankfully, stayed with them." It's just not cool to be bleeding on the hood of a crashed car.

Leaving It up to the Parents

In areas where there is no organized effort to deter drinking and driving on prom night, parents may be required to tackle the issue themselves.

Barbara Mullins of North Little Rock Arkansas says her daughter's school does nothing she's aware of about the issue of drinking and driving. Mullins isn't worried about her daughter as much as she's worried about the other kids who may be drinking and driving. "We've invited her boyfriend [who lives across the state] to come for the weekend and I'll drive them or they'll go with other kids in a rented limo." Mullins hopes there won't be drinking, but fears there may be, so she involves herself and makes sure her daughter knows she is there for her. "Apparently, [school officials] feel that holding the prom is enough."

Section 52.4

Drowsy Driving

This section contains text from "Educating Youth about Sleep and Drowsy Driving Strategy Development Workshop Report," http://www.nhlbi.nih.gov/ health/prof/sleep/dwydrv_y.pdf, September 1998, and "Awake at the Wheel," http:/ /www.nhlbi.nih.gov/health/public/sleep/aaw/brochure.pdf, National Heart, Lung, and Blood Institute (NHLBI), National Institutes of Health (NIH).

It is now recognized that sleep is obligatory and getting optimal sleep enhances performance, cognition, and mood. Major developmental trends occur during adolescence, including (1) a decrease in the amount of sleep obtained, (2) a delay in the timing of sleep (going to bed later), and (3) an increase in the school night/ weekend night discrepancy in the sleep schedule. Numerous psychosocial and biological factors influence the sleep patterns of adolescents, including parents, peers, jobs, and school:

- Parents' role changes during their child's teen years. Parents of pre-adolescents usually set bedtimes. By the time their children are of high school age, parents retreat from setting bedtimes and instead focus on waking them in the morning. Parents may think that older children need less sleep than they did previously, when in fact they need at least as much or more sleep.

- Peers may influence the amount of sleep obtained relative to social activities, television viewing, and the Internet.

- Careful sociological studies indicate that most teens work to buy personal consumables (such as clothing) and to pay for entertainment, rather than to contribute to family income. Most are employed in entry-level positions or in jobs requiring unskilled labor. Many teens work on the weekends and on weeknights after school. Those who work 20 or more hours per week tend to have a later bedtime, shorter sleep periods, more falling asleep in class, and more oversleeping.

- For most teens, the school start time means a nonnegotiable wake-up time. Most adolescents would sleep significantly longer if they could. Preliminary data indicate a trend over the past 25 years toward earlier school start times, with high schools starting earlier than middle and elementary schools.

New studies show that the well-known adolescent sleep patterns of going to bed later and rising later may have a biological as well as a psychosocial basis. A study with sixth graders showed a preference for phase delay that is related to puberty. Recent data indicate that the circadian clock in adolescence is "ticking" somewhat slower than that in adults, thereby accounting for the phase-delay preference.

One field study showed that many 10th graders attending school at 7:20 a.m. were sleepy, and some had sleep abnormalities similar to those seen in narcolepsy. Another recent study evaluated the amount that teens slept during the school week. The average amount of sleep was about 61/ 2 hours, with the longest sleeper getting less than 8 hours. There was some increase in weekend sleep, but not enough to compensate fully.

When a person does not get enough sleep, even on one night, a "sleep debt" begins to build and increases until enough sleep is obtained. Problem sleepiness occurs as the debt accumulates. If too much sleep has been lost, sleeping in on the weekend may not completely reverse the effects of not getting enough sleep during the week. In general, pre-adolescents may be getting sufficient sleep, particularly if parents help "protect" sleep times. Older adolescents, however, are staying up later, rising earlier, and incurring sleep debts. As a result, teachers end up with sleepy students, and teens live under a "dark cloud of insufficient sleep" that may include microsleeps, attention lapses, decreased reaction times, impaired divergent thinking skills, impaired mental functioning, low mood, and a higher rate of accidents and injuries.

Drowsy Driving and Teens

There is a discrepancy between police-reported crash data and self-reported data. Police-reported data show that drowsy driving-related crashes comprise 1 percent of all crashes and 4 percent of crashes in which a fatality occurs. The number of self-reported drowsy driving-related crashes is much higher. Some of the factors that likely contribute to this discrepancy include:

- Not all sleep-related crashes are reported to the police, since many are drive-off-the-road crashes.

- Police may not recognize the crash as drowsy-driving related.

- Police may be reluctant to code a crash as the "fall-asleep" sort without physical evidence to support it in court.

- Standardized reporting for drowsy driving does not exist.

Data from a 1995 study conducted in North Carolina showed the following characteristics of crashes that police attributed to the driver falling asleep:

- Crashes were predominantly drive-off-the-road types.

- Crashes were often serious because no corrective action was taken.

- The times of occurrence were late at night and mid-afternoon (siesta time).

The data from this study further showed that most of the crashes were predominantly among young people. Fifty-five percent of all crashes occurred among those under age 26. There was a difference in the time of occurrence of these crashes among drivers of different ages. A major risk group that was identified comprises young males driving alone at night.

Awake at the Wheel

Advice for Teens

You have school and homework. Sports and clubs. Friends and family. And an after-school job. Who has time for sleep? Who needs sleep anyway? Believe it or not, you do. As a teen, you actually need more sleep than younger kids: about nine hours every night. Like most teens, you probably sleep only about six. You wake up tired, and you stay that way. Do you think that's okay—that you'll be fine, just like everyone else? No way! Here's why: When you don't get the sleep you need, you start to get drowsy in class, at work, at parties, and behind the wheel of your car. That's where lack of sleep can really hurt you and others. The solution is simple—crash in bed, not on the road. Go to bed earlier. Take a nap if you're sleepy. Sleep late when you can.

Top Five Reasons to Get Enough Sleep

- Drowsy drivers can crash their cars. Crashes disfigure, disable, and kill drivers, passengers, or pedestrians.

- Drowsy teens react more slowly and perform worse in sports than well-rested teens.

- Drowsy teens do poorly in school and have problems socially.

- Drowsy teens have trouble making good decisions.

- Drowsy teens don t look their best.

Many teens need at least 9 hours of sleep per night. More than younger kids, and more than adults. But most teens get less than 6.5 hours of sleep. If most teens is you, you're probably sleepy most of the time.

When kids hit puberty, their internal clocks change: that's why teens just naturally want to go to bed late and sleep late in the morning! Teenagers have more responsibilities than younger kids. And, between school, homework, jobs, sports and a social life, it is difficult for them to get enough sleep.

Brianne

Brianne is a 17-year-old junior who lives in the suburbs. She's a good student, a member of the high school basketball team, and is very socially active. She stayed up late studying for mid-terms, got to school at 7:30 a.m., finished basketball practice at 4:00 p.m., then drove a friend home from practice. Now it s 6:00 p.m., and she's heading home on the freeway. After a 20-minute drive, she suddenly realizes she missed the exit to her house and doesn't remember driving the last few miles.

What could have happened to Brianne while she was on auto-pilot? How could she have avoided this dangerous situation?

Pete

Pete is 18, and thinking about graduation. He works after school at the mall to make money for college. His older brother is at the state university, about two hours from home; and Pete's planning a weekend road trip starting tonight. After a short night of sleep he goes to school, works for about 4 hours at his job, and grabs a bite to eat. Then, he and his girlfriend, Shelley, jump in the car and head toward the university. It's already 8:00 p.m. Shelley falls asleep, and after about 30 minutes, Pete realizes that he's exhausted, too. A few minutes later, he's startled into alertness as he hits the rumble strips along the shoulder of the highway. How could Pete have avoided this dangerous situation? What should he do now?

Adam

Adam is 17, and has just received his license. His parents have given him a strict 11:00 p.m. curfew. It s now 1:30 a.m., and after a long day, he's about to leave a party at a friend's house. Feeling alert, he jumps behind the wheel of the family car with his best friend Chris in the passenger seat. A few minutes later, Chris yells, "Hit the brakes!" just as Adam, with his eyes closed, is about to drift through a red light.

Teenagers Should Know

- The only way to prevent drowsy driving is to get enough sleep on a regular basis.

- It's possible to build up a big sleep debt by sleeping too few hours for too many days on end. You can't pay off the sleep debt in just one night or day. It can take days to get back to normal.

- Most sleepiness-related crashes happen between 2 a.m. and 6 a.m. (during normal sleeping hours).

- There is only one sure-fire way to wake yourself up when you're sleepy: take a 15–20 minute nap before driving.

- Getting a good night's sleep before a long drive can save your life.

- Traveling with a friend who's awake can help keep you awake. But, a sleeping friend is no help at all.

- Rolling down a window to get some air, stretching your legs, or even cranking up the radio are almost useless when you're trying to stay awake.

- One beer, when someone is sleep-deprived, will hit as hard as two or three beers when one is well rested.

- Drinking caffeine (a caffeinated soft drink, coffee, or tea) before hitting the road may help for a short time, but it can also be a problem. Caffeine can make you lose sleep, which leads to more sleepiness!

Section 52.5

Motorcycle Transportation Safety

This section includes text from "A Comprehensive Approach to Motorcycle Safety," http://www.nhtsa.dot.gov/people/injury/pedbimot/safebike/approach.html, and "Motorcycle Helmets Are Effective in Preventing Serious Brain Injuries," http://www.nhtsa.dot.gov/people/injury/pedbimot/safebike/preventing.html, National Highway Traffic Safety Administration (NHTSA), February 1999, and "Transportation Safety" Brain Injury Association Inc., http://www.biausa.org/transportation_factsheet_10-01.pdf, April 2001. Reprinted with permission.

A Comprehensive Approach to Motorcycle Safety

Traffic crashes are a leading cause of death and disability in the United States. Motorcycle crashes claim the lives of over 2,100 riders each year. Per mile traveled, motorcyclists are 16 times more likely than passenger car occupants to die in a traffic crash and about four times as likely to be injured. While only 20 percent of car crashes result in injury or death, that figure jumps to an astounding 80 percent for motorcycle crashes.

Injury Prevention Components

Despite the best prevention efforts, motorcycle crashes do occur. The majority of the crashes with other vehicles are not the motorcyclist's fault. During a crash, the most important factor in reducing injury is personal protection for the motorcyclist. Leather jackets, gloves, trousers, proper footwear, eye protection, and helmets provide this personal protection. Helmets are by far the motorcycle rider's most important safety equipment because they protect against injuries to the head and brain.

Why Is Injury Prevention Important During a Crash?

- More than 80 percent of all reported motorcycle crashes result in injury or death to the motorcyclist.

- Head injury is a leading cause of death and serious injury in motorcycle crashes, which is why helmets that meet or exceed federal safety standards should always be worn.

- Research studies show that motorcycle helmets are 29 percent effective in preventing fatal injuries and 67 percent effective in preventing serious brain injury.

Clearly riders need protection when a crash occurs! However, a helmet only works if a motorcyclist wears it, and the most effective means of increasing helmet usage is by enacting helmet laws that cover all riders—universal motorcycle helmet laws.

Rapid Emergency Response

After a crash has occurred, an injured rider's life can depend on rapid and appropriate emergency medical response. Emergency medical service personnel provide life support at the scene and during transport to the optimal emergency care facility. Injury severity and time are critical to survival. Wearing a motorcycle helmet lessens the severity of head injuries and may give the emergency response team the extra time needed to save a life.

Motorcycle Helmets Are Effective in Preventing Serious Brain Injuries

Helmets prevent brain injury. Motorcycle helmets save lives and prevent devastating and debilitating head injuries. Motorcyclists who ride without helmets run a significantly greater risk of death or permanent injury. The U.S. General Accounting Office (GAO) has the data that prove it.

Motorcycle Safety

- In 1996, 51% of motorcycle drivers between the ages of 15 to 20 who were fatally injured in crashes were not wearing helmets.

- In 1999, 2,470 motorcyclists were killed and an additional 50,000 were injured in traffic crashes in the United States.

- More than 80% of all motorcycle crashes result in injury or death to the motorcyclist.

- Brain injury is the leading cause of death in motorcycle crashes. Wearing a helmet can substantially reduce the severity of or prevent these injuries.

- A single motorcyclist who sustains a brain injury can cost a state more than $2 million for care and support services over a lifetime.

Chapter 53

Helping Adolescents Cope with Violence and Disasters

The National Institute of Mental Health has joined with other Federal agencies to address the issue of reducing school violence and assisting children who have been victims of or witnesses to violent events. Nationally reported school shootings such as those that occurred in Bethel, Alaska; Pearl, Mississippi; West Paducah, Kentucky; Jonesboro, Arkansas; Edinboro, Pennsylvania; Springfield, Oregon; and Littleton, Colorado have shocked the country. Many questions are being asked about how these tragedies could have been prevented, how those directly involved can be helped, and how we can avoid such events in the future.

Research has shown that both adults and children who experience catastrophic events show a wide range of reactions. Some suffer only worries and bad memories that fade with emotional support and the passage of time. Others are more deeply affected and experience long-term problems. Research on post-traumatic stress disorder (PTSD) shows that some soldiers, survivors of criminal victimization, torture and other violence, and survivors of natural and man-made catastrophes suffer long-term effects from their experiences. Children who have witnessed violence in their families, schools, or communities are also vulnerable to serious long-term problems. Their emotional reactions, including fear, depression, withdrawal or anger, can occur immediately or some time after the tragic event. Youngsters who have experienced a

Excerpted from "Helping Children and Adolescents Cope with Violence and Disasters" National Institute of Mental Health (NIMH), National Institutes of Health (NIH), NIH Pub. No. 99-3518, http://www.nimh.nih.gov/publicat/violence.cfm, page last updated January 13, 2000.

catastrophic event often need support from parents and teachers to avoid long-term emotional harm. Most will recover in a short time, but the minority who develop PTSD or other persistent problems need treatment.

The school shootings caught the Nation's attention, but these events are only a small fraction of the many tragic episodes that affect children's lives. Each year many children and adolescents sustain injuries from violence, lose friends or family members, or are adversely affected by witnessing a violent or catastrophic event. Each situation is unique, whether it centers upon a plane crash where many people are killed, automobile accidents involving friends or family members, or natural disasters such as Hurricane Andrew where deaths occur and homes are lost. But these events have similarities as well, and cause similar reactions in children. Helping young people avoid or overcome emotional problems in the wake of violence or disaster is one of the most important challenges a parent, teacher, or mental health professional can face. The purpose of this chapter is to tell what is known about the impact of violence and disasters on children and suggest steps to minimize long-term emotional harm.

Trauma—What Is It?

Trauma includes emotional as well as physical experiences and injuries. Emotional injury is essentially a normal response to an extreme event. It involves the creation of emotional memories, which arise through a long-lasting effect on structures deep within the brain. The more direct the exposure to the traumatic event, the higher the risk for emotional harm. Thus in a school shooting, the student who is injured probably will be most severely affected emotionally. And the student who sees a classmate shot, even killed, probably will be more emotionally affected than the student who was in another part of the school when the violence occurred. But even second-hand exposure to violence can be traumatic. For this reason, all children and adolescents exposed to violence or a disaster, even if only through graphic media reports, should be watched for signs of emotional distress. In addition to this psychiatric definition, trauma also has a medical definition, which refers to a serious or critical bodily injury, wound, or shock, often treated with trauma medicine practiced in emergency rooms.

How Adolescents React to Trauma

Reactions to trauma may appear immediately after the traumatic event or days and even weeks later. Loss of trust in adults and fear of the event occurring again are responses seen in many children and adolescents who have been exposed to traumatic events. Other reactions vary according to age:

Children 6 to 11 years old may show extreme withdrawal, disruptive behavior, and/or inability to pay attention. Regressive behaviors, nightmares, sleep problems, irrational fears, irritability, refusal to attend school, outbursts of anger and fighting are also common in traumatized children of this age. Also the child may complain of stomach aches or other bodily symptoms that have no medical basis. School work often suffers. Depression, anxiety, feelings of guilt and emotional numbing or "flatness" are often present as well.

Adolescents 12 to 17 years old may exhibit responses similar to those of adults, including flashbacks, nightmares, emotional numbing, avoidance of any reminders of the traumatic event, depression, substance abuse, problems with peers, and anti-social behavior. Also common are withdrawal and isolation, physical complaints, suicidal thoughts, school avoidance, academic decline, sleep disturbances, and confusion. The adolescent may feel extreme guilt over his or her failure to prevent injury or loss of life, and may harbor revenge fantasies that interfere with recovery from the trauma.

Some youngsters are more vulnerable to trauma than others, for reasons scientists don't fully understand. It has been shown that the impact of a traumatic event is likely to be greatest in the child or adolescent who previously has been the victim of child abuse or some other form of trauma, or who already had a mental health problem. And the youngster who lacks family support is more at risk for a poor recovery.

Helping the Child or Adolescent Trauma Victim

Early intervention to help children and adolescents who have suffered trauma from violence or a disaster is critical. Parents, teachers and mental health professionals can do a great deal to help these youngsters recover. Help should begin at the scene of the traumatic event. According to the National Center for Post-Traumatic Stress Disorder of the Department of Veterans Affairs, workers in charge of a disaster scene should:

- Find ways to protect children from further harm and from further exposure to traumatic stimuli. If possible, create a safe haven for them. Protect children from onlookers and the media covering the story.

- When possible, direct children who are able to walk away from the site of violence or destruction, away from severely injured survivors, and away from continuing danger. Kind but firm direction is needed.

- Identify children in acute distress and stay with them until initial stabilization occurs. Acute distress includes panic (marked by trembling, agitation, rambling speech, becoming mute, or erratic behavior) and intense grief (signs include loud crying, rage, or immobility).

- Use a supportive and compassionate verbal or non-verbal exchange (such as a hug, if appropriate) with the child to help him or her feel safe. However brief the exchange, or however temporary, such reassurances are important to children.

After violence or a disaster occurs, the family is the first-line resource for helping. Among the things that parents and other caring adults can do are:

- Explain the episode of violence or disaster as well as you are able.

- Encourage the children to express their feelings and listen without passing judgment. Help younger children learn to use words that express their feelings. However, do not force discussion of the traumatic event.

- Let children and adolescents know that it is normal to feel upset after something bad happens.

- Allow time for the youngsters to experience and talk about their feelings. At home, however, a gradual return to routine can be reassuring to the child.

- If your children are fearful, reassure them that you love them and will take care of them. Stay together as a family as much as possible.

- If behavior at bedtime is a problem, give the child extra time and reassurance. Let him or her sleep with a light on or in your room for a limited time if necessary.

- Reassure children and adolescents that the traumatic event was not their fault.

- Do not criticize regressive behavior or shame the child with words like "babyish."

- Allow children to cry or be sad. Don't expect them to be brave or tough.

- Encourage children and adolescents to feel in control. Let them make some decisions about meals, what to wear, etc.

- Take care of yourself so you can take care of the children.

When violence or disaster affects a whole school or community, teachers and school administrators can play a major role in the healing process. Some of the things educators can do are:

- If possible, give yourself a bit of time to come to terms with the event before you attempt to reassure the children. This may not be possible in the case of a violent episode that occurs at school, but sometimes in a natural disaster there will be several days before schools reopen and teachers can take the time to prepare themselves emotionally.

- Don't try to rush back to ordinary school routines too soon. Give the children or adolescents time to talk over the traumatic event and express their feelings about it.

- Respect the preferences of children who do not want to participate in class discussions about the traumatic event. Do not force discussion or repeatedly bring up the catastrophic event; doing so may re-traumatize children.

- Hold in-school sessions with entire classes, with smaller groups of students, or with individual students. These sessions can be very useful in letting students know that their fears and concerns are normal reactions. Many counties and school districts have teams that will go into schools to hold such sessions after a disaster or episode of violence. Involve mental health professionals in these activities if possible.

- Offer art and play therapy for children in primary school.

- Be sensitive to cultural differences among the children. In some cultures, for example, it is not acceptable to express negative emotions. Also, the child who is reluctant to make eye contact with a teacher may not be depressed, but may simply be exhibiting behavior appropriate to his or her culture.

- Encourage children to develop coping and problem-solving skills and age-appropriate methods for managing anxiety.

- Hold meetings for parents to discuss the traumatic event, their children's response to it, and how they and you can help. Involve mental health professionals in these meetings if possible.

Most children and adolescents, if given support such as that described above, will recover almost completely from the fear and anxiety caused by a traumatic experience within a few weeks. However, some children and adolescents will need more help over a longer period of time in order to heal. Grief over the loss of a loved one, teacher, friend, or pet may take months to resolve, and may be reawakened by reminders such as media reports or the anniversary of the death.

In the immediate aftermath of a traumatic event, and in the weeks following, it is important to identify the youngsters who are in need of more intensive support and therapy because of profound grief or some other extreme emotion. Children who show avoidance and emotional numbing may need the help of a mental health professional, while more common reactions such as re-experiencing the event and hyperarousal (including sleep disturbances and a tendency to be easily startled) may respond to help from parents and teachers.

Post-Traumatic Stress Disorder

As stated earlier, some children and adolescents will have prolonged problems after a traumatic event. These potentially chronic conditions include depression and prolonged grief. Another serious and potentially long-lasting problem is post-traumatic stress disorder (PTSD). This condition is diagnosed when the following symptoms have been present for longer than one month:

- Re-experiencing the event through play or in trauma-specific nightmares or flashbacks, or distress over events that resemble or symbolize the trauma.

- Routine avoidance of reminders of the event or a general lack of responsiveness (e.g., diminished interests or a sense of having a foreshortened future).

- Increased sleep disturbances, irritability, poor concentration, startle reaction and regressive behavior.

Rates of PTSD identified in child and adult survivors of violence and disasters vary widely. For example, estimates range from 2% after a natural disaster (tornado), 28% after an episode of terrorism (mass shooting), and 29% after a plane crash. The disorder may arise weeks or months after the traumatic event. PTSD may resolve without treatment, but some form of therapy by a mental health professional is often required in order for healing to occur. Fortunately, it is more common for a traumatized child or adolescent to have some of the symptoms of PTSD than to develop the full-blown disorder. People differ in their vulnerability to PTSD, and the source of this difference is not known in its entirety.

Research has shown that PTSD clearly alters a number of fundamental brain mechanisms. Because of this, abnormalities have been detected in brain chemicals that affect coping behavior, learning, and memory among people with the disorder. Recent brain imaging studies have detected altered metabolism and blood flow as well as anatomical changes in people with PTSD. Further information on PTSD and research concerning it may be found in the "Additional Help and Information" section of this *Sourcebook*.

Treatment of PTSD

People with PTSD are treated with specialized forms of psychotherapy and sometimes with medications or a combination of the two. One of the forms of psychotherapy shown to be effective is cognitive/behavioral therapy, or CBT. In CBT, the patient is taught methods of overcoming anxiety or depression and modifying undesirable behaviors such as avoidance. The therapist helps the patient examine and re-evaluate beliefs that are interfering with healing, such as the belief that the traumatic event will happen again. Children who undergo CBT are taught to avoid "catastrophizing." For example, they are reassured that dark clouds do not necessarily mean another hurricane, that the fact that someone is angry doesn't necessarily mean that another shooting is imminent, etc. Play therapy and art therapy also can help younger children to remember the traumatic event safely and express their feelings about it. Other forms of psychotherapy that have been found to help persons with PTSD include group and exposure therapy. A reasonable period of time for treatment of PTSD is 6 to 12 weeks with occasional follow-up sessions, but treatment may be longer depending on a patient's particular circumstances. Research has shown that support from family and friends can be an important part of recovery and that involving people in group discussion very soon after a catastrophic event may reduce some of the symptoms of PTSD.

There has been a good deal of research on the use of medications for adults with PTSD, including research on the formation of emotionally charged memories and medications that may help to block the development of symptoms. Medications appear to be useful in reducing overwhelming symptoms of arousal (such as sleep disturbances and an exaggerated startle reflex), intrusive thoughts, and avoidance; reducing accompanying conditions such as depression and panic; and improving impulse control and related behavioral problems. Research is just beginning on the use of medications to treat PTSD in children and adolescents. There is preliminary evidence that psychotherapy focused on trauma and grief, in combination with selected medications, can be effective in alleviating PTSD symptoms and accompanying depression. More medication treatment research is needed to increase our knowledge of how best to treat children who have PTSD.

A mental health professional with special expertise in the area of child and adolescent trauma is the best person to help a youngster with PTSD. Organizations on the accompanying resource list may help you to find such a specialist in your geographical area.

What Are Scientists Learning about Trauma in Children and Adolescents?

The National Institute of Mental Health (NIMH), a part of the Federal Government's National Institutes of Health, supports research on the brain and a wide range of mental disorders, including PTSD and related conditions. The Department of Veterans Affairs also conducts research in this area with adults and their family members.

Recent research findings include:

- Some studies show that counseling children very soon after a catastrophic event may reduce some of the symptoms of PTSD. A study of 12,000 schoolchildren who lived through a hurricane in Hawaii found that those who got counseling early on were doing much better two years later than those who did not.

- Parents' responses to a violent event or disaster strongly influence their children's ability to recover. This is particularly true for mothers of young children. If the mother is depressed or highly anxious, she may need to get emotional support or counseling in order to be able to help her child.

- Community violence can have a profound effect on teachers as well as students. One study of Head Start teachers who lived through the 1992 Los Angeles riots showed that 7% had severe post-traumatic stress symptoms, and 29% had moderate symptoms. Children also were acutely affected by the violence and anxiety around them. They were more aggressive and noisy and less likely to be obedient or get along with each other.

- PTSD is often accompanied by depression. In a group of teenage school students who survived a terrorist shooting in Brooklyn, New York, 4 of the 11 survivors interviewed had both PTSD and depression. In another study, this one involving adults, depression occurred in 44.5% of PTSD patients at 1 month after the traumatic event and in 43.2% at 4 months. Depression must be treated along with PTSD in these instances, and early treatment is best.

- Either being exposed to violence within the home for an extended period of time or exposure to a one-time event like an attack by a dog can cause PTSD in a child. Some scientists believe that younger children are more likely to develop the disorder than older ones.

- Inner-city children experience the greatest exposure to violence. A study of young adolescent boys from inner-city Chicago showed that 68% had seen someone beaten up and 22.5% had seen someone shot or killed. Youngsters who had been exposed to community violence were more likely to exhibit aggressive behavior or depression within the following year.

NIMH-supported scientists are continuing to conduct research into the impact of violence and disaster on children and adolescents. For example, one study will follow 6,000 Chicago children from 80 different neighborhoods over a period of several years. It will examine the emotional, social and academic effects of exposure to violence. In some of the children, the researchers will look at the role of stress hormones in a child or adolescent's response to traumatic experiences. Another study will deal specifically with the victims of school violence, attempting to determine what places children at risk for victimization at school and what factors protect them. It is particularly important to conduct research to discover which individual, family, school and community interventions work best for children and adolescents exposed to violence or disaster, and to find out whether it is possible for a well-intended but ill-designed intervention to set the youngsters back by keeping the trauma alive in their minds. Through research, NIMH hopes to gain knowledge to lessen the suffering that violence and disasters impose on children and adolescents and their families.

Chapter 54

Physical Abuse

Chapter Contents

Section 54.1

A Guide to Understanding Abuse and Harassment

Excerpted from "Fair Play Means Safety for All, A Parents' and Guardians' Guide to Understanding Abuse & Harassment," Canadian Hockey Association, 2001. Contributors to this text include Judi Fairholm, National Coordinator of the Canadian Red Cross Abuse Prevention Services, and Sally Spilhaus, Advisor, Rights and Responsibilities, Concordia University in Montreal Quebec. Reprinted with permission.

What Does Safety for My Child Mean?

We all want our children to be safe—keeping them safe means putting the child's best interests first. This means ensuring that the young player is treated with respect and integrity—emotionally, socially, intellectually, physically, culturally, and spiritually.

When Is My Child Unsafe?

Young people are unsafe when someone uses his or her power or position to harm them either emotionally, physically and/or sexually— this is ABUSE!! Your child's safety is also at risk when she or he is threatened, intimidated, taunted or subjected to racial slurs by a peer—this is HARASSMENT! Harassment can also occur when an adult discriminates against a youth.

What Is Emotional Abuse?

Emotional abuse is a chronic attack on a child's self esteem; it is psychologically destructive behavior by a person in a position of power, authority or trust. It can take the form of name calling, threatening, ridiculing, intimidating, isolating, hazing, or ignoring a child's needs! It is not:

- benching a player for disciplinary reasons
- cutting a player from a team after tryouts

498

- refusing to transfer a player
- limiting ice time
- yelling instructions from the bench

What Is Physical Abuse?

Physical abuse is when a person in a position of power or trust purposefully injures or threatens to injure a child or youth. This may take the form of slapping, hitting, shaking, kicking, pulling hair or ears, striking, shoving, grabbing, hazing or excessive exercise as a form of punishment.

What Is Neglect?

Neglect is the chronic inattention to the basic necessities of life such as clothing, shelter, nutritious diet, education, good hygiene, supervision, medical and dental care, adequate rest, safe environment, moral guidance and discipline, exercise, and fresh air. This may occur when injuries are not adequately treated, players are made to play with injuries, equipment is inadequate or unsafe, or road trips are not properly supervised.

What Is Sexual Abuse?

Sexual abuse is when a young person is used by an older child, adolescent, or adult for his or her own sexual stimulation or gratification. There are two categories:

Contact

- touched and fondled in sexual areas
- forced to touch another person's sexual areas
- kissed or held in a sexual manner
- forced to perform oral sex
- vaginal or anal intercourse
- vaginal or anal penetration with object or finger
- sexually oriented hazing

Non Contact

- obscene calls/obscene remarks on computer or in notes
- voyeurism

- shown pornography
- forced to watch sexual acts
- sexually intrusive questions or comments
- indecent exposure
- forced to pose for sexual photographs or videos
- forced to self-masturbate
- forced to watch others masturbate

What Is Harassment?

Harassment is a behavior which is insulting, humiliating, malicious, degrading or offensive. Harassment can be a pattern of behavior, a "chilly" or "hostile" environment or a single event. Dealing with harassment can sometimes be difficult, as what is viewed as harassment by one person may be viewed as a joke by another person. But it is the impact of the behavior on the victim that is the most critical, not the intention of the person who is doing the harassing.

Like abuse, harassment is the misuse of power. Harassment can be non-criminal or criminal and falls into three categories: personal, sexual, or abuse of power and authority.

Personal Harassment

Personal harassment is any unwelcome behavior that degrades, demeans, humiliates, or embarrasses a person, and that a reasonable person should have known would be unwelcome. Examples are written or verbal abuse or threats, practical jokes which cause embarrassment or endanger a person's safety, discriminating against a person, or use of degrading words to describe someone.

Sexual Harassment

Sexual harassment is unwelcome behavior of a sexual nature that negatively affects the person or the environment. Examples are questions about one's sex life, sexual staring, sexual comments, unwanted touching, persistence in asking someone for a date even after they have said "No," and sexual assault.

Abuse of Power or Authority

Abuse of power or authority is when someone uses the power of their position or authority to negatively control, influence, discriminate or embarrass another person. Examples are displays of favoritism or dis-favoritism, subtle put-downs, or ostracism.

What Is Hazing?

Hazing is a humiliating and degrading initiation rite in which a player is forced to participate in order to be accepted.

How Do I Know When My Children Are Being Abused or Harassed?

- by listening to them
- by believing them
- by observing them
- by watching their interactions with others
- by being aware of sudden changes in their behavior and/or anger in them
- by questioning unexplained bruises, marks on their faces, back, thighs, upper arms, heads, buttocks, genital areas

Recognizing Abusive and Vulnerable Situations

Who Would Hurt My Child?

Unfortunately, it is usually someone both you and your child know and trust.

- Harassers are usually peers who are insecure and want to feel power.
- Emotional and physical abusers have limited interpersonal skills and use their anger against children and youth.
- Sexual offenders "groom" children and youth by establishing trust relationships and then using them for sexual gratification.

Sexual offenders are/can be:

- most often male but may be female
- heterosexual, homosexual, or bisexual

- an older child, adolescent, or adult
- found in all levels of society and in all cultures
- either infrequent offenders or pedophiles who are fixated on children as sexual objects
- prone to rationalize and minimize their abusive behavior

Where is my child most at risk for all types of abuse? Basically your child is most vulnerable when he/she is alone with another person—this could be in the sports arena, dressing room, car, bus, home, office, outside—anywhere!! In some situations, such as hazing, they are vulnerable in a group setting where there is inadequate supervision.

Recognizing Coping Mechanisms

How Do Children and Youth Cope with the Trauma of Abuse and Harassment?

- some pretend it never happened
- others convince themselves that it wasn't so terrible
- many find excuses as to why it happened
- some blame themselves
- some develop physiological defenses—headaches, body pains, and illnesses
- others escape through drugs, alcohol, food, or sex
- a few try to hide from their pain by being perfect

Why Do Kids Not Tell?

They may:

- be frightened
- believe they are responsible
- not want to get the offender into trouble
- be embarrassed and ashamed
- think no-one will believe them
- worry that they will not be allowed to play hockey

Identifying Parents' and Guardians' Role

What Do I Do If a Child or Youth Tells Me He/She Is Being Harassed?

- listen
- believe
- talk with your coach or officials
- help the young person to learn effective ways of responding
- if it is mild harassment, try to resolve the situation informally
- if it is moderate or serious harassment, refer the complaint as specified in your organization's policy
- give the child or youth continuous support

How Do I Protect My Child or Youth against Hazing?

- talk with him/her about hazing; discuss peer pressure
- explain that he/she does not have to submit to hazing
- report it

What Do I Do If a Child or Youth Tells Me about an Abusive Situation?

Do:

- listen—take the time to hear what he/she is saying
- believe—"I believe you"
- reassure—"It's not your fault!"
- report—contact the appropriate authorities and make a report
- support—provide ongoing support to help the child or youth deal with the trauma of abuse
- take action—do not let the child or youth stay in a vulnerable situation

Don't:

- react with shock, horror or disbelief—even though you may feel like it

- promise to keep a secret—you are legally bound to report
- promise "everything will be fine"—there are many problems to resolve, it will take time
- assume the child or youth hates the abuser—there may be conflicting feelings
- put the responsibility of reporting on someone else—they may not do it
- press the child or youth for details—the matter may go to court, so it is important that evidence is not contaminated

What Do I Do If I Suspect My Child Is Being Abused?

- document your observations
- record behaviors, dates, times and people involved
- identify vulnerable situations and be there to protect your child
- seek advice or information about abuse from a knowledgeable person
- tell your child your concerns
- listen to your child's fears about the situation
- do not promise that "everything will be fine"
- report if your suspicions are strong
- keep it confidential; do not get caught in the "rumor mill"
- support your child

Recognizing Legal Responsibilities

What Is My Legal Responsibility in Reporting Abuse?

Anyone who has reasonable grounds to suspect that a youth is, or may be suffering, or may have suffered from emotional, physical abuse and neglect and/or sexual abuse should immediately report the suspicion and the information on which it is based to the local child protection agency and/or the local police detachment.

When I Report, What Questions Will Be Asked?

- the child's name, address, age, sex, and birth date
- parents'/guardians' names and addresses

- the name and address of alleged offender
- details of the incident(s) that prompted your report
- your name and address

What Happens When a Report Is Made?

- A social worker or police officer will decide if an investigation is needed.
- If the child is "at risk" and needs protection, an investigation is started as soon as possible.
- An experienced interviewer will conduct the interview.
- The primary concern is safety of the child.
- The social worker and/or police officer will decide what further action is required.

Why Don't People Report?

They don't report because they:

- are unaware of the reporting laws
- believe that they can take care of the problem themselves—it's their own business
- are fearful of retaliation from the abuser—or are friends with the abuser
- find it hard to believe
- assume someone else will make a report
- don't want "to tell" on someone
- want to protect their child from questions and embarrassment
- are not sure where or how to make a report
- just want it "all to go away"
- forget that the child's best interests are the priority

Do Children Ever Make False Allegations?

Yes, sometimes it happens. Some of the research shows that about 8% of disclosures are false. Most of the false allegations by children are encouraged by adults—e.g. custody cases, and others have been by adolescents who wanted "to get even." It is important to reinforce the truth—false allegations are devastating to the person accused!

Proactive Roles

How Do I Keep My Children Safe?

There are five essentials to keeping your child safe.

1. Communication

    - Listen, talk, believe and reassure your children.
    - Provide opportunities for conversations with your children.
    - Be open to any questions; nothing is off limits.
    - Be open to discussing difficult subjects such as sexuality.
    - Develop frank and open communication with the coaches.
    - If you have concerns, communicate them to the appropriate persons.
    - If you see or hear harassing or abusive behavior, speak out!

2. Knowledge

    - Make your children aware of vulnerable situations in a matter-of-fact way.
    - Review abuse and harassment policy and procedures.
    - Be aware of the screening and selection process for staff and volunteers.
    - Get to know the adults who are interacting with your children.
    - Discuss with the coaches their expectations and the setting of boundaries: physical, sexual and social.

3. Skills

    - Teach your children specific ways to handle difficult situations.
    - Help your children define their personal boundaries.

- Teach your children how to be assertive when their boundaries are crossed.

4. Build a safety plan

    - Develop check-ins, contingency plans, family codes.
    - Attend practices and games.
    - Be wary of regular private closed practices.
    - Be concerned of time spent alone with adults beyond training and game times.

5. Advocate

    - You are your children's strongest supporter.
    - Evaluate situations according to the "best interest of your child."

Acknowledgements

The Canadian Hockey Association would like to thank the following individuals for their generous assistance in producing this text: Judi Fairholm, National Coordinator, Abuse Prevention Services, Canadian Red Cross Society, Vancouver, BC. Sally Spilhaus, Advisor, Rights and Responsibilities, Concordia University, Montreal, QC.

Section 54.2

Managing Your Anger: Time Out

Excerpted from "Anger And Your Kids: Time Out," an undated document
from the Family Support Network, cited September 2000. See http://
www.familysupport.org or call 1-800-CHILDREN for more information about
the Family Support Network.

To find out if anger is becoming a problem for you, ask yourself a
few questions:

- Have you ever been so angry that you truly didn't care what you
said or did?

- Do you scream at your children to prevent yourself from hitting
them?

- Do you find yourself getting angry "at the drop of a hat?"

- Do you believe that your children do things on purpose just to
aggravate you?

If you answered yes to any of these questions, you may have a problem managing your anger.

Parenting is the hardest job in the world. With all the demands
on us as parents, it is often natural to feel overwhelmed, stressed, and
angry. Anger serves an extremely important purpose: it's a normal
release of stress. Anger momentarily blocks intolerable stress levels.
Anger is a healthy emotion. What we choose to do with it can get us
into trouble, especially when kids are involved.

Three Strategies to Follow

Strategy One: Tune into the Warning Signs

Effective anger management begins with our ability to recognize
the signs our bodies give us when a "storm" is approaching. Think back
to the last time you were really angry. What did you feel like?

Some warning signs are:

- increased heart rate
- flushed face, feeling hot
- sweatiness
- butterflies in the stomach
- shortness of breath
- light seems brighter or dimmer
- sounds seem louder of softer
- tenseness

After this point:

- Try deep breathing exercises to release stress before it becomes intolerable.
- Punch a pillow.
- Go into the bathroom and let out a scream.

Strategy Two: Changing How You Think

Anger is usually rooted in our thinking. Stressful situations trigger thoughts which can be irrational, faulty, or extreme. These triggers contain words like must, always, should, have to, must not, deliberately, purposely, and any other "absolute" words. Some examples or "trigger thoughts" are:

- You are doing this to annoy me.
- You are defying me on purpose.
- This always happens to me.
- You are taking advantage of me.
- You never listen.
- You never do anything right.
- I knew this was going to happen.
- Here we go again.
- This is a manipulation.
- You don't care (what happens, about me, how I feel).
- You are so (stupid, lazy, manipulative, controlling, bratty, etc.).

You can change the way you think. "Talk back" to irrational thoughts and defy them by replacing them with a more realistic thinking:

- Assess the real cause of your child's behavior. Is this his/her temperament? Does this behavior have something to do with his/her developmental stage?

- Realistically assess the size of the problem. We often magnify the size of a situation by using "big" words to describe it. Try not to magnify the problem by thinking it's outrageous, ridiculous, out-of-control, etc.

- Replace negative labels. Don't describe your child as stupid, lazy, cruel, spoiled, etc.

- Take an honest look at your values: what you hold in the highest regard. Are any of your values making you push your children towards activities, interests, or images that they are not interested in or capable of achieving?

- Take an inventory of your expectations of you as a parent and/or your child. Are your expectations of your child age-appropriate? Are your expectations of yourself realistic?

- Remind yourself that you can stay calm and cool. Most of the time, we remain in control of our tempers. However, it can be easy to lose it with kids. Tell yourself that you can stay in control. Repeat the affirmation out loud.

- Keep a sense of humor! Laughing is healthy and it can effectively diffuse a potentially explosive situation.

Strategy Three: Develop Coping Thoughts

Use these positive affirmations and repeat them out loud:

- I can control my temper.

- Children are naturally impulsive.

- I don't have to take this seriously. I can use humor to diffuse the situation.

- I don't need to scream to get my point across.

- Parenting can be a frustrating job. It doesn't mean I'm no good at it. I probably need to learn more about this "job."

- I can use this energy (from stress and anger) to re-direct my child's behavior.

Chapter 55

Youth Violence

Chapter Contents

Section 55.1

Facts about Youth Violence in the United States

Excerpted from "Youth Violence in the United States," National Center for Injury Prevention and Control, Centers for Disease Control and Prevention (CDC), http://www.cdc.gov/ncipc/factsheets/yvfacts.htm, page last reviewed January 27,2000.

Introduction

Violence is a public health issue because of its tremendous impact on the health and well-being of our youth. Violent injury and death disproportionately affect children, adolescents, and young adults in the United States. In response to the toll violence exacts on our nation's youth, the Division of Violence Prevention in the National Center for Injury Prevention and Control is committed to preventing such violence through its research, program evaluation, and dissemination of information.

Magnitude of the Problem

Rates of homicide among youths 15–19 years of age reached record-high levels in the latter half of the 1980s and continue to be among the highest ever recorded in the US for this age group. Between 1985 and 1991, annual homicide rates among males 15–19 years old increased 154 percent (from 13 to 33/100,000), surpassing the rates of youths in the 25–29 and 30–34 year age groups. Homicide rates for young males began to decline in 1994 and dropped 34% between 1993 and 1997 (from 34.0 to 22.6/100,000). In 1997, the rate of homicide among males 15–19 years of age was 22.6/100,000—a decline of 12.4% in one year. Despite this encouraging trend, rates are still unacceptably high.

- In 1997, 6,146 young people 15–24 years old were victims of homicide. This amounts to an average of 17 youth homicide victims per day in the US.

- Homicide is the second leading cause of death for persons 15–24 years of age and is the leading cause of death for African-Americans. In this age-group, homicide is the second leading cause of death for Hispanic youths.

- In each year since 1988, more than 80% of homicide victims 15 to 19 years of age were killed with a firearm. In 1997, 85% of homicide victims 15 to 19 years of age were killed with a firearm.

- Arrest rates for weapons offenses among youths 10 to 17 years of age doubled between 1987 and 1993, then dropped 24% by 1997.

- In 1997, 5.9% of students in a national survey reported carrying a firearm at least once in the previous 30 days. In 1995, this was true of 7.6% of students—a decline of 22.4% over the two year period.

Table 55.1. Risk factors which increase the probability of adolescent violence.

INDIVIDUAL

history of early aggression
beliefs supportive of violence
social cognitive deficits

FAMILY

poor monitoring or supervision of children
exposure to violence
parental drug/alcohol abuse
poor emotional attachment to parents or caregivers

PEER/SCHOOL

associate with peers engaged in high-risk or problem behavior
low commitment to school
academic failure

NEIGHBORHOOD

poverty and diminished economic opportunity
high levels of transiency and family disruption
exposure to violence

Between July 1992 and June 1994, 105 violent deaths occurred on or near school grounds or at school-associated events. The majority (81%) were homicides and firearms were used in most (77%) of the deaths. The violent deaths occurred in communities of all sizes in 25 states.

Key Risk Factors for Violence

One of the first steps toward preventing violence, according to the public health approach, is to identify and understand the factors that place young people at risk for violent victimization and perpetration. Previous research shows that there are a number of individual and social factors that increase the probability of violence during adolescence and young adulthood. Some of these factors clustered in four areas are listed in Table 55.1.

Determining "What Works"

Understanding the factors that place young people at risk for violence is an important first step in preventing violence. The next important step is to design interventions or programs to address these risk factors and evaluate their effectiveness. As the lead agency in injury control, Centers for Disease Control and Prevention (CDC) has funded a number of projects to get a better sense of what works to prevent violence and aggression among our nation's youth. [A few of these are listed below.]

- In 1999, CDC funded four multi-site projects to develop, implement, and evaluate a common violence prevention program in middle schools. These school-based projects will assess the effectiveness of violence prevention among this age group of students. The projects are affiliated with Virginia Commonwealth University, University of Illinois Chicago, University of Georgia, and Duke University to develop a state of the art intervention protocol, a common evaluation design, and a common plan for data collection and analysis.

- In 1998, CDC in collaboration with the Office of Juvenile Justice and Delinquency Prevention (OJJDP) and the Center for the Study and Prevention of Violence University of Colorado at Boulder supported the replication and evaluation of promising prevention program targeting children ages 12–18.

- In 1998, CDC funded projects located in three cities (Birmingham, AL, Oakland, CA, and Boston, MA) targeting high school aged youth at increased risk for violence. Two projects are targeting youths enrolled in alternative or continuation high schools. The third project is hospital-based and targets youths who have been victims of violence-related assaults. It is designed to reduce rates of re-injury and utilizes a model that connects youths to community-based programming.

Section 55.2

Preventing Youth Violence

Excerpted from "Preventing Youth Violence," from the SAFEusa website, Centers for Disease Control and Prevention (CDC), http://www.cdc.gov/safeusa/youthviolence.htm, page last updated May 24, 2000.

Introduction

Violence is a learned behavior that can be changed. Parents, students, and school officials can take steps toward reducing violence in schools by responding to children's emotional and psychological needs and by implementing violence prevention programs.

Preventing Youth Violence

For Parents

- Give your children consistent love and attention. Every child needs a strong, loving relationship with a parent or other adult to feel safe and secure and to develop a sense of trust.

- Children learn by example, so show your children appropriate behavior by the way you act. Settle arguments with calm words, not with yelling, hitting, and slapping.

- Talk with your children about the violence they see on TV, in video games, at school, at home, or in the neighborhood. Discuss

why violence exists in these contexts and what the consequences of this violence are.

- Try to keep your children from seeing too much violence: limit
their TV time, and screen the programs they watch. Seeing a lot
of violence can lead children to behave aggressively.

- Make sure your children do not have access to guns. If you own
firearms or other weapons, unload them and lock them up separately from the bullets. Never store firearms where children can
find them, even if unloaded. Also, talk with your children a bout
how dangerous weapons can be.

- Involve your children in setting rules for appropriate behavior
at home; this will help them understand why the rules should
be followed. Also ask your children what they think an appropriate punishment would be if a rule were broken.

- Teach your children nonaggressive ways to solve problems by
discussing problems with them, asking them to consider what
might happen if they use violence to solve problems, and talking
about what might happen if they solve problems without violence.

- Listen to your children and respect them. They will be more
likely to listen and respect others if they are listened to and
treated with respect.

- Note any disturbing behaviors in your child such as angry outbursts, excessive fighting, cruelty to animals, fire-setting, lack
of friends, or alcohol/drug use. These can be signs of serious
problems. Don't be afraid to get help for your child if such behaviors exist, and talk with a trusted professional in the community.

For Students

- Be a role model by never physically or verbally harming, bullying, teasing, or intimidating others.

- If your friends tell you about troubling feelings or thoughts, listen well and let them know you care. Encourage them to get
help from a trusted adult. If you are very concerned, talk to an
adult you trust.

- When you are angry, take a few deep breaths and imagine your-self on a lake or at the beach or anywhere that makes you feel peaceful. After you are more calm, identify what is making you upset. Decide on your options for handling the problem, such as talking the problem out calmly with the people involved, avoid-ing the problem by staying away from certain people, or diffus-ing the problem by resolving to take it less seriously. After you decide what to do (or not do) and act on your decision, be sure to look back and decide if what you did helped the situation.

- Work with your school to create a process for students to safely report threats, intimidation, weapon possession, drug selling, gang activity, and vandalism.

- Help develop and participate in activities to promote under-standing and respecting differences.

- Volunteer to be a mentor for younger students and/or provide tutoring for your peers.

- If you feel intensely angry, fearful, anxious, or depressed, talk about it with an adult you trust.

- Get involved in your school's violence prevention and response plan. If a plan does not exist, suggest starting one.

For School Officials

- Develop a comprehensive violence prevention plan that does not label or stigmatize children. Involve staff, parents, students, and members of the community in the creation and implemen-tation of this plan.

- Create a school environment that is safe and responsive to all children. Students should be able to share their needs, fears, concerns, and anxieties, and also safely report threats.

- Ensure that opportunities exist for adults to spend quality per-sonal time with children. A positive relationship with an adult who is available to provide support is one of the most critical factors in preventing school violence.

- Discuss safety issues openly. Schools can reduce the risk of vio-lence by teaching children about the dangers of firearms as well as appropriate ways to resolve conflicts and express anger.

- Offer supervised, school-based before- and after-school programs that provide children with support and a range of options, such as counseling, tutoring, clubs, community service, and help with homework.

- Be prepared for a crisis or violent act. Provide in-service training for all faculty and staff to explain what to do in a crisis, including the evacuation procedure, communication plan, and how to contact help.

Who Is Affected?

School-associated violence is a major concern for most Americans. Such violence not only affects the individuals involved, but also has an enormous impact on their families, the entire school population, and the community at large. School-associated violence includes nonfatal events, such as fighting, as well as deaths.

Of high school students nationwide in 1997:

- 15.0% were in one or more physical fights on school property.

- 3.5% were treated by a doctor or a nurse for injuries sustained in a fight.

- 4.0% had missed one or more days of school in the past month because they felt unsafe traveling to or from school.

From an ongoing study of school-associated violent deaths (a school-associated death is one that occurs on school property, at a school-sponsored event, or on the way to or from a school-sponsored event):

- 58 school-associated deaths occurred during the 1997–98 school year.

- The average number of school-associated violent events with multiple victims has increased from one event per school year in 1992 to five events per year in 1998.

Chapter 56

Media Violence

Children and Media Violence

Did you know?

- By the time an average child (one who watches two to four hours of television daily) leaves elementary school, he or she will have witnessed 8,000 murders and over 100,000 other acts of violence.

- By the time a child is 18 years old, he or she will witness (with average viewing time) 200,000 acts of violence including 40,000 murders.

- On an individual day, there are about 5 to 6 violent acts per hour on prime-time television, and 20 to 25 acts of violence on Saturday morning children's television.

- Weekly, in the United States, this adds up to about 188 hours of violent programs or about 15% of the program time.

This chapter contains text from "Children and Media Violence," National Institute on Media and Family, http://www.mediafamily.org/research/fact/ vlent.shtml, updated in 2000, and the following fact sheets from American Academy of Child and Adolescent Psychology (AACAP): "Children and TV Violence," http://www.aacap.org/publications/factsfam/violence.htm, updated April 1999, "Children and the News," http://www.aacap.org/publications/factsfam/ 67.htm, November 1998, and "The Influence of Music and Music Videos," http://www.aacap.org/publications/factsfam/musicvid.htm, updated May 2000, copyright 1997 AACAP. Reprinted with permission.

- Cable can add to the violence by rerunning old shows and the showing of more violent new ones.

- Many popular R-rated films available on video contain far more violence than seen on commercial television.

- Children with VCR or cable access have seen more R-rated films than their non-cable, non-VCR counterparts.

- Since 1955, reports, studies, and congressional testimonies by experts in the field have overwhelmingly concluded that "the mass media are significant contributors to the aggressive behavior and aggression related attitudes of many children, adolescents and adults."

- Two large meta analysis studies have been conducted on research linking media violence to aggression in children. One looked at 67 studies and over 30,000 subjects. The other looked at 230 studies and almost 100,000 subjects. Both supported a number of conclusions: "First, there is a positive association between televised violence exposure and behavior. Second, exposure to violent programming not only increases aggressive behavior, but is associated with lower levels of prosocial behavior."

Many factors in the portrayal of media violence contribute to its affect on teens:

- Is the aggressive behavior on screen rewarded or punished?

- Is the violence gratuitous, is it justified or does it lack consequences?

- Does the viewer identify with the aggressor or the victim?

- Does the viewer become engaged with or aroused by the violence on screen?

- What is the age of the child? Although violence affects children of all ages, middle childhood, ages 8 to 12, seem particularly sensitive.

- What is the total amount of television watched?

- Does the child see television violence as realistic?

Children and TV Violence

American children watch an average of three to fours hours of television daily. Television can be a powerful influence in developing value systems and shaping behavior. Unfortunately, much of today's television programming is violent. Hundreds of studies of the effects of TV violence on youth and teenagers have found that children may:

- become "immune" to the horror of violence

- gradually accept violence as a way to solve problems

- imitate the violence they observe on television

- identify with certain characters, victims and/or victimizers

Extensive viewing of television violence by youth causes greater aggressiveness. Sometimes, watching a single violent program can increase aggressiveness. Children who view shows in which violence is very realistic, frequently repeated, or unpunished, are more likely to imitate what they see. Youth with emotional, behavioral, learning or impulse control problems may be more easily influenced by TV violence. The impact of TV violence may be immediately evident in the youth's behavior or may surface years later, and young people can even be affected when the family atmosphere shows no tendency toward violence.

While TV violence is not the only cause of aggressive or violent behavior, it is clearly a significant factor.

Parents can protect children from excessive TV violence in the following ways:

- pay attention to the programs their children are watching and watch some with them

- set limits on the amount of time they spend with the television; consider removing the TV set from their bedroom

- point out that although the actor has not actually been hurt or killed, such violence in real life results in pain or death

- refuse to let them see shows known to be violent, and change the channel or turn off the TV set when offensive material comes on, with an explanation of what is wrong with the program

- disapprove of the violent episodes in front of the children, stressing the belief that such behavior is not the best way to resolve a problem

- to offset peer pressure among friends and classmates, contact other parents and agree to enforce similar rules about the length of time and type of program the children may watch

Parents can also use these measures to prevent harmful effects from television in other areas such as racial or sexual stereotyping. The amount of time youth watch TV, regardless of content, should be moderated because it decreases time spent on more beneficial activities such as reading, playing with friends, and developing hobbies. If parents have serious difficulties setting limits, or have ongoing concerns about how their child is reacting to television, they should contact a child and adolescent psychiatrist for consultation and assistance.

Children and the News

Youth often see or hear the news many times a day through television, radio, newspapers, magazines, and the Internet. Seeing and hearing about local and world events, such as natural disasters, catastrophic events, and crime reports, may cause children to experience stress, anxiety, and fears.

There have also been several changes in how news is reported that have given rise to the increased potential for children to experience negative effects. These changes include the following:

- television channels and Internet services and sites which report the news 24 hours a day

- television channels broadcasting live events as they are unfolding, in "real time"

- increased reporting of the details of the private lives of public figures and role models

- pressure to get news to the public as part of the competitive nature of the entertainment industry

- detailed and repetitive visual coverage of natural disasters and violent acts

While there has been great public debate about providing television ratings to warn parents about violence and sex in programming, news shows have only recently been considered in these discussions. Research has shown, however, that children and adolescents are prone to imitate what they see and hear in the news, a kind of contagion effect described as "copy cat" events. Chronic and persistent exposure to such violence can lead to fear, desensitization (immunity), and in some children an increase in aggressive and violent behaviors. Studies also show that media broadcasts do not always choose to show things that accurately reflect local or national trends.

For example, statistics report a decrease in the incidence of crime, yet, the reporting of crime in the news has increased 240%. Local news shows often lead with or break into programming to announce crime reports and devote as much as 30% of the broadcast time to detailed crime reporting.

The possible negative effects of news can be lessened by parents, teachers, or other adults by watching the news with the youth and talking about what has been seen or heard. The child's age, maturity, developmental level, life experiences, and vulnerabilities should guide how much and what kind of news the child watches.

Guidelines for minimizing the negative effects of watching the news include:

- make sure you have adequate time and a quiet place to talk if you anticipate that the news is going to be troubling or upsetting to the youth

- ask the youth what he/she has heard and what questions he/she may have

- provide reassurance regarding his/her own safety in simple words emphasizing that you are going to be there to keep him/her safe

- look for signs that the news may have triggered fears or anxieties such as sleeplessness, fears, bedwetting, crying, or talking about being afraid

Parents should remember that it is important to talk to the child or adolescent about what he/she has seen or heard. This allows parents to lessen the potential negative effects of the news and to discuss their own ideas and values. While children cannot be completely protected from outside events, parents can help them feel safe and help them to better understand the world around them.

The Influence of Music and Music Videos

Singing and music have always played an important role in learning and the communication of culture. Youth learn from the role models what they see and hear. For the past 35 years, some children's television has very effectively used the combination of words, music, and fast-paced animation to achieve learning.

Most parents are concerned about what their young children see and hear, but as children grow older, parents pay less attention to the music and videos that hold their children's interest.

The sharing of musical tastes between generations in a family can be a pleasurable experience. Music also is often a major part of a teenager's separate world. It is quite common for teenagers to get pleasure from keeping adults out and causing adults some distress.

A concern to many interested in the development and growth of teenagers is the negative and destructive themes of some rock and other kinds of music, including best-selling albums promoted by major recording companies. The following troublesome themes are prominent:

- advocating and glamorizing abuse of drugs and alcohol

- pictures and explicit lyrics presenting suicide as an "alternative" or "solution"

- graphic violence

- rituals in concerts

- sex which focuses on control, sadism, masochism, incest, children devaluing women, and violence toward women

Parents can help their teenagers by paying attention to their teenager's purchasing, downloading, listening, and viewing patterns, and by helping them identify music that may be destructive. An open discussion without criticism may be helpful.

Music is not usually a danger for a teenager whose life is happy and healthy. But if a teenager is persistently preoccupied with music that has seriously destructive themes, and there are changes in behavior such as isolation, depression, alcohol or other drug abuse, a psychiatric evaluation should be considered.

Chapter 57

Gun Violence at School

Violence is not a single problem amenable to a single solution; all violent youth do not conform to the same profile. A comprehensive approach must address factors in the individual, the family, and society.

Immediate Actions at School

Talk to students about gun violence:

- acknowledge youth violence as a serious, but preventable problem
- explain school policies and safety procedures
- obtain student input on their safety concerns
- encourage students to report threats of violence

Identify youth at risk for gun violence at school:

- students who threaten others or hint about violence
- students with a history of carrying guns, fighting, destroying property, or cruelty to animals
- students who are preoccupied with violent fantasies, movies, games, and music

Excerpted from "Gun Violence at School, Recommendations for Prevention," Virginia Youth Violence Project, http://curry.edschool.Virginia.edu/curry/centers/youthvio/latebreaking/news.html, 1998.

- students, including suicidal students, who feel rejected, humiliated, bullied, or mistreated

Take all threats seriously. Evaluate threatening students following standards comparable to those for suicidal students:

- assess student's intentions and plans, mental state and motivation

- review student's recent stresses and history of violence

- consult with other professionals, estimate risk, and if necessary, take reasonable steps to protect potential victims

- develop a plan of action, including non-violence contracts, parent consultation, and follow-up services

Long-Term Strategies

What schools can do:

- Review and maintain clear written policies on school discipline, building security, and crisis response. Enforce school discipline and security policies. Work to maintain a climate of respect for authority and concern for others.

- Initiate school-wide programs starting in the elementary grades to teach students social competence skills and peaceful methods of resolving conflict. Implement programs to identify and stop bullying.

- Promote student involvement in projects, organizations, and activities which emphasize non-violence, personal responsibility, and service to others.

- Encourage troubled students to seek help. Use school psychologists and counselors to work with troubled, at-risk students and coordinate efforts with community services.

What parents can do:

- Talk to your children about their problems, fears, and concerns. Take them seriously and give them your support.

- Supervise your children. Know where they are and what they are doing.

- Lock up your guns and ammunition. Talk about gun violence with your children.

- Limit your children's exposure to media violence as a form of entertainment. Discuss with them how media violence desensitizes us to violence and portrays violence unrealistically as a glamorous and effective solution to problems.

- Educate your children in moral values and principles, including personal responsibility and respect for others.

- When in doubt about your child's behavior, consult with school or community professionals.

What community agencies and law enforcement can do:

- Work collaboratively with schools to provide them with well-trained school resource officers.

- Expect and encourage schools to assist in enforcement of laws against violence, weapon-carrying, and use of drugs and alcohol.

- Vigorously enforce gun laws and conduct campaigns to get guns off the streets and out of the hands of juveniles.

- Support after-school programs, supervised recreation, youth employment, and community service activities. Establish mentoring as a standard program component.

- Provide comprehensive family services programs, including Head Start, multisystemic family therapy, and parent education.

Assessment of a Potentially Violent Youth

Assessments should be conducted by a qualified mental health professional. These suggestions are not intended to substitute for a comprehensive evaluation.

Identify all potentially relevant sources of information.

- youth self-report
- parent interview
- potential victim
- other as appropriate (peers, law enforcement, professionals)

Assess youth's intent.

- Has youth made verbal threats?
- Has youth been aggressive toward victim?
- Is there a plan? Available weapon?
- Does the youth identify contingencies that would provoke him or her to act?

Review present stress.

- Has there been recent provocation or conflict?
- Any extraneous stresses or life changes?
- Any anticipated negative events?

Assess mental state.

- anger, injustice, over-controlled hostility
- depression, hopelessness, despair
- psychotic or distorted thinking

Check personal risk factors.

- past aggression toward others
- aggressive role models
- fantasy involvement with violence through games, movies, novels, etc.
- substance abuse

Assess coping ability.

- Is youth willing to communicate with you when stressed?
- Can youth engage in a non-violent coping plan?
- Can you elicit youth empathy for victims?

Take appropriate action.

- Can you elicit youth concern for legal and personal consequences?

- Consult with other professionals about your findings and conclusions.

- Document your process, conclusions, and actions with timely notes.

- Take appropriate precautions, including warning potential victims, notifying relevant parties (law enforcement, parents, school personnel, and others as appropriate to the situation).

- Follow up on treatment recommendations and referrals.

- Professional responsibility continues after the assessment.

Chapter 58

Your Adolescent and Gangs

Chapter Contents

Section 58.1

Facts and Figures about Youth Gangs

Virginia Youth Violence Project, http://curry.edschool.virginia.edu/curry/
centers/youthvio/subpages/current/gangva/facts/slideshow.html, 1999.

A law enforcement survey of the National Youth Gang Center documented the prevalence of youth gangs throughout the United States. Out of 3,440 Police and Sheriff's departments, 58 % reported active youth gangs in all 50 states. Half of agencies reporting gangs are in small localities (less than 25,000 people). 63% of cities and 48% of counties have a unit to respond to youth gangs.

A 1996 Virginia law enforcement survey found 260 youth gangs distributed across 32 localities. Over half of the youth gangs were identified in urban and suburban Northern Virginia. Nearly 1/3 were in the heavily populated tidewater region of eastern Virginia. No region was completely free of youth gang activity. The survey was of 125 sheriffs, 180 police chiefs, 35 directors, and 260 youth gangs in 32 (24%) of the cities and counties.

The State Commission on Youth conducted face-to-face anonymous, confidential interviews with 737 of 757 youth in all Virginia detention centers, 97% of the state detained population. Most youth were cooperative and willing to describe their gang involvement, although some declined to answer specific questions (such as the name of their gang). Approximately 9% of the surveys were omitted from analyses because the interviewers judged the youth to be unreliable or uncooperative. Even with these precautions, there is no assurance that all responses were truthful. Some youth may have denied gang involvement and others may have falsely claimed gang involvement.

Youth were asked "Have you ever joined or been a member of a gang?" and if they replied no, were asked, "Have you ever joined or been a member of any other type of youth group such as a crew, clique, posse or something else?" Forty-one percent reported some involvement in a gang or gang-like group.

Typically, youth reported that their gangs had between 20 and 100 members. Some youth reporting larger memberships claimed to be members of national gangs or asserted that almost all youth in their neighborhood belonged to their group.

Most youth referred to their group as a gang, but some used terms such as crew, clique, or posse. Groups were classified based on the terms used by the youth. In some data analyses we compared gang members to the combined membership of all other gang-like groups.

Youth were asked, "Does your (gang or group) have any of the following identifiers?" and presented with a list. Those youth who had described their group as a "gang" reported their group to have more characteristics of formal organization and identity than those belonging to other gang-like groups.

Youth were asked why they joined a gang and presented with a list of possible reasons. Most youth chose more than one reason, with peer involvement and excitement leading the list.

What Can We Do about Gangs?

General Strategies

We need a coordinated, comprehensive response to youth gangs. This includes working to prevent the conditions which lead to gangs, teaching youth skills and values which make them less vulnerable to gangs, providing alternatives to gang involvement, and taking steps to stop gang activity and recruitment of gang members.

School Strategies

Schools should not overlook or minimize the deleterious effects of gang activity on the school learning environment as well as the development of law-abiding and prosocial values. Schools should take proactive steps to prevent gang development by developing and implementing gang policies.

Section 58.2

What's a Parent to Do about Gangs?

"What's a Parent to Do About Gangs?" undated document from National
Crime Prevention Council, from www.ncpc.org/10ad2.htm,
accessed November 2001.

Once found only in large cities, gangs have invaded communities
of all sizes across the United States. Gangs bring drugs, fear, and violence to neighborhoods; destroy property; and drive out businesses.
Gangs draw young people away from school and home and into a life
of violence.

Learn about Gangs

- Gangs can be organized around race or ethnic group, money-
  making activities, or territory.

- Most gang members are male. They range in age from 8 to 22
  years.

- Young people give various reasons for joining gangs. Among the
  most common: to belong to a group, for protection, to earn
  money, for excitement, and to be with friends. For some, it's
  even a family tradition.

- Gangs signal their existence and solidarity through clothing
  and head coverings, a special vocabulary, tattoos, hand signs,
  and tagging their territory with graffiti.

- "Gangsta" rap paints a realistic picture of daily gang activity.
  The lyrics glorify violence, abuse of women, and disrespect for
  authority, especially the police. Its popularity among the young
  has helped spread the culture of gangs, cutting across class,
  economic, racial, and geographic lines.

Signs That Your Child Might Be in a Gang

- changes in type of friends

- changes in dress habits, such as wearing the same color combination all the time
- gang symbols on books or clothing
- tattoos
- secretiveness about activities
- extra cash from unknown sources
- carrying a weapon
- declining interest in school and family
- being arrested or detained by the police

If you notice these patterns, get help. Contact the school counselor or the gang crimes unit of your police department.

Make Sure Your Child Doesn't Need a Gang

- Show your child love with lots of hugs and reassurances. Talk with and listen to your child.

- Supervise your children's activities. Help them get involved in athletics or other activities that interest them.

- Put a high value on education and help your child to do his or her best in school. Do everything possible to prevent dropping out.

- Talk about your values and why you think gangs are dangerous. Discuss the violence, drug dealing, hatred of other groups for no reason, and the likelihood of being arrested and imprisoned.

- And don't forget to listen.

What Communities Can Do to Keep Gangs out

- Develop positive alternatives—after-school, weekend, and summer activities where children and teens can learn, expand their world, and have fun.

- Encourage parents to talk to one another through school forums, social events, networks, parenting classes, and support groups.

- Cooperate with police and other agencies. Report suspicious activity, set up a Neighborhood Watch or citizen patrol, volunteer to clean up graffiti.

- Get organized and show gangs that your neighborhood has zero tolerance for their activities. Your community has many resources who can work together against gangs, including law enforcement, civic groups, religious congregations, schools, youth agencies, Boys & Girls Clubs, YMCA and YWCA, Girl Scouts and Boy Scouts, drug treatment services, and community centers.

Chapter 59

Adolescent Criminals

Adolescent Criminals: Where Do They Come from, Where Do They Go?

When watching television news on any given day, we might see a gruesome account of a man who has just killed his wife and then turned the gun on himself, while his four-year-old son watches. "My God," we say with great compassion. "What must that child be thinking? How can he live through something like this? Whatever will become of that poor child'?"

Now, fast-forward about 12 years. Picture that boy, now 16 years old, standing in a courtroom with that characteristic posture that veritably screams, "I could care less about anything." Now we don't view him with compassion or think of him as a traumatized patient. Rather we see him as a prime example of a psychopath, macho thug, heartless animal or the embodiment of evil. "My God," we say with outrage, "Sixteen years old and already a list of offenses as long as his arm. What's wrong with him?"

This chapter contains text from Thomas J. Cottle, "Adolescent Criminals: Where Do They Come from, Where Do They Go?" *Brown University Child and Adolescent Behavior Letter*, November 1998, copyright 1998 Manisses Communications Group, Inc., reprinted with permission of Manisses Communications Group and Thomas Cottle, and "Children Who Steal" American Academy of Child and Adolescent Psychiatry (AACAP), www.aacap.org/publications/factsfam/steal.htm, April 1999, reprinted with permission.

It's sobering to realize that quite possibly the most dangerous person in America is the 16 year old boy drifting about after school with no place to go and access to a gun. He is not yet old enough to drink (legally) or join the army, but he is old enough to drive, drop out of school, and most definitely to kill if he has the opportunity, the inclination and the desire.

Obviously, we must do something about criminal offenders, be they young or old. They represent a risk to us personally, as well as to the desired civil order. However, the debate on exactly what to do has never reached a conclusion. All it takes for this debate to escalate is the sort of grizzly schoolyard murders we witnessed in Massachusetts, Kentucky and Arkansas. At times such as these, our outrage toward youthful offenders causes us to reconsider the juvenile justice system, the methods of adjudication and the punishments that ought to be meted out in cases of serious crime.

The debate swings between those who argue that crime is crime whether it be committed by a 13-year-old or a 40-year-old, and those who believe that something horrendous must have gone wrong for a child who commits a murder or rape. Surely, they argue, this child is immature, underdeveloped, neglected, or abused, but not evil. Quite possibly, they argue, because he is young, he may be rehabilitated. Besides, they ask, what is prison going to do for the child other than permanently galvanize his furious impulses and turn the still malleable youngster into a hardened life long criminal?

What a society elects to do with its young offenders depends on how that society chooses to perceive them. Tragically, crime is one of the ways that traumatized children react to earlier wounds. It will take a great deal of work to get them in touch with their pain, humiliation, and sense of shame that stems from their perception—not that they have done bad—that they know themselves to be bad.

Something must be done, not to, but for all these children at risk. If a child is immoral, then so too are the conditions that spawn that immorality. The whole notion of a child at risk rests in great measure on the notion of immorality in the society. When it's a matter of a child in trouble here or there, or every now and then, we just take another philosophical position. But generation after generation of offenders tells us that pathology and immorality must breed this condition.

Trauma rarely shows. We see only its ugly, frightening repercussions.

Children Who Steal

When a child or teenager steals, parents are naturally concerned. They worry about what caused their child to steal, and they wonder whether their son or daughter is a "juvenile delinquent."

It is normal for a very young child to take something which excites his or her interest. This should not be regarded as stealing until the youngster is old enough, usually three to five years old, to understand that taking something which belongs to another person is wrong. Parents should actively teach their children about property rights and the consideration of others. Parents are also role models. If you come home with stationary or pens from the office or brag about a mistake at the supermarket checkout counter, your lessons about honesty will be a lot harder for your child to understand.

Although they have learned that theft is wrong, older children or teenagers steal for various reasons. A youngster may steal to make things equal if a brother or sister seems to be favored with affection or gifts. Sometimes, a youth may steal as a show of bravery to friends, or to give presents to family or friends, or to be more accepted by peers. Children may also steal out of a fear of dependency; they don't want to depend on anyone, so they take what they need.

Parents should consider whether the youth has stolen out of a need for more attention. In these cases, the youth may be expressing anger or trying to "get even" with his or her parents; the stolen object may become a substitute for love or affection. The parents should make an effort to give more recognition to the youth as an important family member.

If parents take the proper measures, in most cases the stealing stops as the youth grows older. Child and adolescent psychiatrists recommend that when parents find out their child has stolen, they:

- tell the youth that stealing is wrong

- help the youngster to pay for or return the stolen object

- make sure that the youth does not benefit from the theft in any way

- avoid lecturing, predicting future bad behavior, or saying that they now consider the child to be a thief or a bad person

- make clear that this behavior is totally unacceptable within the family tradition and the community

When the child has paid for or returned the stolen merchandise, the matter should not be brought up again by the parents, so that the youth can begin again with a "clean slate."

If stealing is persistent or accompanied by other problem behaviors or symptoms, the stealing may be a sign of more serious problems in the child's emotional development or problems in the family. Children who repeatedly steal may also have difficulty trusting others and forming close relationships. Rather than feeling guilty, they may blame the behavior on others, arguing that, "Since they refuse to give me what I need, I will take it." These children would benefit from an evaluation by a child and adolescent psychiatrist.

In treating a youth who steals persistently, a child and adolescent psychiatrist will evaluate the underlying reasons for the child's need to steal, and develop a plan of treatment. Important aspects of treatment are helping the youth learn to establish trusting relationships and helping the family to support the youth in changing to a more healthy path of development.

Part Six

Adolescent Education

Chapter 60

What Can Parents and Teachers Do If an Adolescent Begins to Fail in School?

Many teenagers experience times when keeping up with school-work is difficult. These periods may last for several weeks and may result in social problems as well as a decline in academic performance. Some adolescents get through these difficult times with minimal assistance from their parents or teachers. It may be enough for parents to listen to the teenager's problems and suggest coping strategies, provide a supportive home environment, and encourage the teenager's participation in extracurricular school activities. However, when the difficulties last longer than a single grading period or are linked to a long-term pattern of poor school performance or problematic behaviors, parents and teachers may need to intervene. This chapter identifies some characteristics of adolescents at risk for failing in school and offers advice on how parents and teachers can assist them.

Excerpted from "What Can Parents and Teachers Do If an Adolescent Begins to Fail in School?" http://www.accesseric.org/resources/parent/fail.html, prepared by ACCESS ERIC with funding from the Educational Resources Information Center, National Library of Education, Office of Educational Research and Improvement, U.S. Department of Education, under Contract No. RK95188001. Based on the 1997 ERIC Digest *If an Adolescent Begins To Fail in School, What Can Parents and Teachers Do?* by Anne S. Robertson of the National Parent Information Network. Page updated on September 13, 2000. The opinions expressed here do not necessarily reflect the positions of the US Department of Education.

How Can We Identify Students Who Are at Risk for Failure?

Some students may exhibit at-risk behaviors from the early elementary school years on; others may overcome early difficulties but could experience related problems during the middle or high school years. Still others may not exhibit at-risk behaviors until early adolescence. Research suggests that problems are more likely to occur during a transitional year, such as when a student is moving from elementary to middle school or from middle school to high school.

To intervene effectively, parents and teachers need to know some common characteristics of adolescents at risk for school failure. These characteristics include:

- *Attention problems.* The student has a history of attention issues at school.

- *Poor grades.* The student consistently performs at barely average or below average levels.

- *Retentions.* The student has been retained in one or more grade levels.

- *Absenteeism.* The student is absent five or more days per term.

- *Lack of connection with school and community activities.* The student is not involved in sports, music, scouting, or other extracurricular activities.

- *Behavior problems.* The student may be disciplined frequently in school or may show a sudden change in school behavior, such as withdrawing from classroom discussions.

- *Lack of confidence.* The student believes that success is linked to natural intelligence rather than to hard work and that his or her own ability is insufficient and cannot be changed or improved.

- *Limited goals for the future.* The student seems unaware of what career options are available or of how to attain those goals.

When an adolescent exhibits more than one of these characteristics, he or she will likely need assistance from parents and teachers if he or she is to be successful in school. Girls and students from culturally or linguistically diverse groups may be especially at risk for academic failure if they exhibit these behaviors. If parents and teachers step back and let these students "figure it out" or "take responsibility for their own learning," this may lead to a deeper cycle of failure at school.

What Role Does Parenting Style Play?

Parenting style may affect a child's school behavior. Many experts distinguish among permissive, authoritarian, and authoritative parenting styles. These parenting styles are associated with different combinations of warmth and support, and limit-setting and supervision for children. The permissive style tends to emphasize warmth and support, and the authoritarian style tends to emphasize limit-setting and supervision. The authoritative style offers a combination of both warmth and support and limit-setting and supervision, and it has been identified as the parenting style that is more likely to encourage academic success in adolescents. Authoritative parents are warm and responsive but are also able to establish and enforce standards for their children's behavior, to monitor conduct, and to encourage communication. Authoritative parents make it clear that they expect responsible behavior from their children and that they are available to support their children as needed.

How Can Parents and Teachers Respond?

Parents often feel uncertain about how to approach their adolescent or the school when their teenager seems to be having difficulty. However, it is important to remember that adolescents need their parents not only to set appropriate expectations and boundaries, but also to advocate for them. Teachers can ease parents' concerns by including the parents as part of the student's educational support team. When an adolescent is having difficulty, parents and teachers can assist by:

- Making time to listen to the teenager's fears or concerns and trying to understand them.

- Setting appropriate boundaries for behavior that are consistently enforced.

- Emphasizing the importance of study skills, hard work, and follow-through at home and in school.

- Arranging tutoring or study group support for the teenager at the school or in the community through organizations such as the local YMCA or a local college or university.

- Providing a supportive home and school environment in which education is clearly valued.

- Encouraging the teenager to participate in one or more school activities.

- Becoming more involved in school activities by attending school functions, such as sporting events, concerts, science fairs, and plays, to show their support for the school.

- Meeting as a team with the student and a school counselor to share their expectations for the teenager's future and to figure out how they can support his or her learning environment.

- Helping the teenager think about career options by arranging for visits to local companies and colleges, providing information about careers and vocational or college courses, and encouraging the teenager to participate in an internship or a career-oriented part-time job.

- Encouraging the teenager to volunteer in the community or to participate in community groups such as the YMCA, scouting, 4-H, religious organizations, or other service-oriented groups to provide an out-of-school support system.

Conclusion

Understanding the factors that may put an adolescent at risk for academic failure can help parents and teachers to determine if a student is in need of extra help or support. Being aware of common problems can help parents and teachers know when it is important to reach out to the student before a "difficult time" develops into a more serious situation.

Sources

References identified with EJ or ED are abstracted in the ERIC database. EJ references are journal articles available at most research libraries. ED references are documents available in microfiche collections at more than 900 locations or in paper copy and,

546

in some cases, electronically from the ERIC Document Reproduction Service at 800-443-ERIC (3742). Call 800-LET-ERIC (538-3742) for more details.

Debold, E. 1995. "Helping Girls Survive the Middle Grades." *Principal* 74 (3): 22–24. EJ 496–198.

Glasgow, K. L., S. M. Dornbusch, L. Troyer, L. Steinberg, and P. L. Ritter. 1997. "Parenting Styles, Adolescents' Attributions, and Educational Outcomes in Nine Heterogeneous High Schools." *Child Development* 68 (3): 507–29. EJ 549–525.

Jacobsen, T., and V. Hofmann. 1997. "Children's Attachment Representations: Longitudinal Relations to School Behavior and Academic Competency in Middle Childhood and Adolescence." *Developmental Psychology* 33 (4): 703–10. EJ 549–597.

Siegel, J. 1996. "Schools That Work: A Second Chance for Success." *Electronic Learning* 16 (1): 48–51, 67.

Steinberg, L. 1996. "Ethnicity and Adolescent Achievement." *American Educator* 20 (2): 28–35. EJ 531–782.

Chapter 61

Information on Youth Who Drop Out: Why They Leave and What Happens to Them

It has been known for many years that young people who don't complete high school face many more problems in later life than do people who graduate. But, while national leaders have demanded that schools, communities, and families make a major effort to retain students, the dropout rate remains high.

Students drop out for many reasons, some which may even seem like good ones at the time—to help out their families or to start new ones, for example—and their decisions may be supported by the people closest to them in the belief that they have no choice. But the consequences of leaving can be great, and there are many concrete things that schools and families can do to help students stay in school, or get an alternative education, and also meet their personal responsibilities. Several studies recently conducted by the Federal government and private organizations have produced new information about dropouts. Some update statistics regularly kept on these youth. Another reports on a survey on the school and personal lives of both graduates and dropouts who began high school in 1988 to find out the differences between the two groups. Finally, a study on the value to dropouts of color of getting a General Educational Development (GED)

Wendy Schwartz, "New Information on Youth Who Drop Out: Why They Leave and What Happens to Them," Educational Resources Information Center (ERIC) Clearinghouse on Urban Education, http://ericps.ed.uiuc.edu/npin/library/1998/n00064/n00064.html, 1995. Despite the age of this document, readers seeking information about youth who drop out will find this information useful.

alternative high school diploma leads to some surprising, and encouraging, conclusions.

Findings from these studies are presented below so that parents can have up-to-date information when talking to their children about dropping out.

Facts about Dropouts

Who Is at Risk of Dropping out

The following information shows certain groups of young people whose members are more likely than others to leave school before graduating. While not everyone in these categories drops out, paying special attention to the needs of students from these groups can keep some of them in school.

- Students in large cities are twice as likely to leave school before graduating than non-urban youth.

- More than one in four Hispanic youth drop out, and nearly half leave by the eighth grade.

- Hispanics are twice as likely as African Americans to drop out. White and Asian American students are least likely to drop out.

- More than half the students who drop out leave by the tenth grade, 20% quit by the eighth grade, and 3% drop out by the fourth grade.

Earnings and Opportunities for Dropouts

The gap between dropouts and more educated people is widening as opportunities increase for higher skilled workers and all but disappear for the less skilled.

- In the last 20 years the earnings level of dropouts doubled, while it nearly tripled for college graduates.

- Recent dropouts will earn $200,000 less than high school graduates, and over $800,000 less than college graduates, in their lives.

- Dropouts make up nearly half the heads of households on welfare.

- Dropouts make up nearly half the prison population.

Earnings and Opportunities for GED Holders

In the past it was thought that returning to school to get a GED certificate didn't have much effect on a person's job opportunities. Regardless, each year nearly half a million people get a GED. A recent study shows, however, that there are large differences between those who drop out and those who get a GED, not only in the ability to find a job but also in the wages they earn:

- Men who got a GED earned 21% more than male dropouts; women GED holders earned 18% more than female dropouts.

- While only slightly more than half the dropouts were either working or looking for work (called "in the labor force,") over 80% of those who had gotten a GED were in the labor force.

- Twice as many women GED holders were in the labor force as women dropouts. In fact, nearly two out of three female GED holders were in the labor force.

- For African American men, 85% of GED holders were in the labor force, compared with 60% of dropouts.

- For Hispanics, 93% of GED holders were in the labor force, compared with 77% of dropouts.

The Lives of Dropouts

In a recent survey, dropouts, approximately 18-years-old, were asked to tell about their lives before they decided to leave school. They said that both their personal and schools lives were very hard. Experiences like the following ones, which they revealed, can be considered a warning sign that a student is a dropout risk:

- 20% were married, living as married, or divorced, with females more likely than males to be married. Nearly 40% percent had a child or were expecting one.

- Nearly 25% changed schools two or more times, with some changing for disciplinary reasons.

- 12% ran away from home.

- Almost 20% were held back a grade, and almost half failed a course.

- Almost one-half missed at least 10 days of school, one-third cut class at least 10 times, and one-quarter were late at least 10 times.

- One-third were put on in-school suspension, suspended, or put on probation, and more than 15% were either expelled or told they couldn't return.

- 11% were arrested.

- 8% spent time in a juvenile home or shelter.

Reasons Why Youth Drop out

Dropouts listed both school problems and personal factors as reasons for dropping out:

- Didn't like school in general or the school they were attending.

- Were failing, getting poor grades, or couldn't keep up with school work.

- Didn't get along with teachers and/or students.

- Had disciplinary problems, were suspended, or expelled.

- Didn't feel safe in school.

- Got a job, had a family to support, or had trouble managing both school and work.

- Got married, got pregnant, or became a parent.

- Had a drug or alcohol problem.

What Parents Can Do to Prevent Dropping out

Despite leaving high school, many dropouts said that they expected to continue their education. Most planned to finish high school eventually, and some were interested in a career education school, college, and even graduate school. Since they had these goals, it is even more unfortunate that they couldn't be helped to stay in school. But many youth thought that schools didn't do very much to try to keep them, and that their families didn't try much harder. While it is possible that these youth didn't recognize some offers of help, it is important for youth to realize that the adults in their lives do want them to remain in school and are willing to do a lot to make it possible.

Here are some ways that parents, working with school administrators, counselors, and teachers, can help their children remain in high school:

- Arrange for help with making up missed work, tutoring, placement in a special program, and/or a transfer to another school.

- Help them with personal problems, and/or arrange for professional help.

- Help them schedule work and family obligations so that there is also time to attend school.

- Help them understand that the choices they make like marrying, becoming parents, failing courses, or behaving badly enough to get suspended can seriously disrupt their ability to finish school.

- If students do become pregnant or parents, help them find school and social programs that will meet their special needs.

- If all else fails, help them find a GED program and encourage them to stay with it until they get an alternative high school diploma.

Chapter 62

General Information on Learning Disabilities

Introduction

Imagine having important needs and ideas to communicate, but being unable to express them. Perhaps feeling bombarded by sights and sounds, unable to focus your attention. Or trying to read or add but not being able to make sense of the letters or numbers.

You may not need to imagine. You may be the parent or teacher of a child experiencing academic problems, or have someone in your family diagnosed as learning disabled. Or possibly as a child you were told you had a reading problem called dyslexia or some other learning handicap.

Although different from person to person, these difficulties make up the common daily experiences of many learning disabled children, adolescents, and adults. A person with a learning disability may experience a cycle of academic failure and lowered self-esteem. Having these handicaps—or living with someone who has them—can bring overwhelming frustration.

But the prospects are hopeful. It is important to remember that a person with a learning disability can learn. The disability usually only affects certain limited areas of a child's development. In fact, rarely

Excerpted from "Learning Disabilities," National Institute of Mental Health (NIMH), National Institutes of Health (NIH), NIH Publication No. 93-3611, http://www.pueblo.gsa.gov/cic_text/children/leardis/learndis.htm, 1993. Reviewed and revised in July, 2001 by Dr. David A. Cooke, MD, Diplomate, American Board of Internal Medicine.

are learning disabilities severe enough to impair a person's potential to live a happy, normal life.

Understanding the Problem

What Is a Learning Disability?

Unlike other disabilities, such as paralysis or blindness, a learning disability (LD) is a hidden handicap. A learning disability doesn't disfigure or leave visible signs that would invite others to be understanding or offer support.

LD is a disorder that affects people's ability to either interpret what they see and hear or to link information from different parts of the brain. These limitations can show up in many ways—as specific difficulties with spoken and written language, coordination, self-control, or attention. Such difficulties extend to schoolwork and can impede learning to read or write, or to do math.

Learning disabilities can be lifelong conditions that, in some cases, affect many parts of a person's life: school or work, daily routines, family life, and sometimes even friendships and lay. In some people, many overlapping learning disabilities may be apparent. Other people may have a single, isolated learning problem that has little impact on other areas of their lives.

What Are the Types of Learning Disabilities?

"Learning disability" is not a diagnosis in the same sense as "chickenpox" or "mumps." Chickenpox and mumps imply a single, known cause with a predictable set of symptoms. Rather, LD is a broad term that covers a pool of possible causes, symptoms, treatments, and outcomes. Partly because learning disabilities can show up in so many forms, it is difficult to diagnose or to pinpoint the causes. And no one knows of a pill or remedy that will cure them.

Not all learning problems are necessarily learning disabilities. Many children are simply slower in developing certain skills. Because children show natural differences in their rate of development, sometimes what seems to be a learning disability may simply be a delay in maturation. To be diagnosed as a learning disability, specific criteria must be met.

The criteria and characteristics for diagnosing learning disabilities appear in a reference book called the *DSM* (short for the *Diagnostic and Statistical Manual of Mental Disorders*). The *DSM* diagnosis is commonly used when applying for health insurance coverage of diagnostic and treatment services.

Learning disabilities can be divided into three broad categories:

- Communication Disorders

- Learning Disorders

- "Other," a catch-all that includes certain coordination disorders and learning handicaps not covered by the other terms.

Each of these categories includes a number of more specific disorders.

Communication Disorders

Speech and language problems are often the earliest indicators of a learning disability. People with developmental speech and language disorders have difficulty producing speech sounds, using spoken language to communicate, or understanding what other people say. Depending on the problem, the specific diagnosis may be:

- Phonological Disorder

- Expressive Language Disorder

- Mixed Receptive-Expressive Language Disorder

Phonological Disorder (formerly Developmental Articulation Disorder). Children with this disorder may have trouble controlling their rate of speech. Or they may lag behind playmates in learning to make speech sounds. Phonological disorders are common. About 2% of children 6 to 7 years old have moderate to severe forms. Fortunately, articulation disorders can often be outgrown or successfully treated with speech therapy.

Expressive Language Disorder (formerly Developmental Expressive Disorder). Some children with language impairments have problems expressing themselves in speech. Their disorder is called, therefore, Expressive Language Disorder. Someone who often calls objects by the wrong names has an Expressive Language Disorder. Of course, an expressive language disorder can take other forms. A 4-year-old who speaks only in two-word phrases and a 6-year-old who can't answer simple questions also have an expressive language disability. Expressive Language Disorder frequently occurs in combination with Phonological Disorder.

Mixed Receptive-Expressive Language Disorder (formerly Developmental Receptive Language Disorder). Some people have trouble understanding certain aspects of speech. It's as if their brains are set to a different frequency and the reception is poor. There's the toddler who doesn't respond to his name, a preschooler who hands you a bell when you asked for a ball, or the worker who consistently can't follow simple directions. Their hearing is fine, but they can't make sense of certain sounds, words, or sentences they hear. They may even seem inattentive. These people have a receptive language disorder. Because using and understanding speech are strongly related, almost all people with receptive language disorders also have an expressive language disorder, although it may not be as obvious as the receptive disorder.

Of course, in preschoolers, some misuse of sounds, words, or grammar is a normal part of learning to speak. It's only when these problems persist that there is any cause for concern.

Learning Disorders

Students with learning disorders are often years behind their classmates in developing reading, writing, or arithmetic skills. The diagnoses in this category include:

- Reading Disorder
- Disorder of Written Expression
- Mathematics Disorder

Reading Disorder (formerly Developmental Reading Disorder). This type of disorder, also known as dyslexia, is quite widespread. In fact, reading disabilities affect 4 percent of elementary school children.

When you think of what is involved in the "three R's"—reading, 'riting, and 'rithmetic—it's astounding that most of us do learn them. Consider that to read, you must simultaneously:

- focus attention on the printed marks and control eye movements across the page
- recognize the sounds associated with letters
- understand words and grammar
- build ideas and images

- compare new ideas to what you already know
- store ideas in memory

Such mental juggling requires a rich, intact network of nerve cells that connect the brain's centers of vision, language, and memory.

A person can have problems in any of the tasks involved in reading. However, scientists found that a significant number of people with dyslexia share an inability to distinguish or separate the sounds in spoken words. Children with dyslexia may have trouble with rhyming games, such as rhyming "cat" with "bat." Yet scientists have found these skills fundamental to learning to read. Fortunately, remedial reading specialists have developed techniques that can help many children with dyslexia acquire these skills.

However, there is more to reading than recognizing words. If the brain is unable to form images or relate new ideas to those stored in memory, the reader can't understand or remember the new concepts. So other types of reading disabilities can appear in the upper grades when the focus of reading shifts from word identification to comprehension.

Reading Disorder is frequently associated with Disorder of Written Expression and Mathematics Disorder. In fact, the latter two disorders rarely occur without Reading Disorder.

Disorder of Written Expression (formerly Developmental Writing Disorder). Writing, too, involves several brain areas and functions. The brain networks for vocabulary, grammar, hand movement, and memory must all be in good working order. So a disorder of written expression may result from problems in any of these areas. A child with a writing disability, particularly an expressive language disorder, might be unable to compose complete, grammatical sentences. As noted above, it is rare for a person to have a disorder of written expression without also having a reading disorder.

Mathematics Disorder (formerly Developmental Arithmetic Disorder). If you doubt that arithmetic is a complex process, think of the steps you take to solve this simple problem: 25 divided by 3 equals ?

Arithmetic involves recognizing numbers and symbols, memorizing facts such as the multiplication table, aligning numbers, and understanding abstract concepts like place value and fractions. Any of these may be difficult for children with developmental arithmetic disorders. Problems with numbers or basic concepts are likely to show up early. Disabilities that appear in the later grades are more often tied to problems in reasoning. About 80% of children with Mathematics Disorder also have a reading disorder.

Many aspects of speaking, listening, reading, writing, and arithmetic overlap and build on the same brain capabilities. So it's not surprising that people can be diagnosed as having more than one area of learning disability. For example, the ability to understand language underlies learning speak. Therefore, any disorder that hinders the ability to understand language will also interfere with the development of speech, which in turn hinders learning to read and write. A single gap in the brain's operation can disrupt many types of activity.

"Other" Learning Disabilities

The DSM also lists additional categories, such as "motor skills disorders" and "specific developmental disorders not otherwise specified." These diagnoses include delays in acquiring language, academic, and motor skills that can affect the ability to learn, but do not meet the criteria for a specific learning disability. Also included are coordination disorders that can lead to poor penmanship, as well as certain spelling and memory disorders.

Attention Disorders

Nearly 4 million school-age children have learning disabilities. Of these, at least 20 percent have a type of disorder that leaves them unable to focus their attention.

Some children and adults who have attention disorders appear to daydream excessively. And once you get their attention, they're often easily distracted.

In a large proportion of affected children—mostly boys—the attention deficit is accompanied by hyperactivity. They act impulsively, running into traffic or toppling desks. Hyperactive children can't sit still. They blurt out answers and interrupt. In games, they can't wait their turn. These children's problems are usually hard to miss. Because of their constant motion and explosive energy, hyperactive children often get into trouble with parents, teachers, and peers.

By adolescence, physical hyperactivity usually subsides into fidgeting and restlessness. But the problems with attention and concentration often continue into adulthood. At work, adults with ADHD often have trouble organizing tasks or completing their work. They don't seem to listen to or follow directions. Their work may be messy and appear careless.

Attention disorders, with or without hyperactivity, are not considered learning disabilities in themselves. However, because attention problems can seriously interfere with school performance, they often accompany academic skills disorders.

What Causes Learning Disabilities

Understandably, one of the first questions parents ask when they learn their child has a learning disorder is "Why? What went wrong?"

Mental health professionals stress that since no one knows what causes learning disabilities, it doesn't help parents to look backward to search for possible reasons. There are too many possibilities to pin down the cause of the disability with certainty. It is far more important for the family to move forward in finding ways to get help.

Scientists, however, do need to study causes in an effort to identify ways to prevent learning disabilities.

Once, scientists thought that all learning disabilities were caused by a single neurological problem. But research supported by the National Institute of Mental Health (NIMH) has helped us see that the causes are more diverse and complex. New evidence seems to show that most learning disabilities do not stem from a single, specific area of the brain, but from difficulties in bringing together information from various brain regions.

Today, a leading theory is that learning disabilities stem from subtle disturbances in brain structures and functions. Some scientists believe that, in many cases, the disturbance begins before birth.

Errors in Fetal Brain Development

Throughout pregnancy, this brain development is vulnerable to disruptions. If the disruption occurs early, the fetus may die, or the infant may be born with widespread disabilities and possibly mental retardation. If the disruption occurs later when the cells are becoming specialized and moving into place, it may leave errors in the cell makeup, location, or connections. Some scientists believe that these errors may later show up as learning disorders.

Other Factors That Affect Brain Development

Through experiments with animals, scientists at NIMH and other research facilities are tracking clues to determine what disrupts brain development. By studying the normal processes of brain development, scientists can better understand what can go wrong. Some of these studies are examining how genes, substance abuse, pregnancy problems, and toxins may affect the developing brain.

Figure 62.1. *Brain development. By birth, all the basic structures of the brain are present.*

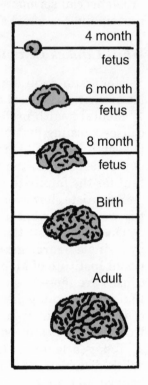

4 month
fetus

6 month
fetus

8 month
fetus

Birth

Adult

Getting Help

How Are Learning Disabilities First Identified?

The first step in solving any problem is realizing there is one. When a baby is born, the parents eagerly wait for the baby's first step, first word, a myriad of other "firsts." During routine checkups, the pediatrician, too, watches for more subtle signs of development. The parents and doctor are watching for the child to achieve developmental milestones.

Parents are usually the first to notice obvious delays in their child reaching early milestones. The pediatrician may observe more subtle signs of minor neurological damage, such as a lack of coordination.

But the classroom teacher, in fact, may be the first to notice the child's persistent difficulties in reading, writing, or arithmetic. As school tasks become more complex, a child with a learning disability may have problems mentally juggling more information.

The learning problems of children who are quiet and polite in school may go unnoticed. Children with above average intelligence, who manage to maintain passing grades despite their disability, are even less likely to be identified. Children with hyperactivity, on the other hand, will be identified quickly by their impulsive behavior and excessive movement. Hyperactivity usually begins before age 4 but may not be recognized until the child enters school.

What should parents, doctors, and teachers do if critical developmental milestones haven't appeared by the usual age? Sometimes it's best to allow a little more time, simply for the brain to mature a bit. But if a milestone is already long delayed, if there's a history of learning disabilities in the family, or if there are several delayed kills, the child should be professionally evaluated as soon as possible. An educator or a doctor who treats children can suggest where to go for help.

How Are Learning Disabilities Formally Diagnosed?

By law, learning disability is defined as a significant gap between a person's intelligence and the skills the person has achieved at each age. This means that a severely retarded 10-year-old who speaks like a 6-year-old probably doesn't have a language or speech disability. He has mastered language up to the limits of his intelligence. On the other hand, a fifth grader with an IQ of 100 who can't write a simple sentence probably does have LD.

Learning disorders may be informally flagged by observing significant delays in the child's skill development. A 2-year delay in the primary grades is usually considered significant. For older students, such a delay is not as debilitating, so learning disabilities aren't usually suspected unless there is more than a 2-year delay. Actual diagnosis of learning disabilities, however, is made using standardized tests that compare the child's level of ability to what is considered normal development for a person of that age and intelligence.

Test outcomes depend not only on the child's actual abilities, but on the reliability of the test and the child's ability to pay attention and understand the questions. Children with poor attention or hyperactivity may score several points below their true level of ability. Testing a child in an isolated room can sometimes help the child concentrate and score higher.

Each type of LD is diagnosed in slightly different ways. To diagnose speech and language disorders, a speech therapist tests the child's pronunciation, vocabulary, and grammar and compares them to the developmental abilities seen in most children that age. A psychologist tests the child's intelligence. A physician checks for any ear infections, and an audiologist may be consulted to rule out auditory problems. If the problem involves articulation, a doctor examines the child's vocal cords and throat.

In the case of academic skills disorders, academic development in reading, writing, and math is evaluated using standardized tests. In addition, vision and hearing are tested to be sure the student can see words clearly and can hear adequately. The specialist also checks if the child has missed much school. It's important to rule out these other possible factors. After all, treatment for a learning disability is very different from the remedy for poor vision or missing school.

ADHD is diagnosed by checking for the long-term presence of specific behaviors, such as considerable fidgeting, losing things, interrupting, and talking excessively. Other signs include an inability to remain seated, stay on task, or take turns. A diagnosis of ADHD is made only if the child shows such behaviors substantially more than other children of the same age.

If the school fails to notice a learning delay, parents can request an outside evaluation. Parents should stay abreast of each step of the school's evaluation. Parents also need to know that they may appeal the school's decision if they disagree with the findings of the diagnostic team. Also, parents always have the option of getting a second opinion.

Some parents feel alone and confused when talking to learning specialists. Such parents may find it helpful to ask someone they like and trust to go with them to school meetings. The person may be the child's clinician or caseworker, or even a neighbor. It can help to have someone along who knows the child and can help understand the child's test scores or learning problems.

What Are the Education Options?

Although obtaining a diagnosis is important, even more important is creating a plan for getting the right help. Because LD can affect the child and family in so many ways, help may be needed on a variety of fronts: educational, medical, emotional, and practical.

In most ways, children with learning disabilities are no different from children without these disabilities. At school, they eat together and share sports, games, and after-school activities. But since children with learning disabilities do have specific learning needs, most public schools provide special programs.

Schools typically provide special education programs either in a separate all-day classroom or as a special educçtion class that the student attends for several hours each week. Some parents hire trained tutors to work with their child after school. If the problems are severe, some parents choose to place their child in a special school for the learning disabled.

If parents choose to get help outside the public schools, they should select a learning specialist carefully. The specialist should be able to explain things in terms that the parents can understand. Whenever possible, the specialist should have professional certification and experience with the learner's specific age group and type of disability.

Planning a special education program begins with systematically identifying what the student can and cannot do. The specialist looks for patterns in the child's gaps. For example, if the child fails to hear the separate sounds in words, are there other sound discrimination problems? If there's a problem with handwriting, are there other motor delays? Are there any consistent problems with memory?

Special education teachers also identify the types of tasks the child can do and the senses that function well. By using the senses that are intact and bypassing the disabilities, many children can develop needed skills. These strengths offer alternative ways the child can learn.

After assessing the child's strengths and weaknesses, the special education teacher designs an Individualized Educational Program (IEP). The IEP outlines the specific skills the child needs to develop as well as appropriate learning activities that build on the child's strengths. Many effective learning activities engage several skills and senses. For example, in learning to spell and recognize words, a student may be asked to see, say, write, and spell each new word. The student may also write the words in sand, which engages the sense of touch. Many experts believe that the more senses children use in learning a skill, the more likely they are to retain it.

An individualized, skill-based approach—like the approach used by speech and language therapists—often succeeds in helping where regular classroom instruction fails. Therapy for speech and language disorders focuses on providing a stimulating but structured environment for hearing and practicing language patterns. For example, the therapist may help a child who has an articulation disorder to produce specific speech sounds. During an engaging activity, the therapist may talk about the toys, then encourage the child to use the same sounds or words. In addition, the child may watch the therapist make the sound, feel the vibration in the therapist's throat, then practice making the sounds before a mirror.

Researchers are also investigating nonstandard teaching methods. Some create artificial learning conditions that may help the brain receive information in nonstandard ways. For example, in some language disorders, the brain seems abnormally slow to process verbal information. Scientists are testing whether computers that talk can help teach children to process spoken sounds more quickly. The computer starts slowly, pronouncing one sound at a time. As the child gets better at recognizing the sounds and hearing them as words, the sounds are gradually sped up to a normal rate of speech.

Is Medication Available?

For nearly six decades, many children with attention disorders have benefitted from being treated with medication. Three rugs, Ritalin (methylphenidate), Dexedrine (dextroamphetamine), and Cylert (pemoline), have been used successfully. Although these drugs are stimulants in the same category as "speed" and "diet pills," they seldom make children "high" or more jittery. Rather, they temporarily improve children's attention and ability to focus. They also help children control their impulsiveness and other hyperactive behaviors.

The effects of medication are most dramatic in children with ADHD. Shortly after taking the medication, they become more able to focus their attention. They become more ready to learn. Studies by NIMH scientists and other researchers have shown that at least 90 percent of hyperactive children can be helped by either Ritalin or Dexedrine. If one medication does not help a hyperactive child to calm down and pay attention in school, the other medication might.

In trying to do everything possible to help their children, many parents have been quick to try new treatments. Most of these treatments sound scientific and reasonable, but a few are pure quackery. Many are developed by reputable doctors or specialists—but when tested scientifically, cannot be proven to help. Following are types of therapy that have not proven effective in treating the majority of children with learning disabilities or attention disorders:

- megavitamins
- colored lenses
- special diets

- sugar-free diets
- body stimulation or manipulation

Although scientists hope that brain research will lead to new medical interventions and drugs, at present there are no medicines for speech, language, or academic disabilities.

How Do Families Learn to Cope?

The effects of learning disabilities can ripple outward from the disabled child or adult to family, friends, and peers at school or work.

Children with LD often absorb what others thoughtlessly say about them. They may define themselves in light of their disabilities, as "behind," "slow," or "different."

Sometimes they don't know how they're different, but they know how awful they feel. Their tension or shame can lead them to act out in various ways—from withdrawal to belligerence. They may get into fights. They may stop trying to learn and achieve and eventually drop out of school or they may become isolated and depressed.

Children with learning disabilities and attention disorders may have trouble making friends with peers. For children with ADHD, this may be due to their impulsive, hostile, or withdrawn behavior. Some children with delays may be more comfortable with younger children who play at their level. Social problems may also be a product of their disability. Some people with LD seem unable to interpret tone of voice or facial expressions. Misunderstanding the situation, they act inappropriately, turning people away.

Without professional help, the situation can spiral out of control. The more that children or teenagers fail, the more they may act out their frustration and damage their self-esteem. The more they act out, the more trouble and punishment it brings, further lowering their self-esteem.

Having a child with a learning disability may also be an emotional burden for the family. Parents often sweep through a range of emotions: denial, guilt, blame, frustration, anger, and despair. Brothers and sisters may be annoyed or embarrassed by their sibling, or jealous of all the attention the child with LD gets.

Counseling can be very helpful to people with LD and their families. Counseling can help affected children, teenagers, and adults develop greater self-control and a more positive attitude toward their own abilities. Talking with a counselor or psychologist also allows family members to air their feelings as well as get support and reassurance.

Many parents find that joining a support group also makes a difference. Support groups can be a source of information, practical suggestions, and mutual understanding. Self-help books written by educators and mental health professionals can also be helpful.

Behavior modification also seems to help many children with hyperactivity and LD. In behavior modification, children receive immediate, tangible rewards when they act appropriately. Receiving an immediate reward can help children learn to control their own actions, both at home and in class. A school or private counselor can explain behavior modification and help parents and teachers set up appropriate rewards for the child.

Parents and teachers can help by structuring tasks and environments for the child in ways that allow the child to succeed. They can find ways to help children build on their strengths and work around their disabilities. This may mean deliberately making eye contact before speaking to a child with an attention disorder. For a teenager with a language problem, it may mean providing pictures and diagrams for performing a task. For students with handwriting or spelling problems a solution may be to provide a word processor and software that checks spelling. A counselor or school psychologist can help identify practical solutions that make it easier for the child and family to cope day by day.

Every child needs to grow up feeling competent and loved. When children have learning disabilities, parents may need to work harder at developing their children's self-esteem and relationship-building skills. But self-esteem and good relationships are as worth developing as any academic skill.

Sustaining Hope

Can Learning Disabilities Be Outgrown or Cured?

Even though most people don't outgrow their brain dysfunction, people do learn to adapt and live fulfilling lives. Even though a learning disability doesn't disappear, given the right types of educational experiences, people have a remarkable ability to learn. The brain's flexibility to learn new skills is probably greatest in young children and may diminish somewhat after puberty. This is why early intervention is so important. Nevertheless, we retain the ability to learn throughout our lives.

Even though learning disabilities can't be cured, there is still cause for hope. Because certain learning problems reflect delayed development, many children do eventually catch up. Of the speech and language disorders, children who have an articulation or an expressive language disorder are the least likely to have long-term problems. Despite initial delays, most children do learn to speak.

For people with dyslexia, the outlook is mixed. But an appropriate remedial reading program can help learners make great strides.

With age, and appropriate help from parents and clinicians, children with ADHD become better able to suppress their hyperactivity and to channel it into more socially acceptable behaviors. The problem may take less disruptive forms, such as fidgeting.

Can an adult be helped? For example, can an adult with dyslexia still learn to read? In many cases, the answer is yes. It may not come as easily as for a child. It may take more time and more repetition, and it may even take more diverse teaching methods. But we know more about reading and about adult learning than ever before. We know that adults have a wealth of life experience to build on as they learn. And because adults choose to learn, they do so with a determination that most children don't have. A variety of literacy and adult education programs sponsored by libraries, public schools, and community colleges are available to help adults develop skills in reading, writing, and math. Some of these programs, as well as private and nonprofit tutoring and learning centers, provide appropriate programs for adults with LD.

Chapter 63

Preparing Your Adolescent for College

What Types of Colleges Exist?

More than half of all recent high school graduates in the United States pursue some type of postsecondary education. In many other countries, a smaller percentage of students go on for more schooling after high school. However, in America, recent surveys show that most parents want their children to get some college education. There is a wide range of higher education options in the United States. For this reason, your child is likely to find a college well-suited to his or her needs.

Throughout this document, the term "college" is used to refer to all post-secondary institutions—technical colleges, junior colleges, community colleges, other two-year colleges, and four-year colleges and universities.

There are two basic types of post-secondary education institutions:

- Community, technical, and junior colleges. Many kinds of colleges offer programs that are less than four years in length. Most of these schools offer education and training programs that are two years in length or shorter. The programs often lead to a license, a certificate, an associate of arts (A.A.) degree, an associate of science (A.S.) degree, or an associate of applied science (A.A.S.) degree.

Excerpted from "Preparing Your Child For College, A Resource Book for Parents, 1996–97 Edition," US Department of Education, http://www.ed.gov/pubs/Prepare/index.html.

- Four-year colleges and universities. These schools usually offer a bachelor of arts (B.A.) or bachelor of science (B.S.) degree. Some also offer graduate and professional degrees.

What Can My Child Do to Prepare Academically for College?

Take Courses Recommended for College-Bound Students

To prepare for college, there is no substitute for your child getting a solid and broad academic education. This means your child should take challenging courses in academic subjects and maintain good grades in high school. Your child's transcript will be an important part of his or her college application.

A college education builds on the knowledge and skills acquired in earlier years. It is best for your child to start planning a high school course schedule early, in the seventh or eighth grade. Students who don't plan ahead may have difficulty completing all the required or recommended courses that will help them qualify for college.

Most selective colleges (those with the highest admissions requirements) prefer to admit students who have taken courses in certain subject areas. For example, many colleges prefer that high school students take at least geometry and trigonometry, rather than only general math and algebra. Basic computer skills are now essential, and some colleges prefer three or four years of a foreign language. Your child's guidance counselor can help your child determine the high school courses required or preferred by different types of colleges. If your child is interested in specific colleges, he or she can contact those schools and ask about their admissions requirements.

Many high schools offer Advanced Placement (AP) courses and exams. AP courses are college-level courses in approximately 16 different subjects; they help students prepare for college-level work while they are still in high school. Students who take AP courses are often more prepared for the academic challenges presented in college. In addition, a student who takes an AP course, and who scores a grade of 3 or higher on an AP exam, can often receive advanced placement in college and/or credit for a college course. Talk to one of your child's teachers, your child's guidance counselor, or the principal of your child's school to find out if AP courses are offered at your child's high school.

This can result in significant cost savings. However, not all colleges and universities give credit or advanced placement for earning a grade of 3 or higher on an AP exam. Write to the admissions office of the colleges that are of interest to your child to find out if they give credit for an AP exam grade of 3 or higher. Ask to obtain the college's AP policy in writing, or look for a discussion of the policy in the institution's catalog.

Below is a list of the high school courses that many higher education associations and guidance counselors recommend for a college-bound student. These courses are especially recommended for students who want to attend a four-year college. Even if your child is interested in attending a junior college, community college, or technical college, he or she should take most of these courses since they provide the preparation necessary for all kinds of post-secondary education (in addition, many students who attend two-year colleges go on to earn a B.A. or B.S. degree at a four-year college or university).

High School Courses Recommended for College

English — 4 Years; Types of Classes

- composition
- English literature
- American literature
- world literature

Mathematics — 3 to 4 Years; Types of Classes

- algebra I
- geometry
- precalculus
- algebra II
- trigonometry
- calculus

History & Geography — 2 to 3 Years; Types of Classes

- geography
- US government
- world cultures
- US history
- world history
- civics

Laboratory Science — 2 to 3 Years; Types of Classes

- biology
- chemistry
- earth science
- physics

Foreign Language — 2 to 3 Years; Types of Classes

- French
- Spanish
- Russian
- German
- Latin
- Japanese

Visual & Performing Arts — 1 Year; Types of Classes

- art
- drama

- dance
- music

Appropriate Electives — 1 to 3 Years; Types of Classes

- economics
- statistics
- communications

- psychology
- computer science

Things You and Your Child Can Do to Prepare for a Technical Program at a Community, Junior, or Technical College

If your child is interested in pursuing a technical program in a community, junior, or technical college, he or she may want to supplement or substitute some of the courses listed in the chart with some vocational or technical courses in his or her field of interest. Look especially for more advanced technology courses in the junior and senior years of high school. However, your child should at least take the suggested courses in the core areas of English, math, science, history, and geography.

Talking to an administrator or professor from a community, junior, or technical college is a good way to find out about the best high school courses to take in order to prepare for a specific technical program offered at that college. The dean of a particular technical program will also be able to tell you about the entry requirements for the program.

Make Sure That All Courses Meet High Standards

It is not only important for your child to enroll in the courses recommended for college-bound students; it is also essential that the material taught in those courses reflect high academic standards and high expectations for what students should know and be able to do. Research indicates that high expectations and high standards improve achievement and positively influence student learning.

Efforts are under way in states and communities across the country to answer the question: "What is it that our children ought to know and be able to do... to participate fully in today's and tomorrow's economy?" Many states and local communities have been developing or revising their standards (sometimes called "curriculum frameworks") in core subject areas such as math, science, English, history, geography, foreign languages, civics, and the arts. These standards help provide parents with answers to questions such as: "Is my child learning?" and "What is it that my child should know by the end of each grade?"

Many school districts are not waiting for their states to complete standards. In many local communities, groups of citizens—parents, teachers, administrators, business leaders, clergy, representatives from colleges, curriculum experts, and other community members—are working together to develop or revise standards. In creating their own standards, many States and local communities are drawing on model voluntary standards developed by national professional associations.

In order to make sure that the curriculum in your child's school meets high academic standards, call your child's school to find out if State or local standards are being developed. Ask how you can get involved in the standard-setting process. Join with other parents, teachers, and your child's principal and compare your school's standards against the best schools and the best State standards. You can also learn about the voluntary standards developed by national professional associations by contacting the professional organizations listed in the back of the book.

Take the Standardized Tests That Many Colleges Require

Many of the courses recommended for college-bound students (such as geometry and rigorous English courses) are also essential preparation for the college entrance examinations—the SAT I (Scholastic Assessment Test) or the ACT Assessment (American College Test). The SAT I measures verbal and mathematical reasoning abilities. The ACT Assessment measures English, mathematics, reading, and science reasoning abilities. Students applying to colleges in the East and West usually take the SAT I exam. Students applying to schools in the South and Midwest often take the ACT (however, students should check the admission requirements at each school to which they are applying).

Usually, the tests are offered in the junior and senior years of high school and can be taken more than once if a student wishes to try to improve his or her score. Students can get books at libraries or bookstores to help them to prepare for all of the tests. Some of these books are listed at the back of this resource book. In addition, some private organizations and companies offer courses that help students prepare for these exams.

575

Many schools offer the Preliminary Scholastic Assessment Test/ National Merit Scholarship Qualifying Test (PSAT/NMSQT) to their students. This practice test helps students prepare for the Scholastic Assessment Test (SAT I). The PSAT is usually administered to tenth or eleventh grade students. A student who does very well on this test and who meets many other academic performance criteria may qualify for the National Merit Scholarship Program. You and your child can find out more about the PSAT/NMSQT and the National Merit Scholarship Program by talking to your child's guidance counselor or by calling or writing to the number or address provided in the back of this handbook.

Some colleges also require that an applicant take one or more SAT II Subject Tests in major areas of study. It is a good idea for a student to consult a guidance counselor about this early in high school; often the best time to take an SAT II Test is right after the student has taken a course in that subject. For example, many students take the Biology SAT II Test right after they have completed a course in biology. This could mean that your child would take his or her first SAT II Test as a freshman or sophomore in high school.

At the back of this *Sourcebook*, in the section that lists places where you can get additional information, you will find the address and phone number where you can write or call for more information about the SAT I and the SAT II Tests. You will also find the address and phone number for the organization that administers the ACT.

Knowing what will be required for college is important; by taking the right courses and examinations from the beginning of high school, your child may avoid admission problems later on. In addition, students who do not prepare well enough academically in high school, if admitted to college, may be required to take remedial courses. Most colleges do not offer credit for these courses, and students may have to pay for these extra courses and spend extra time in college to earn their degrees. The following lists some questions that you or your child may want to ask your child's guidance counselor.

Questions to Ask Guidance Counselors

- What basic academic courses do they recommend for students who want to go to college?

- How many years of each academic subject does the high school require for graduation?

- What elective courses do they recommend for college-bound students?

- How does a student go about completing recommended courses before graduating from high school?

- Can students who are considering college get special help or tutoring?

- What activities can students do at home and over the summers to strengthen their preparation for college?

- How much homework is expected of students preparing for college?

- What kinds of high school grades do different colleges require?

What Can My Child Do outside the Classroom to Prepare for College?

Interpersonal and leadership skills, interests and goals are all important for college preparation. Independent reading and study, extracurricular activities, and work experience will all help your child develop his or her skills, interests, and goals.

Independent Reading and Study

Independent reading and study will help your child to prepare academically for college. This is a good way to develop interests, expand knowledge, and improve the vocabulary and reading comprehension skills needed for college and the SAT I or ACT. Encourage your child to read all kinds of books for fun—fiction and non-fiction. The school library and the local public library are good sources of books, magazines, and newspapers.

Creating a Good Place to Study

Your child needs a quiet and comfortable place to study. Here are a few things that you can do:

- Help him or her find a quiet place with some privacy.

- Set up a desk or large table with good light and place reference books such as a dictionary on the desk or nearby.

- Make sure your child studies there on a regular basis.

Extracurricular Activities

Many school, community, and religious organizations enable high school students to explore their interests and talents by providing activities outside the classroom. Colleges are often interested in a student's extracurricular activities such as school clubs, the student newspaper, athletics, musical activities, arts, drama, and volunteer work, especially if a student has excelled in one or more of these areas.

Work Experience and Community Service

Work experience—paid or volunteer—can teach students discipline, responsibility, reliability, teamwork, and other skills. Some students participate in community service activities such as tutoring elementary school children or volunteering in a local hospital. Such activities make valuable contributions to society and also help students to identify their career interests and goals, gain workplace skills, and apply classroom learning to real-world problem solving. Many colleges view community service as a valuable experience that enhances a student's college application.

Some schools offer academic credit for volunteer work through "service-learning." This is a teaching method that integrates hands-on learning (through service to the community) into the school curriculum. To find out if your child's school offers "service-learning," talk to your child's teacher, guidance counselor, or school principal. For information on how to start a "service-learning" program, contact the Learn and Serve America Clearinghouse at 1-800-808-SERVE.

A summer job is also a good way to gain experience and earn money for college as well. If your child works during the school year, he or she should not work so many hours that the job interferes with school work.

How Can My Child Go about Choosing a College?

Colleges are located in big cities, suburbs, and small towns throughout the country. Some enroll tens of thousands of students; others enroll only a few hundred. Some are public; others are private. Some private institutions are affiliated with religious institutions; others are not. Some schools enroll only women, others only men.

The type of institution best suited to your child depends on his or her individual needs and talents. Your child can begin focusing on the choice of a college by considering the following questions:

- Why do I want to go to college?

- What do I hope to achieve in college?

- Do I have some idea of what I want to study or for which job I want to prepare?

- Do I want to live at home or go away to school?

- Do I prefer an urban or suburban environment?

- Would I be happier in a small college or at a large university?

In order to choose a college, you and your child should ask the following questions about the nature and quality of the schools in which your child has an interest. Ask these questions when you meet staff in the admissions office of the colleges. You may also find answers to these questions in the colleges' catalogs or in reference books on colleges.

College Inquiries

Help your child list the colleges he or she knows about and might be interested in attending. Write down whether they are two-year or four-year colleges or universities. Ask your child why these schools are appealing to him or her. You and your child may want to contact the colleges to get more information.

How Much Does a College Education Cost?

Many people overestimate the cost of college or believe that all schools are expensive. For example, a recent Gallup survey indicated that 13- to 21-year-olds overestimated the average cost of public two- and four-year colleges by more than three times the actual figure. The same group estimated that the costs of private four-year colleges were one-third higher than they actually were. Although some colleges are expensive, costs vary from institution to institution. In addition, the availability of financial aid—money available from various sources to help students pay for college—can make even an expensive college affordable for a qualified student.

Tuition at Public and Private Colleges

It is important to know the difference between public and private institutions. A school's private or public status has a lot to do with its tuition.

Public institutions. Over three-quarters of all students in two- and four-year colleges attend State or other public colleges. Since these schools receive a large proportion of their budgets from State or local government, they can charge students who live in that State (in-State students) relatively low tuition. Students from other States (out-of-State students) usually pay higher tuition.

Private institutions. Private (sometimes called "independent") institutions charge the same tuition for both in-State and out-of-State students. Private college tuitions tend to be higher than those of public colleges because private schools receive less financial support from States and local governments.

Most private colleges are "non-profit." Other private post-secondary schools—mostly vocational and trade schools—are "proprietary." Such institutions are legally permitted to make a profit.

Future College Costs

Because there are many factors that affect the costs of a college education, it is impossible to know exactly how much colleges will charge when your child is ready to enroll. Be cautious when people tell you a particular amount; no one can be sure how much costs will change over time. In addition, as college costs increase, the amount of money you earn, and thus the amount you will have available to pay for college, will also rise.

How Can I Afford to Send My Child to College?

Saving Money

Saving money is the primary way to prepare for the costs of college. Setting aside a certain amount every month or each payday will help build up a fund for college. If you and your child begin saving early, the amount you have to set aside each month will be smaller.

In order to set up a savings schedule, you'll need to think about where your child might attend college, how much that type of college might cost, and how much you can afford to save. Keep in mind that colleges of the same type have a range of costs and your child may be able to attend one that is less expensive.

Financial Aid

Financial aid can help many families meet college costs. Every year millions of students apply for and receive financial aid. In fact, almost one-half of all students who go on for more education after high school receive financial aid of some kind. In school year 1994–95, post-secondary students received about $47 billion in financial aid.

There are three main types of financial assistance available to qualified students at the college level:

- grants and scholarships
- loans
- work-study

Grants and Scholarships

Grants and scholarships provide aid that does not have to be repaid. However, some require that recipients maintain certain grade levels or take certain courses.

Loans

Loans are another type of financial aid and are available to both students and parents. Like a car loan or a mortgage for a house, an education loan must eventually be repaid. Often, payments do not begin until the student finishes school, and the interest rate on education loans is commonly lower than for other types of loans. For students with no established credit record, it is usually easier to get student loans than other kinds of loans.

There are many different kinds of education loans. Before taking out any loan, be sure to ask the following kinds of questions:

- What are the exact provisions of the loan?
- What is the interest rate?
- Exactly how much has to be paid in interest?
- What will the monthly payments be?
- When will the monthly payments begin?
- How long will the monthly payments last?
- What happens if you miss one of the monthly payments?
- Is there a grace period for paying back the loan?

In all cases, a loan taken to pay for a college education must be repaid, whether or not a student finishes school or gets a job after graduation. Failure to repay a student loan can ruin a person's credit rating and make finances much more difficult in the future. This is an important reason to consider a college's graduation and job placement rates when you help your child choose a school.

Work-Study Programs

Many students work during the summer and/or part time during the school year to help pay for college. Although many obtain jobs on their own, many colleges also offer work-study programs to their students. A work-study job is often part of a student's financial aid package. The jobs are usually on campus and the money earned is used to pay for tuition or other college charges. The types of financial aid discussed above can be merit-based, need-based, or a combination of merit-based and need-based.

Merit-Based Financial Aid

Merit-based assistance, usually in the form of scholarships or grants, is given to students who meet requirements not related to financial needs. For example, a merit scholarship may be given to a student who has done well in high school or one who displays artistic or athletic talent. Most merit-based aid is awarded on the basis of academic performance or potential.

Need-Based Financial Aid

Need-based means that the amount of aid a student can receive depends on the cost of the college and on his or her family's ability to pay these costs. Most financial aid is need-based and is available to qualified students.

What Are the Most Common Sources of Financial Aid?

Student financial aid is available from a number of sources, including the Federal Government, State governments, colleges and universities, and other organizations. Students can receive aid from more than one source.

Federal Financial Assistance

The Federal Government supplies the largest amount of all student aid, about 75 percent or $35 billion annually. Students can get aid from more than one Federal program. For the most up-to-date information about student aid supplied by the Federal Government, call the Federal Student Financial Aid Information Center toll-free at the US Department of Education at 1-800-4FED-AID. You can also obtain a guide to Federal financial aid for students, called The Student Guide, which provides an extensive and annually updated discussion of all Federal student aid programs. You can obtain the Guide by writing to the following address:

Federal Student Aid Information Center
P.O. Box 84
Washington, DC 20044

State Financial Assistance

States generally give portions of state budgets to public colleges and universities. This support lowers tuition for all students attending these schools. Some states also offer financial assistance directly to individual students, which can be need-based or merit-based. To find out about state aid where you live, call or write your State's higher education agency.

College / University Assistance

Colleges themselves provide aid to many of their students. Most of this "institutional aid" is in the form of scholarships or grants. Some is need-based and some is merit-based.

When your child wants financial aid information about specific schools, he or she should contact the financial aid offices of these schools and request information.

Are There Other Ways to Keep the Cost of College Down?

Serve in AmeriCorps

AmeriCorps is a domestic Peace Corps in which thousands of young people are working in community service projects around the country in exchange for a living allowance averaging $7,500 per year; health care; child care when needed; and an education award of $4,725 per year for paying back a student loan or for financing postsecondary education. Under some circumstances a person can serve part time and receive an education award of $2,362 per year.

AmeriCorps projects serve communities throughout the country. All meet at least one of four national priorities: (1) education; (2) public safety; (3) human needs; and (4) the environment. For example,

AmeriCorps members teach state-of-the-art computer skills to teen-agers, tutor grade-school children in basic reading, or organize inno-vative after-school programs in some of the education projects. AmeriCorps members in environmental projects clean up urban streams and inland waterways, monitor dangerous trends in air qual-ity, or test-start city-wide recycling programs.

There are many different points in a person's educational career when participation in AmeriCorps is an option: right after high school; during or after college; and during or after graduate school or occu-pational training. AmeriCorps members are recruited locally and nationally. To find out more about AmeriCorps, call the AmeriCorps Hotline free of charge at 1-800-94-ACORPS (1-800-942-2677) or TDD 1-800-833-3722.

Enroll in a Two-Year College; Then Transfer to a Four-Year College

Local community colleges are usually the least expensive. In ad-dition to charging low tuition, they are located in the area in which the student lives, which makes it possible to save by living at home and commuting to campus.

After completing an associate's degree or certificate in a two-year college, students often can transfer to a four-year college and work toward a bachelor's degree.

If your child chooses this route, he or she needs to take courses in the two-year college that will count toward a bachelor's degree. Cer-tain community college courses may not be transferable to a four-year institution. Community college admissions officers can explain trans-fer terms and opportunities.

Take Advantage of Armed Forces Education Programs

The armed forces offer educational programs during or after ac-tive duty. If your child prefers to work toward a college degree imme-diately after high school, attending one of the military academies or attending a civilian school and enrolling in the Reserve Officers Train-ing Corps (ROTC) program are options. If your child wants to join the armed forces before attending college full time, he or she can attend college after military service by taking advantage of the Montgom-ery GI Bill or by obtaining college credit for some of the military train-ing he or she will receive.

Chapter 64

Keep Colleges Informed about Learning Disabilities

My Son Is Applying to College. What Information Should We Send Them about His Learning Disability?

You don't have to say what your son's learning disability is, but at the level of college admissions, a learning disability is not something to hide or to be ashamed of. Indeed, depending on the severity of his disability, your son may be doing himself a disservice if he is not open with college admissions staff about his learning disability. When the time comes to actually attend college, if the needed academic supports are not in place, he could be setting himself up for failure.

What about College Aptitude Tests?

There are options for students to help them compensate for learning disabilities when applying to college. When taking the college aptitude tests like the SAT or the ACT, some students with learning disabilities are offered modifications that allow for their disabilities.

Some students benefit from having more time to complete the tests. Others find it extremely helpful to have someone read the test to them. The procedures for qualifying for this type of testing are complicated,

Penny Paquette and Cheryl Gerson Tuttle, "Ask the Experts: Keep Colleges in the Loop Re: Learning Disabilities," copyright 1995–1999 Community Newspaper Company. Previously published in Marblehead Reporter, Feb. 13, 1997. Reprinted with permission of Community Newspaper Company.

but for many students with learning disabilities they are well worth the effort.

Be sure to check with your child's high school guidance office to see if your child qualifies for this type of testing. Also, you should know that the testing service will notify the college that the test was modified. Some guidance counselors suggest that students take the test both timed and untimed. That way schools can get a good idea of the student's knowledge base where time is not a factor.

Special Services and Special Education Staff

The admissions director of a small college in Massachusetts bemoaned the fact that a number of students were being admitted based on their high school grade point averages.

The students were successful in high school with the support of a special education staff. Their records did not indicate they had received this type of support. Once they arrived at college, they faltered without help.

Some colleges have support programs for students with learning disabilities, but many don't. If your son has required special services through high school, it is likely he will continue to need them in college. School guidance counselors and your son's teachers can help you and your student decide what type of college is best.

Students with mild learning disabilities have a good chance of succeeding in a college without special services. Those with moderate to severe learning disabilities might be best served at a college that specializes in teaching students with learning disabilities or at a school that provides special support services for learning disabled students.

Your son might be able to get into a college without being identified as learning disabled, but he may have to struggle with course work that places him at a disadvantage in his classes. Without help, he risks failure.

Part Seven

Additional Help and Information

Chapter 65

Glossary of Terms Related to Adolescent Health

acne vulgaris: An eruption, predominantly of the face, upper back, and chest, composed of comedones, cysts, papules, and pustules on an inflammatory base; the condition occurs in a majority of people during puberty and adolescence.

adolescence: The period of life beginning with puberty and ending with completed growth and physical maturity.

agoraphobia: A mental disorder characterized by an irrational fear of leaving the familiar setting of home, or venturing into the open, so pervasive that a large number of external life situations are entered into reluctantly or are avoided; often associated with panic attacks.

attention deficit hyperactivity disorder: A disorder of childhood and adolescence manifested at home, in school, and in social situations by developmentally inappropriate degrees of inattention, impulsiveness, and hyperactivity.

bipolar disorder: An affective disorder characterized by the occurrence of alternating periods of euphoria (mania) and depression. Syn: manic-depressive psychosis.

cocaine: A crystalline alkaloid obtained from the leaves of *Erythroxylon coca* (family *Erythroxylaceae*) and other species of

Erythroxylon, or by synthesis from ecgonine or its derivatives; a potent central nervous system stimulant, vasoconstrictor, and topical anesthetic, widely abused as a euphoriant and associated with the risk of severe adverse physical and mental effects.

conduct disorder: A mental disorder of childhood or adolescence characterized by a persistent pattern of violating societal norms and the rights of others; children with the disorder may exhibit physical aggression, cruelty to animals, vandalism and robbery, along with truancy, cheating, and lying.

drug abuse: Habitual use of drugs not needed for therapeutic purposes, such as solely to alter one's mood, affect, or state of consciousness, or to affect a body function unnecessarily (as in laxative abuse); nontherapeutic use of drugs.

eating disorders: A group of mental disorders including anorexia nervosa, bulimia nervosa, pica, and rumination disorder of infancy.

estrogen: Generic term for any substance, natural or synthetic, that exerts biologic effects characteristic of estrogenic hormones. Estrogens are formed by the ovary, placenta, testes, and possibly the adrenal cortex, as well as by certain plants; they stimulate secondary sexual characteristics, and exert systemic effects, such as growth and maturation of long bones, and are used therapeutically in any disorder attributable to estrogen deficiency or amenable to estrogen therapy, such as menstrual disorders and menopausal problems. They control the course of the menstrual cycle.

hepatitis: Inflammation of the liver, due usually to viral infection but sometimes to toxic agents.

heroin: An alkaloid prepared from morphine by acetylation; rapidly metabolized to morphine in the body; formerly used for the relief of cough. Except for research, its use in the United States is prohibited by federal law because of its potential for abuse.

homosexuality: Erotic attraction or activity, including sexual congress, between individuals of the same sex, especially past puberty.

hypertension: High blood pressure; transitory or sustained elevation of systemic arterial blood pressure to a level likely to induce cardiovascular damage or other adverse consequences.

juvenile arthritis, juvenile rheumatoid arthritis: Chronic arthritis beginning in childhood, most cases of which are pauciarticular, i.e., affecting few joints. Several patterns of illness have been identified: in one subset, primarily affecting girls, iritis is common and antinuclear antibody is usually present; another subset, primarily affecting boys, frequently includes spinal arthritis resembling ankylosing spondylitis; some cases are true rheumatoid arthritis beginning in childhood and characterized by the presence of rheumatoid factor and destructive deforming joint changes, often undergoing remission at puberty.

major depression: A mental disorder characterized by sustained depression of mood, anhedonia, sleep and appetite disturbances, and feelings of worthlessness, guilt, and hopelessness.

menarche: Establishment of the menstrual function; the time of the first menstrual period.

menses: A periodic physiologic hemorrhage, occurring at approximately 4-week intervals, and having its source from the uterine mucous membrane; usually the bleeding is preceded by ovulation and predecidual changes in the endometrium.

menstrual cycle: The period in which an ovum matures, is ovulated, and enters the uterine lumen via the fallopian tubes; ovarian hormonal secretions effect endometrial changes such that, if fertilization occurs, nidation will be possible; in the absence of fertilization, ovarian secretions wane, the endometrium sloughs, and menstruation begins; this cycle lasts an average of 28 days, with day 1 of the cycle designated as that day on which menstrual flow begins.

obsessive-compulsive personality disorder: A pervasive pattern in adulthood characterized by unattainable perfectionism; preoccupation with rules, details, and orderliness; unreasonable attempts to control others; excessive devotion to work; and rumination to the point of indecisiveness, all at the expense of flexibility, openness, and efficiency.

oppositional defiant disorder: A disorder of childhood or adolescence characterized by a recurrent pattern of negativistic, hostile, and disobedient behavior toward authority figures.

precocious puberty: Condition in which pubertal changes begin at an unexpectedly early age.

secondary sex characteristics: Those characteristics peculiar to the male or female that develop at puberty.

schizophrenia: A term coined by Bleuler, synonymous with and replacing dementia praecox; a common type of psychosis, characterized by abnormalities in perception, content of thought, and thought processes (hallucinations and delusions) and by extensive withdrawal of interest from other people and the outside world, with excessive focusing on one's own mental life; now considered a group or spectrum of disorders rather than a single entity, with distinction sometimes made between process schizophrenia and reactive schizophrenia. The "split" personality of schizophrenia, in which individual psychic components or functions split off and become autonomous, is popularly but erroneously identified with multiple personality, in which 2 or more relatively complete personalities dominate by turns the psychic life of an individual.

scoliosis: Abnormal lateral and rotational curvature of the vertebral column.

substance abuse: Maladaptive pattern of use of a drug, alcohol, or other chemical agent that may lead to social, occupational, psychological, or physical problems.

tic: Habitual, repeated contraction of certain muscles, resulting in stereotyped individualized actions that can be voluntarily suppressed for only brief periods, e.g., clearing the throat, sniffing, pursing the lips, excessive blinking; especially prominent when the person is under stress; there is no known pathologic substrate.

Tourette syndrome: A tic disorder appearing in childhood, characterized by multiple motor tics and vocal tics present for more than 1 year. Obsessive-compulsive behavior, attention-deficit disorder, and other psychiatric disorders may be associated; coprolalia and echolalia rarely occur; autosomal dominant inheritance.

venereal disease: Any contagious disease acquired during sexual contact; e.g., syphilis, gonorrhea, chancroid.

Chapter 66

Resources for Parents of Teens

This chapter lists contact information for some of the common ailment-related government agencies, professional organizations, websites, and publications. Information is listed according to the organization of the sections in this sourcebook.

Emotional and Mental Health Issues Affecting Adolescents

Girls Incorporated National Resource Center
441 West Michigan Street
Indianapolis, IN 46202-3287
Phone: 800-374-4475
Website: www.girlsinc.org
E-Mail: hn3580@handsnet.org

National Association of Anorexia Nervosa and Associated Disorders
P.O. Box 7
Highland Park, IL 60035
Phone: 847-831-3438
Fax: 847-433-4632
Website: www.anad.org
E-Mail: info@anad.org

The resources listed in this section were compiled from a wide variety of sources deemed accurate. Contact information was updated and verified in December 2001. Inclusion does not constitute endorsement.

The National Eating Disorders Association (formerly American Anorexia/Bulimia Association, Inc.)
603 Stewart Street
Suite 803
Seattle, WA 98101
Toll Free: 800-931-2237
Phone: 206-382-3587
Fax: 206-829-8501
Website: www.edap.org
E-Mail: info@edap.org

National Institute of Neurological Disorders and Stroke, Brain Resources and Information Network (BRAIN)
P.O. Box 5801
Bethesda, Maryland 20824
Toll Free: 800-352-9424
Phone: 301-496-5751
Website: www.ninds.nih.gov

The Tourette Syndrome Association, Inc.
42-40 Bell Boulevard
Bayside, NY 11361-2861
Phone: 718-224-2999
Fax: 718-279-9596
Website: www.tsa-usa.org
E-Mail: ts@tsa-usa.org

Other Physical Health Issues Affecting Adolescents

Allergy and Asthma Network/Mothers of Asthmatics
2751 Prosperity Ave.
Suite 150
Fairfax, VA 22031
Toll Free: 800-878-4403
Fax: 703-573-7794
Website: www.aanma.org

American Association of Respiratory Care
11030 Ables Lane
Dallas, TX 75229-4593
Phone: 972-243-2272
Fax: 972-484-2720
Website: www.aarc.org
E-Mail: info@aarc.org

American Juvenile Arthritis Organization (AJAO)
1330 West Peachtree Street
Atlanta, GA 30309
Toll Free: 800-283-7800
Phone: 404-872-7100
Fax: 404-872-0457
Website: www.arthritis.org

American Lung Association
1740 Broadway, 14th Floor
New York, NY 10019-4374
Toll Free: 800-LUNG-USA
Phone: 212-315-8700
Website: www.lungusa.org
E-Mail: info@lungusa.org

American Physical Therapy Association
1111 North Fairfax Street
Alexandria, VA 22314-1488
Toll Free: 800-999-2782
Phone: 703-684-2782
TDD: 703-683-6748
Fax: 703-684-7374
Website: www.apta.org

Asthma and Allergy Foundation of America
1125 15th Street, NW, Suite 502
Washington, DC 20005
Toll Free: 800-7-ASTHMA
Phone: 202-466-7643

Healthy Kids: The Key to Basics
79 Elmore Street
Newton, MA 02159-1137
Phone: 617-965-9637
Fax: 617-965-5407
Website: www.information-engineer.com/kids/kidshp.htm
E-Mail: erg@hk.pn.com

National Heart, Lung, and Blood Institute, National Asthma Education and Prevention Program
P.O. Box 30105
Bethesda, MD 20824-0105
Phone: 301-592-8573
Fax: 301-592-8563
Website: www.nhlbi.nih.gov
E-Mail: NHLBIinfo@rover.nhlbi.nih.gov

National Institute of Arthritis and Musculoskeletal and Skin Diseases (NIAMS) Information Clearinghouse, National Institutes of Health
1 AMS Circle
Bethesda, MD 20892-3675
Toll Free: 877-22-NIAMS
Phone: 301-495-4484
Fax: 301-718-6366
TTY: 301-565-2966
Website: www.niams.nih.gov
E-Mail: niamsinfo@mail.nih.gov

NIAMS Fast Facts
Health information available 24 hours a day by fax, call 301/881-2731 from a fax machine telephone.

National Scoliosis Foundation
5 Cabot Place
Stoughton, MA 02072
Toll Free: 800-NSF-MYBACK (800-673-6922)
Phone: 781-341-6333
Fax: 781-341-8333
Website: www.scoliosis.org
E-Mail: NSF@scoliosis.org

The Scoliosis Association, Inc.
P.O. Box 811705
Boca Raton, FL 33481-1705
Toll Free: 800-800-0669
Phone: 561-994-4435
Fax: 561-994-2455
Website: www.scoliosis-assoc.org

The Scoliosis Research Society
6300 North River Rd., Suite 727
Rosemont, IL 60018-4226
Phone: 847-698-1627
Fax: 847-823-0536
Website: www.srs.org

Adolescent Sexual Health

Advocates for Youth
1025 Vermont Avenue N.W.
Suite 200
Washington, D.C. 20005
Phone: 202-347-5700
Fax: 202-347-2263
Website:
www.advocatesforyouth.org
E-Mail:
info@advocatesforyouth.org

Alan Guttmacher Institute (AGI)
120 Wall Street
21st Floor
New York, NY 10005
Phone: 212-248-1111
Fax: 212-248-1951
Website: www.agi-usa.org
E-Mail: info@guttmacher.org

The Alan Guttmacher Institute (AGI) is an independent, non-profit corporation for research, policy analysis, and public education. Committed to enabling all men and women to exercise their rights and responsibilities with regard to reproduction and family formation, AGI protects and enhances the exercise of reproductive choices for those particularly disadvantaged in this regard as a result of poverty, youth, lack of education, racial or ethnic background, or place of residence.

American Social Health Association (ASHA)
P. O. Box 13827
Research Triangle Park, NC 27709-3827
Toll Free: 800-783-9877
Phone: 919-361-8400
Fax: 919-361-8425
Website: www.ashastd.org

Centers for Disease Control and Prevention, Division of Sexually Transmitted Diseases (DSTD)
1600 Clifton Road NE
Atlanta, GE 30333
CDC National STD Hotline:
800-227-8922 or 800-342-2437
En Espanol: 800-344-7432
National Herpes Hotline: 919-361-8488
National HPV and Cervical Cancer Hotline: 919-361-4848
TTY: 800-243-7889
Website: www.cdc.gov/std

Family Resource Coalition (FRC)
20 North Wacker Dr., Suite 1100
Chicago, IL 60606
Phone: 312-341-0900
Fax: 312-338-9361
Website:
www.familysupportamerica.org
E-Mail:
info@familysupportamerica.org

*International
Endometriosis Association*
8585 N. 76th Place
Milwaukee, WI 53223
Toll Free: 800-992-3636
Phone: 414-355-2200
Fax: 414-355-6065
Website:
www.endometriosisassn.org

Kempe Children's Center
1825 Marion Street
Denver, CO 80218
Phone: 303-864-5252
Fax: 303- 864-5302
Website: www.kempecenter.org
E-Mail: kempe@kempecenter.org

The C. Henry Kempe National Center for the Prevention and Treatment of Child Abuse and Neglect provides training, consultation, research and program development on all forms of abuse and neglect.

The National Adolescent Perpetrator Network is housed at the C. Henry Kempe Center. It can provide professionals and parents with a bibliography on juvenile sex offenders and with referrals to treatment programs for adolescent offenders. It also operates a Perpetration Prevention Project which provides training to professionals and paraprofessionals on "Understanding the Sexual Behavior of Children."

*National Adoption
Information Clearinghouse*
330 C Street, SW
Washington, D.C. 20447
Toll Free: 888-251-0075
Phone: 703-352-3488
Fax: 703-385-3206
Website: www.calib.com/naic
E-Mail: naic@calib.com

The National Adoption Information Clearinghouse maintains a list of adoption experts who have expertise in many areas of adoption, including the adoption of children who have experienced sexual abuse.

National Cancer Institute
Cancer Information Service
Toll Free: 800-4 CANCER (800-422-6237)
TTY: 800-332-8615
Website: www.nci.nih.gov

*National Clearinghouse on
Child Abuse and Neglect
Information*
330 C Street, SW
Washington, DC 20447
Toll Free: 800-394-3366
Phone: 703-385-7565
Fax: 703-385-3206
Website: www.calib.com/nccanch

The National Clearinghouse on Child Abuse and Neglect collects and disseminates information on child sexual abuse. It will do research upon request on a particular subject at a very low cost. It also has general publications which you can request.

National HPV and Cervical Cancer Prevention Resource Center, American Social Health Association
P. O. Box 13827
Research Triangle Park, NC 27709-3827
Toll Free: 800-783-9877
Phone: 919-361-8400
Fax: 919-361-8425
www.ashastd.org/hpvccrc/

National Organization on Adolescent Pregnancy, Parenting, and Prevention, Inc. (NOAPPP)
2401 Pennsylvania Ave.
Suite 350
Washington, DC 20037
Phone: 202-293-8370
Fax: 202-293-8805
Website: www.noappp.org
E-Mail: noappp@noappp.org

National Prevention Information Network (NPIN)
Centers for Disease Control and Prevention (CDC)
P.O. Box 6003
Rockville, MD 20849-6003
Toll Free: 800-458-5231
Fax: 888-282-7681
TTY: 800-243-7012
Website: www.cdcnpin.org
E-Mail: info@cdcnpin.org

National Runaway Switchboard
3080 N. Lincoln Ave.
Chicago, IL 60657
Toll Free Crisis Line: 800-621-4000
Phone: 773-880-9860
Fax: 773-929-5150
Website: www.nrscrisisline.org
E-Mail: info@nrscrisisline.org

The National Runaway Switchboard is a 24 hour crisis line for runaway youth and children considering running away. The Switchboard offers limited problem solving in a confidential, non-judgmental manner. It also offers a message service and a referral service for youth in need of shelter.

Social Issues and Other Parenting Concerns Affecting Adolescent Health and Safety

American Academy of Child and Adolescent Psychiatry
3615 Wisconsin Avenue, NW
Washington, DC 20016-3007
Phone: 202-966-7300
Fax: 202-966-2891
Website: www.aacap.org

American Academy of Ophthalmology
EyeNET
P.O. Box 7424
San Francisco, CA 94120
Phone: 415-561-8500
Website: www.aao.org
E-Mail: comm@aao.org

Provides eye safety information for children, including how to prevent sports-related eye injuries.

American Academy of Orthopaedic Surgeons (AAOS)
6300 North River Road
Rosemont, IL 60018
Toll Free: 800-346-AAOS
Phone: 847-823-7186
Fax: 847-823-8125
Website: www.aaos.org

Through the public information link on the AAOS home page (www.aaos.org), you can access fact sheets on injury prevention for many popular sports.

American Academy of Pediatrics (AAP)
141 Northwest Point Boulevard
Elk Grove Village, IL 60007
Phone: 847-434-4000
Fax: 847-434-8000
Website: www.aap.org
E-Mail: erg@aap.org

The AAP offers guidance on sports and your child, including their policy on sports participation for preschool children.

American Psychiatric Association
1400 K Street, NW
Washington, DC 20005
Toll Free: 800-357-7924
Fax: 202-682-6850
Website: www.psych.org
E-Mail: apa@psych.org

American Psychological Association (APA)
750 First Street, NE
Washington, DC 20002
Toll Free: 800-374-2721
TDD/TTY: 202-336-6123
Website: www.apa.org

To help youth proactively address the problem of violence, APA and MTV have teamed up to provide youth with information about identifying the warning signs of violent behavior and how to get help if they recognize these signs in themselves or their peers.

Anxiety Disorders Association of America (ADAA)
11900 Parklawn Drive
Suite 100
Rockville, MD 20852
Phone: 301-231-9350
Website: www.adaa.org

Blueprints for Violence Prevention

The Center for the Study and
Prevention of Violence
University of Colorado at
Boulder
439 UCB
Boulder, CO 80309
Phone: 303-492-8465
Fax: 303-443-3297
Website: www.colorado.edu/cspv
E-Mail: cspv@colorado.edu

Researchers at the Center for the
Study and Prevention of Violence
(CSVP), supported in part by the
U.S. Department of Justice and
Centers for Disease Control and
Prevention (CDC), have generated descriptions of programs
that met evaluation criteria for
youth-violence prevention. In addition, the center provides technical assistance with these
programs. Their Information
House collects research literature
on the causes and prevention of
violence and offers topical bibliographic searches. The center offers a variety of resources from
facts and statistics on youth violence to database searches on
youth violence.

Boys and Girls Clubs of America

1230 W. Peachtree, NW
Atlanta, GA 30309
Phone: 404-487-5700
Website: www.bgca.org
E-Mail: crathburn@bgca.org

Boys & Girls Clubs, neighbor-
hood-based facilities designed
solely for youth programs and
activities, are open every day after school and on weekends
when kids have free time and
need positive, productive outlets. Every Club has full-time,
trained youth development professionals who act as positive
role models and mentors. Volunteers provide key supplemen-
tary support.

Boys Town

Boys Town Center
Boys Town, NE 68010
Toll Free: 800-448-3000
E-Mail:
admissions@boystown.org
Website:
www.girlsandboystown.org

Boys Town is an organization
that cares for troubled children—both boys and girls—and
for families in crisis. The hotline
staff is trained to handle calls
and questions about violence
and suicide.

Brain Injury Association (BIA)

105 North Alfred Street
Alexandria, VA 22314
Family Helpline: 800-444-6443
Phone: 703-236-6000
Fax: 703-236-6443
Website: www.biause.org

BIA's fact sheet about sports and concussion safety (www.biausa.org/sportsfs.htm) provides data on brain injuries for several sports, including football, soccer, and baseball. Call toll-free, 1-800-444-6443.

Bureau of Justice Statistics
810 Seventh Street, NW
Washington, DC 20531
Phone: 202-307-0765
Website: www.ojp.usdoj.gov/bjs
E-Mail: askbjs@ojp.usdoj.gov

Bureau of Justice Statistics, U.S. Department of Justice The Office of Justice Programs provides summary findings about criminal victimization, victim characteristics, and characteristics of crime.

Center for Effective Collaboration and Practice
1000 Thomas Jefferson St., NW
Suite 400
Washington, DC 20007
Toll Free: 888-457-1551
Phone: 202-944-5400
Fax: 202-944-5454
Website: www.air.org/cecp/default.htm
E-Mail: center@air.org

Their web site provides on-line information, electronic interactive discussions, lists of individuals and organizations with expertise in school safety and violence prevention, and links to many resources important to developing safe schools and communities.

Center for Mental Health Services (CMHS)
5600 Fishers Lane, Room 17-99
Rockville, MD 20857
Phone: 301-443-8956
Website: www.samhsa.gov
E-Mail: info@samhsa.gov

Offers basic mental health information, details on services, and information from the Emergency Services and Disaster Relief Branch; the Child, Adolescent, and Family Branch; and the School Violence Prevention Initiative.

Child Welfare League of America (CWLA)
440 First Street, NW
Third Floor
Washington, DC 20001
Phone: 202-638-2952
Fax: 202-638-4004
Website: www.cwla.org

CWLA is an association of nearly 1,000 public and not-for-profit agencies devoted to improving the lives of more than 2.5 million at-risk children and youths and their families. Member agencies are involved with prevention and treatment of child abuse and neglect, and they provide various services in addition to child protection. Their phone number is 202-638-2952, and their web address is www.cwla.org/.

Children's Defense Fund
25 E Street, NW
Washington, DC 20001
Phone: 202-628-8787
Website:
www.childrensdefense.org
E-Mail:
cdfinfo@childrensdefense.org

The Children's Defense Fund provides a strong and effective voice for all children in the US. Their goal is to educate the nation about the needs of children and encourage investment in children before they get sick, drop out of school, suffer family breakdown, or get into trouble.

Children's Safety Network (CSN)
55 Chapel Street
Newton, MA 02458
Phone: 617-969-7100
Fax: 617-969-9186
Website: www.edu.org/HHD/csn

The CSN National Injury and Violence Prevention Resource Center provides resources and technical assistance to maternal and child health agencies and other organizations seeking to reduce unintentional injuries and violence among children and adolescents.

Division of Adolescent and School Health (DASH)
Phone: 770-488-3254
Website: www.cdc.gov/nccdphp/dash
E-Mail: healthyyouth@cdc.gov

Part of the Centers for Disease Control and Prevention (CDC), this division provides information on the following: adolescent health risk behaviors, including violence and unintentional injury; school health policies and programs; CDC-funded programs and research activities; funding opportunities; publications; and links to other school health sites.

Drug Strategies
1575 Eye Street, NW
Suite 210
Washington, DC 20005
Phone: 202-289-9070
Website:
www.drugstrategies.org
E-Mail: dspolicy@aol.com

Drug Strategies is a non-profit research institute that promotes more effective approaches to the nation's drug problems and supports private and public initiatives to reduce the demand for drugs through prevention, treatment, and law enforcement. As drugs are often linked with violence, the institute has produced Safe Schools/Safe Students: A Guide to Violence Prevention Strategies, a publication that assesses more than 80 violence prevention programs created for classroom use.

Federal Emergency Management Agency
FEMA for Kids
500 C Street, SW
Washington, DC 20472
Website: www.fema.gov/kids

International Society for Traumatic Stress Studies (ISTSS)
60 Revere Drive, Suite 500
Northbrook, IL 60062
Phone: 847-480-9028
Fax: 847-480-9292
Website: www.istss.org
E-Mail: istss@istss.org

National Alliance for Safe Schools
Ice Mountain
P.O. Box 290
Slanesville, WV 25444
Toll Free: 888-510-6500
Phone: 304-496-8100
Fax: 304-496-8105
Website: www.safeschools.org
E-Mail: NASS@raven-villages.net

National Athletic Trainers Association
2952 Stemmons Freeway
Dallas, TX 75247
Toll Free: 800-879-6282
Phone: 214-637-6283
Fax: 214-637-2206

National Clearinghouse on Child Abuse and Neglect Information
330 C Street, SW
Washington, DC 20447
Toll Free: 800-394-3366
Phone: 703-385-7565
Fax: 703-385-3206
Website: www.calib.com/nccanch

National Center for Injury Prevention and Control (NCIPC)
Mailstop K65
4770 Buford Highway, NE
Atlanta, GA 30341
Phone: 770-488-1506
Fax: 770-488-1667
Website: www.cdc.gov/ncipc
E-Mail: ohcinfo@cdc.gov

NCIPC's web site provides data on injury and violence epidemiology and prevention, CDC-funded programs and prevention research, funding opportunities, and links to other injury-related sites.

National Conference of State Legislatures School Health Finance Project
444 N. Capitol St., NW, Suite 515
Washington, DC 20001
Phone: 202-624-5400 (Washington, DC)
Phone: 303-830-2200 (Denver, CO)
Fax: 202-737-1069
Website: www.ncsl.org/programs/health/pp/schlfund.htm
E-Mail: info@ncsl.org

This project provides comprehensive funding information on coordinated school health programs, including programs to address teen pregnancy, underage alcohol use, school violence, preventive health care, HIV/AIDS education, substance abuse, and mental health issues.

National Federation of State High School Associations (NFHS)
P.O. Box 690
Indianapolis, IN 46206
Phone: 317-972-6900
Fax: 317-822-5700
Website: www.nfhs.org

On the NFHS home page you can find information about the benefits of high school activities, including sports.

National Governors' Association
Hall of States
444 N. Capitol St.
Washington, DC 20001
Phone: 202-624-5300
Website: www.nga.org

Features programs on making schools safe and preparing kids for success.

National Institute of Mental Health (NIMH)
6001 Executive Boulevard
Room 8184, MSC 9663
Bethesda, MD 20892
Phone: 301-443-4514
TTY: 301-443-8431
Fax: 301-443-429
Website: www.nimh.nih.gov
E-Mail: nimhinfo@nih.gov

NIMH carries out educational activities and publishes and distributes research reports, press releases, fact sheets, and publications intended for researchers, health care providers, and the general public.

National Mental Health and Education Center for Children and Families
4340 East West Highway
Suite 402
Bethesda, MD 20814
Phone: 301-657-0270
Fax: 301-657-0275
TDD: 301-657-4155
Website: www.naspcenter.org

A public service of the National Association of School Psychologists, this center provides resources for safe school programs and crisis response, and information on current issues and programs.

National Organization for Victim Assistance (NOVA)
1730 Park Rd., NW
Washington, DC 20010
Toll Free: 800-try-nova
Phone: 202-232-6682
Fax: 202-462-255
Website: www.try-nova.org

National PTA
330 N. Wabash Avenue
Suite 2100
Chicago, IL 60611
Toll Free: 800-307-4782
Phone: 312-670-6782
Fax: 312-670-6783
Website: www.pta.org
E-Mail: info@pta.org

The National PTA helps identify effective school violence problems, find solutions, and develop action plans. Among their materials is a community violence prevention kit.

National SAFE KIDS Campaign
1301 Pennsylvania Ave., NW
Suite 1000
Washington, DC 20004
Phone: 202-622-0600
Fax: 202-393-2072
Website: www.safekids.org

Visit the SAFE KIDS home page (www.safekids.org) to access fact sheets on sports and recreation injuries.

National School Safety Center
141 Duesenberg Drive
Suite 11
Westlake village, CA 91362
Phone: 805-373-9977
Fax: 805-373-9277
Website: www.nssc1.org
E-Mail: info@nssc1.org

National Youth Sports Safety Foundation
333 Longwood Avenue
Suite 202
Boston, MA 02115
Phone: 617-277-1771
Fax: 617-277-2278
Website: www.nyssf.org
E-Mail: nyssf@aol.com

Office for Victims of Crime Resource Center
National Criminal Justice Reference Service
P.O. Box 6000
Rockville, MD 20850
Toll Free: 800-627-6872
Website: www.ncjrs.org

Work Safe This Summer
US Department of Labor
200 Constitution Avenue, NW
Washington, DC 20210
Toll Free: 866-487-9243
Website: www.dol.gov

Work Safe This Summer (or anytime) is a joint effort of the US Department of Labor, the National Institute for Occupational Safety and Health, the American Academy of Pediatrics, and the National Consumers League. Through the use of a toll-free telephone number (1-866-487-9243), an Internet web site (www.dol.gov), and a variety of education materials, Work Safe This Summer is designed to bring important information about on-the-job safety for working teens to employers, parents, and the teens themselves.

When Teens Turn Violent

National Safety Council
1121 Spring Lake Drive
Itasca, IL 60143
Phone: 630-285-1121
Fax: 630-285-1315
Website: www.nsc.org

Adolescent Education

ACT Registration

P.O. Box 414
Iowa City, IA 52243
Phone: 319-337-1000
Website: www.act.org

The College Board

P.O. Box 6200
Princeton, NJ 08541-6200
Phone: 609-771-7600
Website: www.collegeboard.org

The College Board is a national membership association of schools and colleges whose aim is to facilitate the student transition to higher education.

ERIC Clearinghouse on Elementary and Early Childhood Education

University of Illinois
Children's Research Center
51 Gerty Drive
Champaign, IL 61820
Toll Free: 800-583-4135
Phone: 217-333-1386
Fax: 217-333-3767
Website: www.ericeece.org

Federal Student Aid Information Center

P.O. Box 84
Washington, DC 20044
Toll Free: 800-4FED-AID
Website: www.ed.gov/offices/
OSFAP/Students
E-Mail: SFAmail@ncs.ed.gov

The Illinois Student Aid Commission (ISAC)

1755 Lake Cook Road
Deerfield, IL 60015
Toll Free: 800-899-ISAC
Website: www.isac1.org

The Illinois Student Aid Commission (ISAC) also provides information over the Internet about preparing and paying for college.

National Clearinghouse on Families and Youth

P.O. Box 13505
Silver Spring, MD 20911
Phone: 301-608-8098
Fax: 301-608-8721
Website: www.ncfy.com
E-Mail: info@ncfy.com

National Middle School Association
4151 Executive Pky., Suite 300
Westerville, OH 43081
Toll Free: 800-528-NMSA (6672)
Website: www.nmsa.org
E-Mail: info@NMSA.org

National Tech Prep Network
Center for Occupational
Research and Development
P.O. Box 21689
Waco, TX 76702-1689
Toll Free: 800-972-2766
Phone: 254-772-8756
Fax: 254-772-8972
Website: www.cord.org

PSAT/NMSQT
P.O. Box 6720
Princeton, NJ 08541-6720
Phone: 609-771-7070
Website: www.collegeboard.org

SAT Program
P.O. Box 6200
Princeton, NJ 08541-6200
Phone: 609-771-7600
Website: www.collegeboard.org

School-To-Work Opportunities Information Center
400 Virginia Ave., SW, Room 150
Washington, DC 20024
Toll Free: 800-251-7236
Phone: 202-401-6222
Fax: 202-488-7395
Website: www.stw.ed.gov
E-Mail: stw-lc.gov

The Student Loan Marketing Association
11600 Sallie Mae Drive
Reston, Virginia 20193
Toll Free: 800-239-4269
Website: www.salliemae.com

The Student Loan Marketing Association is a provider of financial services and operational support for higher education.

The Texas Guaranteed Student Loan Corporation (TGSLC)
P.O. Box 201725
Austin, TX 78720
Toll Free: 800-845-6267
Website: www.tgslc.org

The Texas Guaranteed Student Loan Corporation (TGSLC) makes a great deal of information available to help prospective college students prepare for college. Its information includes career planning and college selection information.

U.S. Department of Education
400 Maryland Avenue, SW
Washington DC 20202-1328
Toll Free: 800-USA-LEARN
Fax: 202-401-0689
Website: www.ed.gov
E-Mail:
customerservice@inet.ed.gov

Chapter 67

References and Additional Reading

This chapter lists book titles, brochures, pamphlets, and articles that contain useful information on some of the topics in this *Sourcebook*. For easy reference, the listings are organized in alphabetical order. Email, website, and other contact information is included when available.

A Guide to Safe Schools & Creating Safe and Drug Free Schools. Call the US Department of Education, 1-800-USA-LEARN.

American Academy of Orthopaedic Surgeons. "Play it safe sports: A guide to safety for young athletes, 1995." Available at www.aaos.org/wordhtml/pat_educ/playspor.htm. Accessed July 8, 1999.

American Academy of Pediatrics. "Sports and your child." Available at www.aap.org/family/sports.htm. Accessed July 13, 1999.

American College Testing (ACT). "Realizing the Dream." Call 319-337-1379 or write to:

Program Coordinator, ACT, 2201 North Dodge Street, PO Box 168, Iowa City, IA 52243-0168. Many schools around the country are using this kit to help students identify careers of interest.

American Social Health Association. *Sexually transmitted diseases in America: How many cases and at what cost?* Research Triangle Park, NC, 1998.

Bosworth K, Espelage DL, Simon TR. "Factors Associated with Bullying in Middle School Students." *Journal of Early Adolescence.* 1999; 19(3):341 362.

Brain Injury Association. "Sports and concussion safety." Available at www.biausa.org/sportsfs.htm. Accessed July 23, 1999.

Brener ND, Simon TR, Krug EG, Lowry R. "Recent Trends in Violence-Related Behaviors Among High School Students in the United States." *Journal of the American Medical Association.* 1999; 282(5):440 446.

Budman MV, Powell KE, Everett SA, Anderson MA, Bolen JC, Sleet DA. "The Prevalence of Injury Prevention Activities in American Schools." *Journal of Health Education.* 1999; 30:S34-S41.

Carskadon MA, Acebo C, Richardson GS, Tate BA, Seifer R. "An approach to studying circadian rhythms of adolescent humans." *Journal of Biological Rhythms.* 1997; 12(3): 278 289.

Carskadon MA. "Factors influencing sleep patterns of adolescents." In: Carskadon MA, ed. *Adolescent Sleep Patterns: Biological, Social, and Psychological Influences.* New York: Cambridge University Press, 1998 (in press).

Carskadon MA, Wolfson AR, Acebo C, Tzischinsky O, Seifer R. "Adolescent sleep patterns, circadian timing, and sleepiness at a transition to early school days." *Sleep.* 1998 (in press).

Centers for Disease Control and Prevention. "Firearm-Associated Deaths and Hospitalizations California, 1995–1996." *MMWR.* 1999;48:485 488; June 18.

Carskadon MA. "Sleep disturbances." In: Friedman SB, Fisher M, Schonberg SK, Alderman EM, eds. *Comprehensive Adolescent Health Care.* Second Edition. St. Louis: Mosby, 1997; 805 814.

Centers for Disease Control and Prevention. "1998 guidelines for treatment of sexually transmitted diseases." *MMWR.* 1998; 47(RR-1), 70-74.

Centers for Disease Control and Prevention. "Nonfatal and Fatal Firearm-Related Injuries United States, 1993–1997." *MMWR.* 1999;48:1029 1034; November 19.

College Costs and Financial Aid Handbook, 1996, Sixteenth Edition. The College Board, 1995.

Creating Safe and Drug Free Schools. The Department of Education's action guide for creating safe, orderly, drug-free schools. Available at www.ed.gov/offices/OESE/SDFS/actguid/index.html.

"Firearm-Related Injury Surveillance." *American Journal of Preventive Medicine,* Supplement to Volume 15, Number 3, 1998.

Hillier, S. and Holmes, K. "Bacterial vaginosis." In: K. Holmes, P. Mardh, P. Sparling et al (eds). *Sexually Transmitted Diseases, 3rd Edition.* New York: McGraw-Hill, 1999, 563-586.

Measuring Violence-Related Attitudes, Beliefs, and Behaviors Among Youths: A Compendium of Assessment Tools. Atlanta, GA: Centers for Disease Control and Prevention, National Center for Injury Prevention and Control, 1998.

National Federation of State High School Associations. "The case for high school activities." Available at www.nfhs.org. Accessed August 2, 1999.

National SAFE KIDS Campaign. *Sports and recreational activity injury.* December 1998.

The Occupational Outlook Handbook, 1996-97 Edition. U.S. Department of Labor, Bureau of Labor Statistics, 1996.

Potter LB, Sacks JJ, Kresnow M, Mercy J. "Nonfatal Physical Violence, United States, 1994." *Public Health Reports 1999* (July/August); 114:343 352.

Potter LB. "Understanding the Incidence and Origins of Community Violence: Toward a Comprehensive Perspective of Violence Prevention." In: Gullotta TP, McElhaney SJ, eds. *Violence in Homes and Communities: Prevention, Intervention, and Treatment,* 1999:101 132.

Simon TR, Crosby AE, Dahlberg LL. "Students Who Carry Weapons to High School." *Journal of Adolescent Health.* 1999; 24(5):340 348.

US Department of Education. "A Guide to Safe Schools." Research-based practices designed to assist school communities identify warning signs early and develop prevention, intervention and crisis response plans. Available on the web at www.ed.gov/offices/OSERS/OSEP/earlywrn.html.

What Color Is Your Parachute? Richard Nelson Bolles. Ten Speed Press, 1995.

Zetaruk M, Mitchell W. *Gymnastics injuries*. Sidelines 1998;7(2):1-2.

Index

Index

Page numbers followed by 'n' indicate a footnote. Page numbers in *italics* indicate a table or illustration.

A

615

Q

Health Reference Series
COMPLETE CATALOG

Adolescent Health Sourcebook

Basic Consumer Health Information about Common Medical, Mental, and Emotional Concerns in Adolescents, Including Facts about Acne, Body Piercing, Mononucleosis, Nutrition, Eating Disorders, Stress, Depression, Behavior Problems, Peer Pressure, Violence, Gangs, Drug Use, Puberty, Sexuality, Pregnancy, Learning Disabilities, and More

Along with a Glossary of Terms and Other Resources for Further Help and Information

Edited by Chad T. Kimball. 658 pages. 2002. 0-7808-0248-9. $78.

∎

AIDS Sourcebook, 1st Edition

Basic Information about AIDS and HIV Infection, Featuring Historical and Statistical Data, Current Research, Prevention, and Other Special Topics of Interest for Persons Living with AIDS

Along with Source Listings for Further Assistance

Edited by Karen Bellenir and Peter D. Dresser. 831 pages. 1995. 0-7808-0031-1. $78.

"One strength of this book is its practical emphasis. The intended audience is the lay reader . . . useful as an educational tool for health care providers who work with AIDS patients. Recommended for public libraries as well as hospital or academic libraries that collect consumer materials."
— *Bulletin of the Medical Library Association, Jan '96*

"This is the most comprehensive volume of its kind on an important medical topic. Highly recommended for all libraries." — *Reference Book Review, '96*

"Very useful reference for all libraries."
— *Choice, Association of College and Research Libraries, Oct '95*

"There is a wealth of information here that can provide much educational assistance. It is a must book for all libraries and should be on the desk of each and every congressional leader. Highly recommended."
— *AIDS Book Review Journal, Aug '95*

"Recommended for most collections."
— *Library Journal, Jul '95*

∎

AIDS Sourcebook, 2nd Edition

Basic Consumer Health Information about Acquired Immune Deficiency Syndrome (AIDS) and Human Immunodeficiency Virus (HIV) Infection, Featuring Updated Statistical Data, Reports on Recent Research and Prevention Initiatives, and Other Special Topics of Interest for Persons Living with AIDS, Including New Antiretroviral Treatment Options, Strategies for Combating Opportunistic Infections, Information about Clinical Trials, and More

Along with a Glossary of Important Terms and Resource Listings for Further Help and Information

Edited by Karen Bellenir. 751 pages. 1999. 0-7808-0225-X. $78.

"Highly recommended."
— *American Reference Books Annual, 2000*

"Excellent sourcebook. This continues to be a highly recommended book. There is no other book that provides as much information as this book provides."
— *AIDS Book Review Journal, Dec-Jan 2000*

"Recommended reference source."
— *Booklist, American Library Association, Dec '99*

"A solid text for college-level health libraries."
— *The Bookwatch, Aug '99*

Cited in *Reference Sources for Small and Medium-Sized Libraries, American Library Association, 1999*

∎

Alcoholism Sourcebook

Basic Consumer Health Information about the Physical and Mental Consequences of Alcohol Abuse, Including Liver Disease, Pancreatitis, Wernicke-Korsakoff Syndrome (Alcoholic Dementia), Fetal Alcohol Syndrome, Heart Disease, Kidney Disorders, Gastrointestinal Problems, and Immune System Compromise and Featuring Facts about Addiction, Detoxification, Alcohol Withdrawal, Recovery, and the Maintenance of Sobriety

Along with a Glossary and Directories of Resources for Further Help and Information

Edited by Karen Bellenir. 613 pages. 2000. 0-7808-0325-6. $78.

"This title is one of the few reference works on alcoholism for general readers. For some readers this will be a welcome complement to the many self-help books on the market. Recommended for collections serving general readers and consumer health collections."
— *E-Streams, Mar '01*

"This book is an excellent choice for public and academic libraries."
— *American Reference Books Annual, 2001*

"Recommended reference source."
— *Booklist, American Library Association, Dec '00*

"Presents a wealth of information on alcohol use and abuse and its effects on the body and mind, treatment, and prevention." — *SciTech Book News, Dec '00*

"Important new health guide which packs in the latest consumer information about the problems of alcoholism." — *Reviewer's Bookwatch, Nov '00*

SEE ALSO *Drug Abuse Sourcebook, Substance Abuse Sourcebook*

Allergies Sourcebook, 1st Edition

Basic Information about Major Forms and Mechanisms of Common Allergic Reactions, Sensitivities, and Intolerances, Including Anaphylaxis, Asthma, Hives and Other Dermatologic Symptoms, Rhinitis, and Sinusitis

Along with Their Usual Triggers Like Animal Fur, Chemicals, Drugs, Dust, Foods, Insects, Latex, Pollen, and Poison Ivy, Oak, and Sumac; Plus Information on Prevention, Identification, and Treatment

Edited by Allan R. Cook. 611 pages. 1997. 0-7808-0036-2. $78.

■

Allergies Sourcebook, 2nd Edition

Basic Consumer Health Information about Allergic Disorders, Triggers, Reactions, and Related Symptoms, Including Anaphylaxis, Rhinitis, Sinusitis, Asthma, Dermatitis, Conjunctivitis, and Multiple Chemical Sensitivity

Along with Tips on Diagnosis, Prevention, and Treatment, Statistical Data, a Glossary, and a Directory of Sources for Further Help and Information

Edited by Annemarie S. Muth. 598 pages. 2002. 0-7808-0376-0. $78.

■

Alternative Medicine Sourcebook, First Edition

Basic Consumer Health Information about Alternatives to Conventional Medicine, Including Acupressure, Acupuncture, Aromatherapy, Ayurveda, Bioelectromagnetics, Environmental Medicine, Essence Therapy, Food and Nutrition Therapy, Herbal Therapy, Homeopathy, Imaging, Massage, Naturopathy, Reflexology, Relaxation and Meditation, Sound Therapy, Vitamin and Mineral Therapy, and Yoga, and More

Edited by Allan R. Cook. 737 pages. 1999. 0-7808-0200-4. $78.

"Recommended reference source."
—*Booklist, American Library Association, Feb '00*

"A great addition to the reference collection of every type of library." —*American Reference Books Annual, 2000*

■

Alternative Medicine Sourcebook, Second Edition

Basic Consumer Health Information about Alternative and Complementary Medical Practices, Including Acupuncture, Chiropractic, Herbal Medicine, Homeopathy, Naturopathic Medicine, Mind-Body Interventions, Ayurveda, and Other Non-Western Medical Traditions

Along with Facts about such Specific Therapies as Massage Therapy, Aromatherapy, Qigong, Hypnosis, Prayer, Dance, and Art Therapies, a Glossary, and Resources for Further Information

Edited by Dawn D. Matthews. 650 pages. 2002. 0-7808-0605-0. $78.

Alzheimer's, Stroke & 29 Other Neurological Disorders Sourcebook, 1st Edition

Basic Information for the Layperson on 31 Diseases or Disorders Affecting the Brain and Nervous System, First Describing the Illness, Then Listing Symptoms, Diagnostic Methods, and Treatment Options, and Including Statistics on Incidences and Causes

Edited by Frank E. Bair. 579 pages. 1993. 1-55888-748-2. $78.

"Nontechnical reference book that provides reader-friendly information."
—*Family Caregiver Alliance Update, Winter '96*

"Should be included in any library's patient education section." —*American Reference Books Annual, 1994*

"Written in an approachable and accessible style. Recommended for patient education and consumer health collections in health science center and public libraries." —*Academic Library Book Review, Dec '93*

"It is very handy to have information on more than thirty neurological disorders under one cover, and there is no recent source like it." —*Reference Quarterly, American Library Association, Fall '93*

SEE ALSO Brain Disorders Sourcebook

■

Alzheimer's Disease Sourcebook, 2nd Edition

Basic Consumer Health Information about Alzheimer's Disease, Related Disorders, and Other Dementias, Including Multi-Infarct Dementia, AIDS-Related Dementia, Alcoholic Dementia, Huntington's Disease, Delirium, and Confusional States

Along with Reports Detailing Current Research Efforts in Prevention and Treatment, Long-Term Care Issues, and Listings of Sources for Additional Help and Information

Edited by Karen Bellenir. 524 pages. 1999. 0-7808-0223-3. $78.

"Provides a wealth of useful information not otherwise available in one place. This resource is recommended for all types of libraries."
—*American Reference Books Annual, 2000*

"Recommended reference source."
—*Booklist, American Library Association, Oct '99*

■

Arthritis Sourcebook

Basic Consumer Health Information about Specific Forms of Arthritis and Related Disorders, Including Rheumatoid Arthritis, Osteoarthritis, Gout, Polymyalgia Rheumatica, Psoriatic Arthritis, Spondyloarthropathies, Juvenile Rheumatoid Arthritis, and Juvenile Ankylosing Spondylitis

Along with Information about Medical, Surgical, and Alternative Treatment Options, and Including Strategies for Coping with Pain, Fatigue, and Stress

Edited by Allan R. Cook. 550 pages. 1998. 0-7808-0201-2. $78.

"... accessible to the layperson."
—*Reference and Research Book News, Feb '99*

■

Asthma Sourcebook

Basic Consumer Health Information about Asthma, Including Symptoms, Traditional and Nontraditional Remedies, Treatment Advances, Quality-of-Life Aids, Medical Research Updates, and the Role of Allergies, Exercise, Age, the Environment, and Genetics in the Development of Asthma

Along with Statistical Data, a Glossary, and Directories of Support Groups, and Other Resources for Further Information

Edited by Annemarie S. Muth. 628 pages. 2000. 0-7808-0381-7. $78.

"A worthwhile reference acquisition for public libraries and academic medical libraries whose readers desire a quick introduction to the wide range of asthma information." — *Choice, Association of College & esearch Libraries, Jun '01*

"Recommended reference source."
— *Booklist, American Library Association, Feb '01*

"Highly recommended." — *The Bookwatch, Jan '01*

"There is much good information for patients and their families who deal with asthma daily."
— *American Medical Writers Association Journal, Winter '01*

"This informative text is recommended for consumer health collections in public, secondary school, and community college libraries and the libraries of universities with a large undergraduate population."
— *American Reference Books Annual, 2001*

■

Back & Neck Disorders Sourcebook

Basic Information about Disorders and Injuries of the Spinal Cord and Vertebrae, Including Facts on Chiropractic Treatment, Surgical Interventions, Paralysis, and Rehabilitation

Along with Advice for Preventing Back Trouble

Edited by Karen Bellenir. 548 pages. 1997. 0-7808-0202-0. $78.

"The strength of this work is its basic, easy-to-read format. Recommended."
— *Reference and User Services Quarterly, American Library Association, Winter '97*

■

Blood & Circulatory Disorders Sourcebook

Basic Information about Blood and Its Components, Anemias, Leukemias, Bleeding Disorders, and Circulatory Disorders, Including Aplastic Anemia, Thalas-

semia, Sickle-Cell Disease, Hemochromatosis, Hemophilia, Von Willebrand Disease, and Vascular Diseases

Along with a Special Section on Blood Transfusions and Blood Supply Safety, a Glossary, and Source Listings for Further Help and Information

Edited by Karen Bellenir and Linda M. Shin. 554 pages. 1998. 0-7808-0203-9. $78.

"Recommended reference source."
— *Booklist, American Library Association, Feb '99*

"An important reference sourcebook written in simple language for everyday, non-technical users. "
— *Reviewer's Bookwatch, Jan '99*

■

Brain Disorders Sourcebook

Basic Consumer Health Information about Strokes, Epilepsy, Amyotrophic Lateral Sclerosis (ALS/Lou Gehrig's Disease), Parkinson's Disease, Brain Tumors, Cerebral Palsy, Headache, Tourette Syndrome, and More

Along with Statistical Data, Treatment and Rehabilitation Options, Coping Strategies, Reports on Current Research Initiatives, a Glossary, and Resource Listings for Additional Help and Information

Edited by Karen Bellenir. 481 pages. 1999. 0-7808-0229-2. $78.

"Belongs on the shelves of any library with a consumer health collection." — *E-Streams, Mar '00*

"Recommended reference source."
— *Booklist, American Library Association, Oct '99*

SEE ALSO Alzheimer's, Stroke & 29 Other Neurological Disorders Sourcebook, 1st Edition

■

Breast Cancer Sourcebook

Basic Consumer Health Information about Breast Cancer, Including Diagnostic Methods, Treatment Options, Alternative Therapies, Self-Help Information, Related Health Concerns, Statistical and Demographic Data, and Facts for Men with Breast Cancer

Along with Reports on Current Research Initiatives, a Glossary of Related Medical Terms, and a Directory of Sources for Further Help and Information

Edited by Edward J. Prucha and Karen Bellenir. 580 pages. 2001. 0-7808-0244-6. $78.

"Recommended reference source."
— *Booklist, American Library Association, Jan '02*

"This reference source is highly recommended. It is quite informative, comprehensive and detailed in nature, and yet it offers practical advice in easy-to-read language. It could be thought of as the 'bible' of breast cancer for the consumer." — *E-Streams, Jan '02*

"From the pros and cons of different screening methods and results to treatment options, *Breast Cancer Sourcebook* provides the latest information on the subject."
— *Library Bookwatch, Dec '01*

"This thoroughgoing, very readable reference covers all aspects of breast health and cancer. . . . Readers will find much to consider here. Recommended for all public and patient health collections."
— *Library Journal, Sep '01*

SEE ALSO *Cancer Sourcebook for Women, 1st and 2nd Editions, Women's Health Concerns Sourcebook*

■

Breastfeeding Sourcebook

Basic Consumer Health Information about the Benefits of Breastmilk, Preparing to Breastfeed, Breastfeeding as a Baby Grows, Nutrition, and More, Including Information on Special Situations and Concerns Such as Mastitis, Illness, Medications, Allergies, Multiple Births, Prematurity, Special Needs, and Adoption

Along with a Glossary and Resources for Additional Help and Information

Edited by Jenni Lynn Colson. 388 pages. 2002. 0-7808-0332-9. $78.

SEE ALSO *Pregnancy & Birth Sourcebook*

■

Burns Sourcebook

Basic Consumer Health Information about Various Types of Burns and Scalds, Including Flame, Heat, Cold, Electrical, Chemical, and Sun Burns

Along with Information on Short-Term and Long-Term Treatments, Tissue Reconstruction, Plastic Surgery, Prevention Suggestions, and First Aid

Edited by Allan R. Cook. 604 pages. 1999. 0-7808-0204-7. $78.

"This is an exceptional addition to the series and is highly recommended for all consumer health collections, hospital libraries, and academic medical centers."
— *E-Streams, Mar '00*

"This key reference guide is an invaluable addition to all health care and public libraries in confronting this ongoing health issue."
— *American Reference Books Annual, 2000*

"Recommended reference source."
— *Booklist, American Library Association, Dec '99*

SEE ALSO *Skin Disorders Sourcebook*

■

Cancer Sourcebook, 1st Edition

Basic Information on Cancer Types, Symptoms, Diagnostic Methods, and Treatments, Including Statistics on Cancer Occurrences Worldwide and the Risks Associated with Known Carcinogens and Activities

Edited by Frank E. Bair. 932 pages. 1990. 1-55888-888-8. $78.

Cited in *Reference Sources for Small and Medium-Sized Libraries, American Library Association, 1999*

"Written in nontechnical language. Useful for patients, their families, medical professionals, and librarians."
— *Guide to Reference Books, 1996*

"Designed with the non-medical professional in mind. Libraries and medical facilities interested in patient education should certainly consider adding the *Cancer Sourcebook* to their holdings. This compact collection of reliable information . . . is an invaluable tool for helping patients and patients' families and friends to take the first steps in coping with the many difficulties of cancer."
— *Medical Reference Services Quarterly, Winter '91*

"Specifically created for the nontechnical reader . . . an important resource for the general reader trying to understand the complexities of cancer."
— *American Reference Books Annual, 1991*

"This publication's nontechnical nature and very comprehensive format make it useful for both the general public and undergraduate students."
— *Choice, Association of College and Research Libraries, Oct '90*

■

New Cancer Sourcebook, 2nd Edition

Basic Information about Major Forms and Stages of Cancer, Featuring Facts about Primary and Secondary Tumors of the Respiratory, Nervous, Lymphatic, Circulatory, Skeletal, and Gastrointestinal Systems, and Specific Organs; Statistical and Demographic Data; Treatment Options; and Strategies for Coping

Edited by Allan R. Cook. 1,313 pages. 1996. 0-7808-0041-9. $78.

"An excellent resource for patients with newly diagnosed cancer and their families. The dialogue is simple, direct, and comprehensive. Highly recommended for patients and families to aid in their understanding of cancer and its treatment."
— *Booklist Health Sciences Supplement, American Library Association, Oct '97*

"The amount of factual and useful information is extensive. The writing is very clear, geared to general readers. Recommended for all levels."
— *Choice, Association of College and Research Libraries, Jan '97*

■

Cancer Sourcebook, 3rd Edition

Basic Consumer Health Information about Major Forms and Stages of Cancer, Featuring Facts about Primary and Secondary Tumors of the Respiratory, Nervous, Lymphatic, Circulatory, Skeletal, and Gastrointestinal Systems, and Specific Organs

Along with Statistical and Demographic Data, Treatment Options, Strategies for Coping, a Glossary, and a Directory of Sources for Additional Help and Information

Edited by Edward J. Prucha. 1,069 pages. 2000. 0-7808-0227-6. $78.

"This title is recommended for health sciences and public libraries with consumer health collections."
— *E-Streams, Feb '01*

"... can be effectively used by cancer patients and their families who are looking for answers in a language they can understand. Public and hospital libraries should have it on their shelves."
— *American Reference Books Annual, 2001*

"Recommended reference source."
— *Booklist, American Library Association, Dec '00*

■

Cancer Sourcebook for Women, 1st Edition

Basic Information about Specific Forms of Cancer That Affect Women, Featuring Facts about Breast Cancer, Cervical Cancer, Ovarian Cancer, Cancer of the Uterus and Uterine Sarcoma, Cancer of the Vagina, and Cancer of the Vulva; Statistical and Demographic Data; Treatments, Self-Help Management Suggestions, and Current Research Initiatives

Edited by Allan R. Cook and Peter D. Dresser. 524 pages. 1996. 0-7808-0076-1. $78.

"... written in easily understandable, non-technical language. Recommended for public libraries or hospital and academic libraries that collect patient education or consumer health materials."
— *Medical Reference Services Quarterly, Spring '97*

"Would be of value in a consumer health library. . . . written with the health care consumer in mind. Medical jargon is at a minimum, and medical terms are explained in clear, understandable sentences."
— *Bulletin of the Medical Library Association, Oct '96*

"The availability under one cover of all these pertinent publications, grouped under cohesive headings, makes this certainly a most useful sourcebook."
— *Choice, Association of College and Research Libraries, Jun '96*

"Presents a comprehensive knowledge base for general readers. Men and women both benefit from the gold mine of information nestled between the two covers of this book. Recommended."
— *Academic Library Book Review, Summer '96*

"This timely book is highly recommended for consumer health and patient education collections in all libraries."
— *Library Journal, Apr '96*

SEE ALSO *Breast Cancer Sourcebook, Women's Health Concerns Sourcebook*

■

Cancer Sourcebook for Women, 2nd Edition

Basic Consumer Health Information about Gynecologic Cancers and Related Concerns, Including Cervical Cancer, Endometrial Cancer, Gestational Trophoblastic Tumor, Ovarian Cancer, Uterine Cancer, Vaginal Cancer, Vulvar Cancer, Breast Cancer, and Common Non-Cancerous Uterine Conditions, with Facts about Cancer Risk Factors, Screening and Prevention, Treatment Options, and Reports on Current Research Initiatives

Along with a Glossary of Cancer Terms and a Directory of Resources for Additional Help and Information

Edited by Karen Bellenir. 604 pages. 2002. 0-7808-0226-8. $78.

SEE ALSO *Breast Cancer Sourcebook, Women's Health Concerns Sourcebook*

■

Cardiovascular Diseases & Disorders Sourcebook, 1st Edition

Basic Information about Cardiovascular Diseases and Disorders, Featuring Facts about the Cardiovascular System, Demographic and Statistical Data, Descriptions of Pharmacological and Surgical Interventions, Lifestyle Modifications, and a Special Section Focusing on Heart Disorders in Children

Edited by Karen Bellenir and Peter D. Dresser. 683 pages. 1995. 0-7808-0032-X. $78.

". . . comprehensive format provides an extensive overview on this subject."
— *Choice, Association of College & Research Libraries, Jun '96*

". . . an easily understood, complete, up-to-date resource. This well executed public health tool will make valuable information available to those that need it most, patients and their families. The typeface, sturdy non-reflective paper, and library binding add a feel of quality found wanting in other publications. Highly recommended for academic and general libraries. "
— *Academic Library Book Review, Summer '96*

SEE ALSO *Healthy Heart Sourcebook for Women, Heart Diseases & Disorders Sourcebook, 2nd Edition*

■

Caregiving Sourcebook

Basic Consumer Health Information for Caregivers, Including a Profile of Caregivers, Caregiving Responsibilities and Concerns, Tips for Specific Conditions, Care Environments, and the Effects of Caregiving

Along with Facts about Legal Issues, Financial Information, and Future Planning, a Glossary, and a Listing of Additional Resources

Edited by Joyce Brennfleck Shannon. 600 pages. 2001. 0-7808-0331-0. $78.

"An ideal addition to the reference collection of any public library. Health sciences information professionals may also want to acquire the *Caregiving Sourcebook* for their hospital or academic library for use as a ready reference tool by health care workers interested in aging and caregiving."
— *E-Streams, Jan '02*

"Recommended reference source."
— *Booklist, American Library Association, Oct '01*

Colds, Flu & Other Common Ailments Sourcebook

Basic Consumer Health Information about Common Ailments and Injuries, Including Colds, Coughs, the Flu, Sinus Problems, Headaches, Fever, Nausea and Vomiting, Menstrual Cramps, Diarrhea, Constipation, Hemorrhoids, Back Pain, Dandruff, Dry and Itchy Skin, Cuts, Scrapes, Sprains, Bruises, and More

Along with Information about Prevention, Self-Care, Choosing a Doctor, Over-the-Counter Medications, Folk Remedies, and Alternative Therapies, and Including a Glossary of Important Terms and a Directory of Resources for Further Help and Information

Edited by Chad T. Kimball. 638 pages. 2001. 0-7808-0435-X. $78.

"Will prove valuable to any library seeking to maintain a current, comprehensive reference collection of health resources. . . . Excellent reference."
— The Bookwatch, Aug '01

"Recommended reference source."
— Booklist, American Library Association, July '01

■

Communication Disorders Sourcebook

Basic Information about Deafness and Hearing Loss, Speech and Language Disorders, Voice Disorders, Balance and Vestibular Disorders, and Disorders of Smell, Taste, and Touch

Edited by Linda M. Ross. 533 pages. 1996. 0-7808-0077-X. $78.

"This is skillfully edited and is a welcome resource for the layperson. It should be found in every public and medical library." — Booklist Health Sciences Supplement, American Library Association, Oct '97

■

Congenital Disorders Sourcebook

Basic Information about Disorders Acquired during Gestation, Including Spina Bifida, Hydrocephalus, Cerebral Palsy, Heart Defects, Craniofacial Abnormalities, Fetal Alcohol Syndrome, and More

Along with Current Treatment Options and Statistical Data

Edited by Karen Bellenir. 607 pages. 1997. 0-7808-0205-5. $78.

"Recommended reference source."
— Booklist, American Library Association, Oct '97

SEE ALSO Pregnancy & Birth Sourcebook

■

Consumer Issues in Health Care Sourcebook

Basic Information about Health Care Fundamentals and Related Consumer Issues, Including Exams and Screening Tests, Physician Specialties, Choosing a Doctor, Using Prescription and Over-the-Counter Medica-

tions Safely, Avoiding Health Scams, Managing Common Health Risks in the Home, Care Options for Chronically or Terminally Ill Patients, and a List of Resources for Obtaining Help and Further Information

Edited by Karen Bellenir. 618 pages. 1998. 0-7808-0221-7. $78.

"Both public and academic libraries will want to have a copy in their collection for readers who are interested in self-education on health issues."
— American Reference Books Annual, 2000

"The editor has researched the literature from government agencies and others, saving readers the time and effort of having to do the research themselves. Recommended for public libraries."
— Reference and User Services Quarterly, American Library Association, Spring '99

"Recommended reference source."
— Booklist, American Library Association, Dec '98

■

Contagious & Non-Contagious Infectious Diseases Sourcebook

Basic Information about Contagious Diseases like Measles, Polio, Hepatitis B, and Infectious Mononucleosis, and Non-Contagious Infectious Diseases like Tetanus and Toxic Shock Syndrome, and Diseases Occurring as Secondary Infections Such as Shingles and Reye Syndrome

Along with Vaccination, Prevention, and Treatment Information, and a Section Describing Emerging Infectious Disease Threats

Edited by Karen Bellenir and Peter D. Dresser. 566 pages. 1996. 0-7808-0075-3. $78.

■

Death & Dying Sourcebook

Basic Consumer Health Information for the Layperson about End-of-Life Care and Related Ethical and Legal Issues, Including Chief Causes of Death, Autopsies, Pain Management for the Terminally Ill, Life Support Systems, Insurance, Euthanasia, Assisted Suicide, Hospice Programs, Living Wills, Funeral Planning, Counseling, Mourning, Organ Donation, and Physician Training

Along with Statistical Data, a Glossary, and Listings of Sources for Further Help and Information

Edited by Annemarie S. Muth. 641 pages. 1999. 0-7808-0230-6. $78.

"Public libraries, medical libraries, and academic libraries will all find this sourcebook a useful addition to their collections."
— American Reference Books Annual, 2001

"An extremely useful resource for those concerned with death and dying in the United States."
— Respiratory Care, Nov '00

"Recommended reference source."
— Booklist, American Library Association, Aug '00

"This book is a definite must for all those involved in end-of-life care." — Doody's Review Service, 2000

Diabetes Sourcebook, 1st Edition

Basic Information about Insulin-Dependent and Non-insulin-Dependent Diabetes Mellitus, Gestational Diabetes, and Diabetic Complications, Symptoms, Treatment, and Research Results, Including Statistics on Prevalence, Morbidity, and Mortality

Along with Source Listings for Further Help and Information

Edited by Karen Bellenir and Peter D. Dresser. 827 pages. 1994. 1-55888-751-2. $78.

". . . very informative and understandable for the layperson without being simplistic. It provides a comprehensive overview for laypersons who want a general understanding of the disease or who want to focus on various aspects of the disease."
— *Bulletin of the Medical Library Association, Jan '96*

■

Diabetes Sourcebook, 2nd Edition

Basic Consumer Health Information about Type 1 Diabetes (Insulin-Dependent or Juvenile-Onset Diabetes), Type 2 (Noninsulin-Dependent or Adult-Onset Diabetes), Gestational Diabetes, and Related Disorders, Including Diabetes Prevalence Data, Management Issues, the Role of Diet and Exercise in Controlling Diabetes, Insulin and Other Diabetes Medicines, and Complications of Diabetes Such as Eye Diseases, Periodontal Disease, Amputation, and End-Stage Renal Disease

Along with Reports on Current Research Initiatives, a Glossary, and Resource Listings for Further Help and Information

Edited by Karen Bellenir. 688 pages. 1998. 0-7808-0224-1. $78.

"An invaluable reference." — *Library Journal, May '00*

Selected as one of the 250 "Best Health Sciences Books of 1999." — *Doody's Rating Service, Mar-Apr 2000*

"This comprehensive book is an excellent addition for high school, academic, medical, and public libraries. This volume is highly recommended."
— *American Reference Books Annual, 2000*

"Provides useful information for the general public."
— *Healthlines, University of Michigan Health Management Research Center, Sep/Oct '99*

". . . provides reliable mainstream medical information . . . belongs on the shelves of any library with a consumer health collection." — *E-Streams, Sep '99*

"Recommended reference source."
— *Booklist, American Library Association, Feb '99*

■

Diet & Nutrition Sourcebook, 1st Edition

Basic Information about Nutrition, Including the Dietary Guidelines for Americans, the Food Guide Pyramid, and Their Applications in Daily Diet, Nutritional Advice for Specific Age Groups, Current Nutritional Issues and Controversies, the New Food Label and How to Use It to Promote Healthy Eating, and Recent Developments in Nutritional Research

Edited by Dan R. Harris. 662 pages. 1996. 0-7808-0084-2. $78.

"Useful reference as a food and nutrition sourcebook for the general consumer." — *Booklist Health Sciences Supplement, American Library Association, Oct '97*

"Recommended for public libraries and medical libraries that receive general information requests on nutrition. It is readable and will appeal to those interested in learning more about healthy dietary practices."
— *Medical Reference Services Quarterly, Fall '97*

"An abundance of medical and social statistics is translated into readable information geared toward the general reader." — *Bookwatch, Mar '97*

"With dozens of questionable diet books on the market, it is so refreshing to find a reliable and factual reference book. Recommended to aspiring professionals, librarians, and others seeking and giving reliable dietary advice. An excellent compilation." — *Choice, Association of College and Research Libraries, Feb '97*

SEE ALSO *Digestive Diseases & Disorders Sourcebook, Gastrointestinal Diseases & Disorders Sourcebook*

■

Diet & Nutrition Sourcebook, 2nd Edition

Basic Consumer Health Information about Dietary Guidelines, Recommended Daily Intake Values, Vitamins, Minerals, Fiber, Fat, Weight Control, Dietary Supplements, and Food Additives

Along with Special Sections on Nutrition Needs throughout Life and Nutrition for People with Such Specific Medical Concerns as Allergies, High Blood Cholesterol, Hypertension, Diabetes, Celiac Disease, Seizure Disorders, Phenylketonuria (PKU), Cancer, and Eating Disorders, and Including Reports on Current Nutrition Research and Source Listings for Additional Help and Information

Edited by Karen Bellenir. 650 pages. 1999. 0-7808-0228-4. $78.

"This book is an excellent source of basic diet and nutrition information." — *Booklist Health Sciences Supplement, American Library Association, Dec '00*

"This reference document should be in any public library, but it would be a very good guide for beginning students in the health sciences. If the other books in this publisher's series are as good as this, they should all be in the health sciences collections."
— *American Reference Books Annual, 2000*

"This book is an excellent general nutrition reference for consumers who desire to take an active role in their health care for prevention. Consumers of all ages who select this book can feel confident they are receiving current and accurate information." — *Journal of Nutrition for the Elderly, Vol. 19, No. 4, '00*

"Recommended reference source."
— *Booklist, American Library Association, Dec '99*

SEE ALSO *Digestive Diseases & Disorders Sourcebook, Gastrointestinal Diseases & Disorders Sourcebook*

Digestive Diseases & Disorders Sourcebook

Basic Consumer Health Information about Diseases and Disorders that Impact the Upper and Lower Digestive System, Including Celiac Disease, Constipation, Crohn's Disease, Cyclic Vomiting Syndrome, Diarrhea, Diverticulosis and Diverticulitis, Gallstones, Heartburn, Hemorrhoids, Hernias, Indigestion (Dyspepsia), Irritable Bowel Syndrome, Lactose Intolerance, Ulcers, and More

Along with Information about Medications and Other Treatments, Tips for Maintaining a Healthy Digestive Tract, a Glossary, and Directory of Digestive Diseases Organizations

Edited by Karen Bellenir. 335 pages. 2000. 0-7808-0327-2. $78.

"This title would be an excellent addition to all public or patient-research libraries."
—American Reference Books Annual, 2001

"This title is recommended for public, hospital, and health sciences libraries with consumer health collections." *—E-Streams, Jul-Aug '00*

"Recommended reference source."
—Booklist, American Library Association, May '00

SEE ALSO *Diet & Nutrition Sourcebook, 1st and 2nd Editions, Gastrointestinal Diseases & Disorders Sourcebook*

■

Disabilities Sourcebook

Basic Consumer Health Information about Physical and Psychiatric Disabilities, Including Descriptions of Major Causes of Disability, Assistive and Adaptive Aids, Workplace Issues, and Accessibility Concerns

Along with Information about the Americans with Disabilities Act, a Glossary, and Resources for Additional Help and Information

Edited by Dawn D. Matthews. 616 pages. 2000. 0-7808-0389-2. $78.

"A much needed addition to the Omnigraphics *Health Reference Series*. A current reference work to provide people with disabilities, their families, caregivers or those who work with them, a broad range of information in one volume, has not been available until now. . . . It is recommended for all public and academic library reference collections." *—E-Streams, May '01*

"An excellent source book in easy-to-read format covering many current topics; highly recommended for all libraries." *—Choice, Association of College and Research Libraries, Jan '01*

"Recommended reference source."
—Booklist, American Library Association, Jul '00

"An involving, invaluable handbook."
—The Bookwatch, May '00

Domestic Violence & Child Abuse Sourcebook

Basic Consumer Health Information about Spousal/ Partner, Child, Sibling, Parent, and Elder Abuse, Covering Physical, Emotional, and Sexual Abuse, Teen Dating Violence, and Stalking; Includes Information about Hotlines, Safe Houses, Safety Plans, and Other Resources for Support and Assistance, Community Initiatives, and Reports on Current Directions in Research and Treatment

Along with a Glossary, Sources for Further Reading, and Governmental and Non-Governmental Organizations Contact Information

Edited by Helene Henderson. 1,064 pages. 2001. 0-7808-0235-7. $78.

"This is important information. The Web has many resources but this sourcebook fills an important societal need. I am not aware of any other resources of this type." *—Doody's Review Service, Sep '01*

"Recommended for all libraries, scholars, and practitioners." *—Choice, Association of College & Research Libraries, Jul '01*

"Recommended reference source."
—Booklist, American Library Association, Apr '01

"Important pick for college-level health reference libraries." *—The Bookwatch, Mar '01*

"Because this problem is so widespread and because this book includes a lot of issues within one volume, this work is recommended for all public libraries."
—American Reference Books Annual, 2001

■

Drug Abuse Sourcebook

Basic Consumer Health Information about Illicit Substances of Abuse and the Diversion of Prescription Medications, Including Depressants, Hallucinogens, Inhalants, Marijuana, Narcotics, Stimulants, and Anabolic Steroids

Along with Facts about Related Health Risks, Treatment Issues, and Substance Abuse Prevention Programs, a Glossary of Terms, Statistical Data, and Directories of Hotline Services, Self-Help Groups, and Organizations Able to Provide Further Information

Edited by Karen Bellenir. 629 pages. 2000. 0-7808-0242-X. $78.

"Containing a wealth of information, this book will be useful to the college student just beginning to explore the topic of substance abuse. This resource belongs in libraries that serve a lower-division undergraduate or community college clientele as well as the general public." *—Choice, Association of College and Research Libraries, Jun '01*

"Recommended reference source."
—Booklist, American Library Association, Feb '01

"Highly recommended." *—The Bookwatch, Jan '01*

"Even though there is a plethora of books on drug abuse, this volume is recommended for school, public, and college libraries."
—American Reference Books Annual, 2001

SEE ALSO *Alcoholism Sourcebook, Substance Abuse Sourcebook*

Ear, Nose & Throat Disorders Sourcebook

Basic Information about Disorders of the Ears, Nose, Sinus Cavities, Pharynx, and Larynx, Including Ear Infections, Tinnitus, Vestibular Disorders, Allergic and Non-Allergic Rhinitis, Sore Throats, Tonsillitis, and Cancers That Affect the Ears, Nose, Sinuses, and Throat

Along with Reports on Current Research Initiatives, a Glossary of Related Medical Terms, and a Directory of Sources for Further Help and Information

Edited by Karen Bellenir and Linda M. Shin. 576 pages. 1998. 0-7808-0206-3. $78.

"Overall, this sourcebook is helpful for the consumer seeking information on ENT issues. It is recommended for public libraries."
—*American Reference Books Annual, 1999*

"Recommended reference source."
—*Booklist, American Library Association, Dec '98*

Eating Disorders Sourcebook

Basic Consumer Health Information about Eating Disorders, Including Information about Anorexia Nervosa, Bulimia Nervosa, Binge Eating, Body Dysmorphic Disorder, Pica, Laxative Abuse, and Night Eating Syndrome

Along with Information about Causes, Adverse Effects, and Treatment and Prevention Issues, and Featuring a Section on Concerns Specific to Children and Adolescents, a Glossary, and Resources for Further Help and Information

Edited by Dawn D. Matthews. 322 pages. 2001. 0-7808-0335-3. $78.

"This volume is another convenient collection of excerpted articles. Recommended for school and public library patrons; lower-division undergraduates; and two-year technical program students."
—*Choice, Association of College & Research Libraries, Jan '02*

"Recommended reference source." —*Booklist, American Library Association, Oct '01*

Endocrine & Metabolic Disorders Sourcebook

Basic Information for the Layperson about Pancreatic and Insulin-Related Disorders Such as Pancreatitis, Diabetes, and Hypoglycemia; Adrenal Gland Disorders Such as Cushing's Syndrome, Addison's Disease, and Congenital Adrenal Hyperplasia; Pituitary Gland Disorders Such as Growth Hormone Deficiency, Acromegaly, and Pituitary Tumors; Thyroid Disorders Such as Hypothyroidism, Graves' Disease, Hashimoto's Disease, and Goiter; Hyperparathyroidism; and Other Diseases and Syndromes of Hormone Imbalance or Metabolic Dysfunction

Along with Reports on Current Research Initiatives

Edited by Linda M. Shin. 574 pages. 1998. 0-7808-0207-1. $78.

"Omnigraphics has produced another needed resource for health information consumers."
—*American Reference Books Annual, 2000*

"Recommended reference source."
—*Booklist, American Library Association, Dec '98*

Environmentally Induced Disorders Sourcebook

Basic Information about Diseases and Syndromes Linked to Exposure to Pollutants and Other Substances in Outdoor and Indoor Environments Such as Lead, Asbestos, Formaldehyde, Mercury, Emissions, Noise, and More

Edited by Allan R. Cook. 620 pages. 1997. 0-7808-0083-4. $78.

"Recommended reference source."
—*Booklist, American Library Association, Sep '98*

"This book will be a useful addition to anyone's library." —*Choice Health Sciences Supplement, Association of College and Research Libraries, May '98*

". . . a good survey of numerous environmentally induced physical disorders . . . a useful addition to anyone's library."
—*Doody's Health Sciences Book Reviews, Jan '98*

". . . provide[s] introductory information from the best authorities around. Since this volume covers topics that potentially affect everyone, it will surely be one of the most frequently consulted volumes in the *Health Reference Series*." —*Rettig on Reference, Nov '97*

Ethnic Diseases Sourcebook

Basic Consumer Health Information for Ethnic and Racial Minority Groups in the United States, Including General Health Indicators and Behaviors, Ethnic Diseases, Genetic Testing, the Impact of Chronic Diseases, Women's Health, Mental Health Issues, and Preventive Health Care Services

Along with a Glossary and a Listing of Additional Resources

Edited by Joyce Brennfleck Shannon. 664 pages. 2001. 0-7808-0336-1. $78.

"Recommended for health sciences libraries where public health programs are a priority."
—*E-Streams, Jan '02*

"Recommended reference source."
—*Booklist, American Library Association, Oct '01*

"Will prove valuable to any library seeking to maintain a current, comprehensive reference collection of health resources. . . . An excellent source of health information about genetic disorders which affect particular ethnic and racial minorities in the U.S."
—*The Bookwatch, Aug '01*

Family Planning Sourcebook

Basic Consumer Health Information about Planning for Pregnancy and Contraception, Including Traditional Methods, Barrier Methods, Hormonal Methods, Permanent Methods, Future Methods, Emergency Contraception, and Birth Control Choices for Women at Each Stage of Life

Along with Statistics, a Glossary, and Sources of Additional Information

Edited by Amy Marcaccio Keyzer. 520 pages. 2001. 0-7808-0379-5. $78.

"Recommended reference source."
— *Booklist, American Library Association, Oct '01*

"Will prove valuable to any library seeking to maintain a current, comprehensive reference collection of health resources. . . . Excellent reference."
— *The Bookwatch, Aug '01*

SEE ALSO Pregnancy & Birth Sourcebook

■

Fitness & Exercise Sourcebook, 1st Edition

Basic Information on Fitness and Exercise, Including Fitness Activities for Specific Age Groups, Exercise for People with Specific Medical Conditions, How to Begin a Fitness Program in Running, Walking, Swimming, Cycling, and Other Athletic Activities, and Recent Research in Fitness and Exercise

Edited by Dan R. Harris. 663 pages. 1996. 0-7808-0186-5. $78.

"A good resource for general readers." — *Choice, Association of College and Research Libraries, Nov '97*

"The perennial popularity of the topic . . . make this an appealing selection for public libraries."
— *Rettig on Reference, Jun/Jul '97*

■

Fitness & Exercise Sourcebook, 2nd Edition

Basic Consumer Health Information about the Fundamentals of Fitness and Exercise, Including How to Begin and Maintain a Fitness Program, Fitness as a Lifestyle, the Link between Fitness and Diet, Advice for Specific Groups of People, Exercise as It Relates to Specific Medical Conditions, and Recent Research in Fitness and Exercise

Along with a Glossary of Important Terms and Resources for Additional Help and Information

Edited by Kristen M. Gledhill. 646 pages. 2001. 0-7808-0334-5. $78.

"Highly recommended for public, consumer, and school grades fourth through college."
— *E-Streams, Nov '01*

"Recommended reference source." — *Booklist, American Library Association, Oct '01*

"The information appears quite comprehensive and is considered reliable. . . . This second edition is a welcomed addition to the series."
— *Doody's Review Service, Sep '01*

"This reference is a valuable choice for those who desire a broad source of information on exercise, fitness, and chronic-disease prevention through a healthy lifestyle." — *American Medical Writers Association Journal, Fall '01*

"Will prove valuable to any library seeking to maintain a current, comprehensive reference collection of health resources. . . . Excellent reference."
— *The Bookwatch, Aug '01*

■

Food & Animal Borne Diseases Sourcebook

Basic Information about Diseases That Can Be Spread to Humans through the Ingestion of Contaminated Food or Water or by Contact with Infected Animals and Insects, Such as Botulism, E. Coli, Hepatitis A, Trichinosis, Lyme Disease, and Rabies

Along with Information Regarding Prevention and Treatment Methods, and Including a Special Section for International Travelers Describing Diseases Such as Cholera, Malaria, Travelers' Diarrhea, and Yellow Fever, and Offering Recommendations for Avoiding Illness

Edited by Karen Bellenir and Peter D. Dresser. 535 pages. 1995. 0-7808-0033-8. $78.

"Targeting general readers and providing them with a single, comprehensive source of information on selected topics, this book continues, with the excellent caliber of its predecessors, to catalog topical information on health matters of general interest. Readable and thorough, this valuable resource is highly recommended for all libraries."
— *Academic Library Book Review, Summer '96*

"A comprehensive collection of authoritative information." — *Emergency Medical Services, Oct '95*

■

Food Safety Sourcebook

Basic Consumer Health Information about the Safe Handling of Meat, Poultry, Seafood, Eggs, Fruit Juices, and Other Food Items, and Facts about Pesticides, Drinking Water, Food Safety Overseas, and the Onset, Duration, and Symptoms of Foodborne Illnesses, Including Types of Pathogenic Bacteria, Parasitic Protozoa, Worms, Viruses, and Natural Toxins

Along with the Role of the Consumer, the Food Handler, and the Government in Food Safety; a Glossary, and Resources for Additional Help and Information

Edited by Dawn D. Matthews. 339 pages. 1999. 0-7808-0326-4. $78.

"This book is recommended for public libraries and universities with home economic and food science programs." — *E-Streams, Nov '00*

"Recommended reference source."
— *Booklist, American Library Association, May '00*

"This book takes the complex issues of food safety and foodborne pathogens and presents them in an easily understood manner. [It does] an excellent job of covering a large and often confusing topic."
—*American Reference Books Annual, 2000*

Forensic Medicine Sourcebook

Basic Consumer Information for the Layperson about Forensic Medicine, Including Crime Scene Investigation, Evidence Collection and Analysis, Expert Testimony, Computer-Aided Criminal Identification, Digital Imaging in the Courtroom, DNA Profiling, Accident Reconstruction, Autopsies, Ballistics, Drugs and Explosives Detection, Latent Fingerprints, Product Tampering, and Questioned Document Examination

Along with Statistical Data, a Glossary of Forensics Terminology, and Listings of Sources for Further Help and Information

Edited by Annemarie S. Muth. 574 pages. 1999. 0-7808-0232-2. $78.

"Given the expected widespread interest in its content and its easy to read style, this book is recommended for most public and all college and university libraries."
— *E-Streams, Feb '01*

"Recommended for public libraries."
—*Reference & User Services Quarterly, American Library Association, Spring 2000*

"Recommended reference source."
—*Booklist, American Library Association, Feb '00*

"A wealth of information, useful statistics, references are up-to-date and extremely complete. This wonderful collection of data will help students who are interested in a career in any type of forensic field. It is a great resource for attorneys who need information about types of expert witnesses needed in a particular case. It also offers useful information for fiction and nonfiction writers whose work involves a crime. A fascinating compilation. All levels." — *Choice, Association of College and Research Libraries, Jan 2000*

"There are several items that make this book attractive to consumers who are seeking certain forensic data. . . . This is a useful current source for those seeking general forensic medical answers."
—*American Reference Books Annual, 2000*

Gastrointestinal Diseases & Disorders Sourcebook

Basic Information about Gastroesophageal Reflux Disease (Heartburn), Ulcers, Diverticulosis, Irritable Bowel Syndrome, Crohn's Disease, Ulcerative Colitis, Diarrhea, Constipation, Lactose Intolerance, Hemorrhoids, Hepatitis, Cirrhosis, and Other Digestive Problems, Featuring Statistics, Descriptions of Symptoms, and Current Treatment Methods of Interest for Persons Living with Upper and Lower Gastrointestinal Maladies

Edited by Linda M. Ross. 413 pages. 1996. 0-7808-0078-8. $78.

". . . very readable form. The successful editorial work that brought this material together into a useful and understandable reference makes accessible to all readers information that can help them more effectively understand and obtain help for digestive tract problems."
— *Choice, Association of College and Research Libraries, Feb '97*

SEE ALSO Diet & Nutrition Sourcebook, 1st and 2nd Editions, Digestive Diseases & Disorders

Genetic Disorders Sourcebook, 1st Edition

Basic Information about Heritable Diseases and Disorders Such as Down Syndrome, PKU, Hemophilia, Von Willebrand Disease, Gaucher Disease, Tay-Sachs Disease, and Sickle-Cell Disease, Along with Information about Genetic Screening, Gene Therapy, Home Care, and Including Source Listings for Further Help and Information on More Than 300 Disorders

Edited by Karen Bellenir. 642 pages. 1996. 0-7808-0034-6. $78.

"Recommended for undergraduate libraries or libraries that serve the public."
— *Science & Technology Libraries, Vol. 18, No. 1, '99*

"Provides essential medical information to both the general public and those diagnosed with a serious or fatal genetic disease or disorder." —*Choice, Association of College and Research Libraries, Jan '97*

"Geared toward the lay public. It would be well placed in all public libraries and in those hospital and medical libraries in which access to genetic references is limited." —*Doody's Health Sciences Book Review, Oct '96*

Genetic Disorders Sourcebook, 2nd Edition

Basic Consumer Health Information about Hereditary Diseases and Disorders, Including Cystic Fibrosis, Down Syndrome, Hemophilia, Huntington's Disease, Sickle Cell Anemia, and More; Facts about Genes, Gene Research and Therapy, Genetic Screening, Ethics of Gene Testing, Genetic Counseling, and Advice on Coping and Caring

Along with a Glossary of Genetic Terminology and a Resource List for Help, Support, and Further Information

Edited by Kathy Massimini. 768 pages. 2001. 0-7808-0241-1. $78.

"Recommended for public libraries and medical and hospital libraries with consumer health collections."
—*E-Streams, May '01*

"Recommended reference source."
—*Booklist, American Library Association, Apr '01*

"Important pick for college-level health reference libraries." —*The Bookwatch, Mar '01*

Head Trauma Sourcebook

Basic Information for the Layperson about Open-Head and Closed-Head Injuries, Treatment Advances, Recovery, and Rehabilitation

Along with Reports on Current Research Initiatives

Edited by Karen Bellenir. 414 pages. 1997. 0-7808-0208-X. $78.

■

Headache Sourcebook

Basic Consumer Health Information about Migraine, Tension, Cluster, Rebound and Other Types of Headaches, with Facts about the Cause and Prevention of Headaches, the Effects of Stress and the Environment, Headaches during Pregnancy and Menopause, and Childhood Headaches

Along with a Glossary and Other Resources for Additional Help and Information

Edited by Dawn D. Matthews. 362 pages. 2002. 0-7808-0337-X. $78.

■

Health Insurance Sourcebook

Basic Information about Managed Care Organizations, Traditional Fee-for-Service Insurance, Insurance Portability and Pre-Existing Conditions Clauses, Medicare, Medicaid, Social Security, and Military Health Care

Along with Information about Insurance Fraud

Edited by Wendy Wilcox. 530 pages. 1997. 0-7808-0222-5. $78.

"Particularly useful because it brings much of this information together in one volume. This book will be a handy reference source in the health sciences library, hospital library, college and university library, and medium to large public library."
—*Medical Reference Services Quarterly, Fall '98*

Awarded "Books of the Year Award"
—*American Journal of Nursing, 1997*

"The layout of the book is particularly helpful as it provides easy access to reference material. A most useful addition to the vast amount of information about health insurance. The use of data from U.S. government agencies is most commendable. Useful in a library or learning center for healthcare professional students."
—*Doody's Health Sciences Book Reviews, Nov '97*

■

Health Reference Series Cumulative Index 1999

A Comprehensive Index to the Individual Volumes of the Health Reference Series, Including a Subject Index, Name Index, Organization Index, and Publication Index

Along with a Master List of Acronyms and Abbreviations

Edited by Edward J. Prucha, Anne Holmes, and Robert Rudnick. 990 pages. 2000. 0-7808-0382-5. $78.

"This volume will be most helpful in libraries that have a relatively complete collection of the Health Reference Series." —*American Reference Books Annual, 2001*

"Essential for collections that hold any of the numerous *Health Reference Series* titles."
—*Choice, Association of College and Research Libraries, Nov '00*

■

Healthy Aging Sourcebook

Basic Consumer Health Information about Maintaining Health through the Aging Process, Including Advice on Nutrition, Exercise, and Sleep, Help in Making Decisions about Midlife Issues and Retirement, and Guidance Concerning Practical and Informed Choices in Health Consumerism

Along with Data Concerning the Theories of Aging, Different Experiences in Aging by Minority Groups, and Facts about Aging Now and Aging in the Future; and Featuring a Glossary, a Guide to Consumer Help, Additional Suggested Reading, and Practical Resource Directory

Edited by Jenifer Swanson. 536 pages. 1999. 0-7808-0390-6. $78.

"Recommended reference source."
—*Booklist, American Library Association, Feb '00*

SEE ALSO *Physical & Mental Issues in Aging Sourcebook*

■

Healthy Heart Sourcebook for Women

Basic Consumer Health Information about Cardiac Issues Specific to Women, Including Facts about Major Risk Factors and Prevention, Treatment and Control Strategies, and Important Dietary Issues

Along with a Special Section Regarding the Pros and Cons of Hormone Replacement Therapy and Its Impact on Heart Health, and Additional Help, Including Recipes, a Glossary, and a Directory of Resources

Edited by Dawn D. Matthews. 336 pages. 2000. 0-7808-0329-9. $78.

"A good reference source and recommended for all public, academic, medical, and hospital libraries."
—*Medical Reference Services Quarterly, Summer '01*

"Because of the lack of information specific to women on this topic, this book is recommended for public libraries and consumer libraries."
—*American Reference Books Annual, 2001*

"Contains very important information about coronary artery disease that all women should know. The information is current and presented in an easy-to-read format. The book will make a good addition to any library." —*American Medical Writers Association Journal, Summer '00*

"Important, basic reference."
—*Reviewer's Bookwatch, Jul '00*

SEE ALSO *Cardiovascular Diseases & Disorders Sourcebook, 1st Edition, Heart Diseases & Disorders*

Sourcebook, 2nd Edition, Women's Health Concerns Sourcebook

Heart Diseases & Disorders Sourcebook, 2nd Edition

Basic Consumer Health Information about Heart Attacks, Angina, Rhythm Disorders, Heart Failure, Valve Disease, Congenital Heart Disorders, and More, Including Descriptions of Surgical Procedures and Other Interventions, Medications, Cardiac Rehabilitation, Risk Identification, and Prevention Tips

Along with Statistical Data, Reports on Current Research Initiatives, a Glossary of Cardiovascular Terms, and Resource Directory

Edited by Karen Bellenir. 612 pages. 2000. 0-7808-0238-1. $78.

"This work stands out as an imminently accessible resource for the general public. It is recommended for the reference and circulating shelves of school, public, and academic libraries."
—American Reference Books Annual, 2001

"Recommended reference source."
—Booklist, American Library Association, Dec '00

"Provides comprehensive coverage of matters related to the heart. This title is recommended for health sciences and public libraries with consumer health collections."
—E-Streams, Oct '00

SEE ALSO *Cardiovascular Diseases & Disorders Sourcebook, 1st Edition; Healthy Heart Sourcebook for Women*

Household Safety Sourcebook

Basic Consumer Health Information about Household Safety, Including Information about Poisons, Chemicals, Fire, and Water Hazards in the Home

Along with Advice about the Safe Use of Home Maintenance Equipment, Choosing Toys and Nursery Furniture, Holiday and Recreation Safety, a Glossary, and Resources for Further Help and Information

Edited by Dawn D. Matthews. 606 pages. 2002. 0-7808-0338-8. $78.

Immune System Disorders Sourcebook

Basic Information about Lupus, Multiple Sclerosis, Guillain-Barré Syndrome, Chronic Granulomatous Disease, and More

Along with Statistical and Demographic Data and Reports on Current Research Initiatives

Edited by Allan R. Cook. 608 pages. 1997. 0-7808-0209-8. $78.

Infant & Toddler Health Sourcebook

Basic Consumer Health Information about the Physical and Mental Development of Newborns, Infants, and Toddlers, Including Neonatal Concerns, Nutrition Recommendations, Immunization Schedules, Common Pediatric Disorders, Assessments and Milestones, Safety Tips, and Advice for Parents and Other Caregivers

Along with a Glossary of Terms and Resource Listings for Additional Help

Edited by Jenifer Swanson. 585 pages. 2000. 0-7808-0246-2. $78.

"As a reference for the general public, this would be useful in any library." *—E-Streams, May '01*

"Recommended reference source."
—Booklist, American Library Association, Feb '01

"This is a good source for general use."
—American Reference Books Annual, 2001

Injury & Trauma Sourcebook

Basic Consumer Health Information about the Impact of Injury, the Diagnosis and Treatment of Common and Traumatic Injuries, Emergency Care, and Specific Injuries Related to Home, Community, Workplace, Transportation, and Recreation

Along with Guidelines for Injury Prevention, a Glossary, and a Directory of Additional Resources

Edited by Joyce Brennfleck Shannon. 696 pages. 2002. 0-7808-0421-X. $78.

Kidney & Urinary Tract Diseases & Disorders Sourcebook

Basic Information about Kidney Stones, Urinary Incontinence, Bladder Disease, End Stage Renal Disease, Dialysis, and More

Along with Statistical and Demographic Data and Reports on Current Research Initiatives

Edited by Linda M. Ross. 602 pages. 1997. 0-7808-0079-6. $78.

Learning Disabilities Sourcebook

Basic Information about Disorders Such as Dyslexia, Visual and Auditory Processing Deficits, Attention Deficit/Hyperactivity Disorder, and Autism

Along with Statistical and Demographic Data, Reports on Current Research Initiatives, an Explanation of the Assessment Process, and a Special Section for Adults with Learning Disabilities

Edited by Linda M. Shin. 579 pages. 1998. 0-7808-0210-1. $78.

Named "Outstanding Reference Book of 1999."
—New York Public Library, Feb 2000

"An excellent candidate for inclusion in a public library reference section. It's a great source of information. Teachers will also find the book useful. Definitely worth reading."
— *Journal of Adolescent & Adult Literacy, Feb 2000*

"Readable . . . provides a solid base of information regarding successful techniques used with individuals who have learning disabilities, as well as practical suggestions for educators and family members. Clear language, concise descriptions, and pertinent information for contacting multiple resources add to the strength of this book as a useful tool." — *Choice, Association of College and Research Libraries, Feb '99*

"Recommended reference source."
— *Booklist, American Library Association, Sep '98*

"A useful resource for libraries and for those who don't have the time to identify and locate the individual publications." — *Disability Resources Monthly, Sep '98*

Liver Disorders Sourcebook

Basic Consumer Health Information about the Liver and How It Works; Liver Diseases, Including Cancer, Cirrhosis, Hepatitis, and Toxic and Drug Related Diseases; Tips for Maintaining a Healthy Liver; Laboratory Tests, Radiology Tests, and Facts about Liver Transplantation

Along with a Section on Support Groups, a Glossary, and Resource Listings

Edited by Joyce Brennfleck Shannon. 591 pages. 2000. 0-7808-0383-3. $78.

"A valuable resource."
— *American Reference Books Annual, 2001*

"This title is recommended for health sciences and public libraries with consumer health collections."
— *E-Streams, Oct '00*

"Recommended reference source."
— *Booklist, American Library Association, Jun '00*

Lung Disorders Sourcebook

Basic Consumer Health Information about Emphysema, Pneumonia, Tuberculosis, Asthma, Cystic Fibrosis, and Other Lung Disorders, Including Facts about Diagnostic Procedures, Treatment Strategies, Disease Prevention Efforts, and Such Risk Factors as Smoking, Air Pollution, and Exposure to Asbestos, Radon, and Other Agents

Along with a Glossary and Resources for Additional Help and Information

Edited by Dawn D. Matthews. 678 pages. 2002. 0-7808-0339-6. $78.

Medical Tests Sourcebook

Basic Consumer Health Information about Medical Tests, Including Periodic Health Exams, General Screening Tests, Tests You Can Do at Home, Findings of the U.S. Preventive Services Task Force, X-ray and Radiology Tests, Electrical Tests, Tests of Blood and Other Body Fluids and Tissues, Scope Tests, Lung Tests, Genetic Tests, Pregnancy Tests, Newborn Screening Tests, Sexually Transmitted Disease Tests, and Computer Aided Diagnoses

Along with a Section on Paying for Medical Tests, a Glossary, and Resource Listings

Edited by Joyce Brennfleck Shannon. 691 pages. 1999. 0-7808-0243-8. $78.

"Recommended for hospital and health sciences libraries with consumer health collections."
— *E-Streams, Mar '00*

"This is an overall excellent reference with a wealth of general knowledge that may aid those who are reluctant to get vital tests performed."
— *Today's Librarian, Jan 2000*

"A valuable reference guide."
— *American Reference Books Annual, 2000*

Men's Health Concerns Sourcebook

Basic Information about Health Issues That Affect Men, Featuring Facts about the Top Causes of Death in Men, Including Heart Disease, Stroke, Cancers, Prostate Disorders, Chronic Obstructive Pulmonary Disease, Pneumonia and Influenza, Human Immunodeficiency Virus and Acquired Immune Deficiency Syndrome, Diabetes Mellitus, Stress, Suicide, Accidents and Homicides; and Facts about Common Concerns for Men, Including Impotence, Contraception, Circumcision, Sleep Disorders, Snoring, Hair Loss, Diet, Nutrition, Exercise, Kidney and Urological Disorders, and Backaches

Edited by Allan R. Cook. 738 pages. 1998. 0-7808-0212-8. $78.

"This comprehensive resource and the series are highly recommended."
— *American Reference Books Annual, 2000*

"Recommended reference source."
— *Booklist, American Library Association, Dec '98*

Mental Health Disorders Sourcebook, 1st Edition

Basic Information about Schizophrenia, Depression, Bipolar Disorder, Panic Disorder, Obsessive-Compulsive Disorder, Phobias and Other Anxiety Disorders, Paranoia and Other Personality Disorders, Eating Disorders, and Sleep Disorders

Along with Information about Treatment and Therapies

Edited by Karen Bellenir. 548 pages. 1995. 0-7808-0040-0. $78.

"This is an excellent new book . . . written in easy-to-understand language."
— *Booklist Health Sciences Supplement, American Library Association, Oct '97*

". . . useful for public and academic libraries and consumer health collections."
— *Medical Reference Services Quarterly, Spring '97*

"The great strengths of the book are its readability and its inclusion of places to find more information. Especially recommended." — *Reference Quarterly, American Library Association, Winter '96*

". . . a good resource for a consumer health library."
— *Bulletin of the Medical Library Association, Oct '96*

"The information is data-based and couched in brief, concise language that avoids jargon. . . . a useful reference source." — *Readings, Sep '96*

"The text is well organized and adequately written for its target audience." — *Choice, Association of College and Research Libraries, Jun '96*

". . . provides information on a wide range of mental disorders, presented in nontechnical language."
— *Exceptional Child Education Resources, Spring '96*

"Recommended for public and academic libraries."
— *Reference Book Review, 1996*

Mental Health Disorders Sourcebook, 2nd Edition

Basic Consumer Health Information about Anxiety Disorders, Depression and Other Mood Disorders, Eating Disorders, Personality Disorders, Schizophrenia, and More, Including Disease Descriptions, Treatment Options, and Reports on Current Research Initiatives

Along with Statistical Data, Tips for Maintaining Mental Health, a Glossary, and Directory of Sources for Additional Help and Information

Edited by Karen Bellenir. 605 pages. 2000. 0-7808-0240-3. $78.

"Well organized and well written."
— *American Reference Books Annual, 2001*

"Recommended reference source."
— *Booklist, American Library Association, Jun '00*

Mental Retardation Sourcebook

Basic Consumer Health Information about Mental Retardation and Its Causes, Including Down Syndrome, Fetal Alcohol Syndrome, Fragile X Syndrome, Genetic Conditions, Injury, and Environmental Sources

Along with Preventive Strategies, Parenting Issues, Educational Implications, Health Care Needs, Employment and Economic Matters, Legal Issues, a Glossary, and a Resource Listing for Additional Help and Information

Edited by Joyce Brennfleck Shannon. 642 pages. 2000. 0-7808-0377-9. $78.

"Public libraries will find the book useful for reference and as a beginning research point for students, parents, and caregivers."
— *American Reference Books Annual, 2001*

"The strength of this work is that it compiles many basic fact sheets and addresses for further information in one volume. It is intended and suitable for the general public. This sourcebook is relevant to any collection providing health information to the general public."
— *E-Streams, Nov '00*

"From preventing retardation to parenting and family challenges, this covers health, social and legal issues and will prove an invaluable overview."
— *Reviewer's Bookwatch, Jul '00*

Obesity Sourcebook

Basic Consumer Health Information about Diseases and Other Problems Associated with Obesity, and Including Facts about Risk Factors, Prevention Issues, and Management Approaches

Along with Statistical and Demographic Data, Information about Special Populations, Research Updates, a Glossary, and Source Listings for Further Help and Information

Edited by Wilma Caldwell and Chad T. Kimball. 376 pages. 2001. 0-7808-0333-7. $78.

"This is a very useful resource book for the lay public."
— *Doody's Review Service, Nov '01*

"Well suited for the health reference collection of a public library or an academic health science library that serves the general population." — *E-Streams, Sep '01*

"Recommended reference source."
— *Booklist, American Library Association, Apr '01*

" Recommended pick both for specialty health library collections and any general consumer health reference collection." — *The Bookwatch, Apr '01*

Ophthalmic Disorders Sourcebook

Basic Information about Glaucoma, Cataracts, Macular Degeneration, Strabismus, Refractive Disorders, and More

Along with Statistical and Demographic Data and Reports on Current Research Initiatives

Edited by Linda M. Ross. 631 pages. 1996. 0-7808-0081-8. $78.

Oral Health Sourcebook

Basic Information about Diseases and Conditions Affecting Oral Health, Including Cavities, Gum Disease, Dry Mouth, Oral Cancers, Fever Blisters, Canker Sores, Oral Thrush, Bad Breath, Temporomandibular Disorders, and other Craniofacial Syndromes

Along with Statistical Data on the Oral Health of Americans, Oral Hygiene, Emergency First Aid, In-

formation on Treatment Procedures and Methods of Replacing Lost Teeth

Edited by Allan R. Cook. 558 pages. 1997. 0-7808-0082-6. $78.

"Unique source which will fill a gap in dental sources for patients and the lay public. A valuable reference tool even in a library with thousands of books on dentistry. Comprehensive, clear, inexpensive, and easy to read and use. It fills an enormous gap in the health care literature." — Reference and User Services Quarterly, American Library Association, Summer '98

"Recommended reference source."
— Booklist, American Library Association, Dec '97

■

Osteoporosis Sourcebook

Basic Consumer Health Information about Primary and Secondary Osteoporosis and Juvenile Osteoporosis and Related Conditions, Including Fibrous Dysplasia, Gaucher Disease, Hyperthyroidism, Hypophosphatasia, Myeloma, Osteopetrosis, Osteogenesis Imperfecta, and Paget's Disease

Along with Information about Risk Factors, Treatments, Traditional and Non-Traditional Pain Management, a Glossary of Related Terms, and a Directory of Resources

Edited by Allan R. Cook. 584 pages. 2001. 0-7808-0239-X. $78.

"This would be a book to be kept in a staff or patient library. The targeted audience is the layperson, but the therapist who needs a quick bit of information on a particular topic will also find the book useful."
— Physical Therapy, Jan '02

"Recommended for all public libraries and general health collections, especially those supporting patient education or consumer health programs."
— E-Streams, Nov '01

"Will prove valuable to any library seeking to maintain a current, comprehensive reference collection of health resources. . . . From prevention to treatment and associated conditions, this provides an excellent survey."
— The Bookwatch, Aug '01

"Recommended reference source."
— Booklist, American Library Association, July '01

SEE ALSO Women's Health Concerns Sourcebook

■

Pain Sourcebook, 1st Edition

Basic Information about Specific Forms of Acute and Chronic Pain, Including Headaches, Back Pain, Muscular Pain, Neuralgia, Surgical Pain, and Cancer Pain

Along with Pain Relief Options Such as Analgesics, Narcotics, Nerve Blocks, Transcutaneous Nerve Stimulation, and Alternative Forms of Pain Control, Including Biofeedback, Imaging, Behavior Modification, and Relaxation Techniques

Edited by Allan R. Cook. 667 pages. 1997. 0-7808-0213-6. $78.

"The text is readable, easily understood, and well indexed. This excellent volume belongs in all patient education libraries, consumer health sections of public libraries, and many personal collections."
— American Reference Books Annual, 1999

"A beneficial reference." — Booklist Health Sciences Supplement, American Library Association, Oct '98

"The information is basic in terms of scholarship and is appropriate for general readers. Written in journalistic style . . . intended for non-professionals. Quite thorough in its coverage of different pain conditions and summarizes the latest clinical information regarding pain treatment." — Choice, Association of College and Research Libraries, Jun '98

"Recommended reference source."
— Booklist, American Library Association, Mar '98

■

Pain Sourcebook, 2nd Edition

Basic Consumer Health Information about Specific Forms of Acute and Chronic Pain, Including Muscle and Skeletal Pain, Nerve Pain, Cancer Pain, and Disorders Characterized by Pain, Such as Fibromyalgia, Shingles, Angina, Arthritis, and Headaches

Along with Information about Pain Medications and Management Techniques, Complementary and Alternative Pain Relief Options, Tips for People Living with Chronic Pain, a Glossary, and a Directory of Sources for Further Information

Edited by Karen Bellenir. 650 pages. 2002. 0-7808-0612-3. $78.

■

Pediatric Cancer Sourcebook

Basic Consumer Health Information about Leukemias, Brain Tumors, Sarcomas, Lymphomas, and Other Cancers in Infants, Children, and Adolescents, Including Descriptions of Cancers, Treatments, and Coping Strategies

Along with Suggestions for Parents, Caregivers, and Concerned Relatives, a Glossary of Cancer Terms, and Resource Listings

Edited by Edward J. Prucha. 587 pages. 1999. 0-7808-0245-4. $78.

"An excellent source of information. Recommended for public, hospital, and health science libraries with consumer health collections." — E-Streams, Jun '00

"Recommended reference source."
— Booklist, American Library Association, Feb '00

"A valuable addition to all libraries specializing in health services and many public libraries."
— American Reference Books Annual, 2000

Physical & Mental Issues in Aging Sourcebook

Basic Consumer Health Information on Physical and Mental Disorders Associated with the Aging Process, Including Concerns about Cardiovascular Disease, Pulmonary Disease, Oral Health, Digestive Disorders, Musculoskeletal and Skin Disorders, Metabolic Changes, Sexual and Reproductive Issues, and Changes in Vision, Hearing, and Other Senses

Along with Data about Longevity and Causes of Death, Information on Acute and Chronic Pain, Descriptions of Mental Concerns, a Glossary of Terms, and Resource Listings for Additional Help

Edited by Jenifer Swanson. 660 pages. 1999. 0-7808-0233-0. $78.

"This is a treasure of health information for the layperson." — *Choice Health Sciences Supplement, Association of College & Research Libraries, May 2000*

"Recommended for public libraries."
—*American Reference Books Annual, 2000*

"Recommended reference source."
— *Booklist, American Library Association, Oct '99*

SEE ALSO *Healthy Aging Sourcebook*

Podiatry Sourcebook

Basic Consumer Health Information about Foot Conditions, Diseases, and Injuries, Including Bunions, Corns, Calluses, Athlete's Foot, Plantar Warts, Hammertoes and Clawtoes, Clubfoot, Heel Pain, Gout, and More

Along with Facts about Foot Care, Disease Prevention, Foot Safety, Choosing a Foot Care Specialist, a Glossary of Terms, and Resource Listings for Additional Information

Edited by M. Lisa Weatherford. 380 pages. 2001. 0-7808-0215-2. $78.

Pregnancy & Birth Sourcebook

Basic Information about Planning for Pregnancy, Maternal Health, Fetal Growth and Development, Labor and Delivery, Postpartum and Perinatal Care, Pregnancy in Mothers with Special Concerns, and Disorders of Pregnancy, Including Genetic Counseling, Nutrition and Exercise, Obstetrical Tests, Pregnancy Discomfort, Multiple Births, Cesarean Sections, Medical Testing of Newborns, Breastfeeding, Gestational Diabetes, and Ectopic Pregnancy

Edited by Heather E. Aldred. 737 pages. 1997. 0-7808-0216-0. $78.

"A well-organized handbook. Recommended."
— *Choice, Association of College and Research Libraries, Apr '98*

"Recommended reference source."
— *Booklist, American Library Association, Mar '98*

"Recommended for public libraries."
— *American Reference Books Annual, 1998*

SEE ALSO *Congenital Disorders Sourcebook, Family Planning Sourcebook*

Prostate Cancer Sourcebook

Basic Consumer Health Information about Prostate Cancer, Including Information about the Associated Risk Factors, Detection, Diagnosis, and Treatment of Prostate Cancer

Along with Information on Non-Malignant Prostate Conditions, and Featuring a Section Listing Support and Treatment Centers and a Glossary of Related Terms

Edited by Dawn D. Matthews. 358 pages. 2001. 0-7808-0324-8. $78.

"Recommended reference source."
—*Booklist, American Library Association, Jan '02*

Public Health Sourcebook

Basic Information about Government Health Agencies, Including National Health Statistics and Trends, Healthy People 2000 Program Goals and Objectives, the Centers for Disease Control and Prevention, the Food and Drug Administration, and the National Institutes of Health

Along with Full Contact Information for Each Agency

Edited by Wendy Wilcox. 698 pages. 1998. 0-7808-0220-9. $78.

"Recommended reference source."
— *Booklist, American Library Association, Sep '98*

"This consumer guide provides welcome assistance in navigating the maze of federal health agencies and their data on public health concerns."
— *SciTech Book News, Sep '98*

Reconstructive & Cosmetic Surgery Sourcebook

Basic Consumer Health Information on Cosmetic and Reconstructive Plastic Surgery, Including Statistical Information about Different Surgical Procedures, Things to Consider Prior to Surgery, Plastic Surgery Techniques and Tools, Emotional and Psychological Considerations, and Procedure-Specific Information

Along with a Glossary of Terms and a Listing of Resources for Additional Help and Information

Edited by M. Lisa Weatherford. 374 pages. 2001. 0-7808-0214-4. $78.

"Recommended for health science libraries that are open to the public, as well as hospital libraries that are open to the patients. This book is a good resource for the consumer interested in plastic surgery."
—*E-Streams, Dec '01*

"Recommended reference source."
—*Booklist, American Library Association, July '01*

Rehabilitation Sourcebook

Basic Consumer Health Information about Rehabilitation for People Recovering from Heart Surgery, Spinal Cord Injury, Stroke, Orthopedic Impairments, Amputation, Pulmonary Impairments, Traumatic Injury, and More, Including Physical Therapy, Occupational Therapy, Speech/ Language Therapy, Massage Therapy, Dance Therapy, Art Therapy, and Recreational Therapy

Along with Information on Assistive and Adaptive Devices, a Glossary, and Resources for Additional Help and Information

Edited by Dawn D. Matthews. 531 pages. 1999. 0-7808-0236-5. $78.

"This is an excellent resource for public library reference and health collections."
— *American Reference Books Annual, 2001*

"Recommended reference source."
— *Booklist, American Library Association, May '00*

■

Respiratory Diseases & Disorders Sourcebook

Basic Information about Respiratory Diseases and Disorders, Including Asthma, Cystic Fibrosis, Pneumonia, the Common Cold, Influenza, and Others, Featuring Facts about the Respiratory System, Statistical and Demographic Data, Treatments, Self-Help Management Suggestions, and Current Research Initiatives

Edited by Allan R. Cook and Peter D. Dresser. 771 pages. 1995. 0-7808-0037-0. $78.

"Designed for the layperson and for patients and their families coping with respiratory illness. . . . an extensive array of information on diagnosis, treatment, management, and prevention of respiratory illnesses for the general reader." — *Choice, Association of College and Research Libraries, Jun '96*

"A highly recommended text for all collections. It is a comforting reminder of the power of knowledge that good books carry between their covers."
— *Academic Library Book Review, Spring '96*

"A comprehensive collection of authoritative information presented in a nontechnical, humanitarian style for patients, families, and caregivers."
— *Association of Operating Room Nurses, Sep/Oct '95*

■

Sexually Transmitted Diseases Sourcebook, 1st Edition

Basic Information about Herpes, Chlamydia, Gonorrhea, Hepatitis, Nongonoccocal Urethritis, Pelvic Inflammatory Disease, Syphilis, AIDS, and More

Along with Current Data on Treatments and Preventions

Edited by Linda M. Ross. 550 pages. 1997. 0-7808-0217-9. $78.

Sexually Transmitted Diseases Sourcebook, 2nd Edition

Basic Consumer Health Information about Sexually Transmitted Diseases, Including Information on the Diagnosis and Treatment of Chlamydia, Gonorrhea, Hepatitis, Herpes, HIV, Mononucleosis, Syphilis, and Others

Along with Information on Prevention, Such as Condom Use, Vaccines, and STD Education; And Featuring a Section on Issues Related to Youth and Adolescents, a Glossary, and Resources for Additional Help and Information

Edited by Dawn D. Matthews. 538 pages. 2001. 0-7808-0249-7. $78.

"Every school and public library should have a copy of this comprehensive and user-friendly reference book."
— *Choice, Association of College & Research Libraries, Sep '01*

"This is a highly recommended book. This is an especially important book for all school and public libraries." — *AIDS Book Review Journal, Jul-Aug '01*

"Recommended reference source."
— *Booklist, American Library Association, Apr '01*

"Recommended pick both for specialty health library collections and any general consumer health reference collection." — *The Bookwatch, Apr '01*

■

Skin Disorders Sourcebook

Basic Information about Common Skin and Scalp Conditions Caused by Aging, Allergies, Immune Reactions, Sun Exposure, Infectious Organisms, Parasites, Cosmetics, and Skin Traumas, Including Abrasions, Cuts, and Pressure Sores

Along with Information on Prevention and Treatment

Edited by Allan R. Cook. 647 pages. 1997. 0-7808-0080-X. $78.

". . . comprehensive, easily read reference book."
— *Doody's Health Sciences Book Reviews, Oct '97*

SEE ALSO *Burns Sourcebook*

■

Sleep Disorders Sourcebook

Basic Consumer Health Information about Sleep and Its Disorders, Including Insomnia, Sleepwalking, Sleep Apnea, Restless Leg Syndrome, and Narcolepsy

Along with Data about Shiftwork and Its Effects, Information on the Societal Costs of Sleep Deprivation, Descriptions of Treatment Options, a Glossary of Terms, and Resource Listings for Additional Help

Edited by Jenifer Swanson. 439 pages. 1998. 0-7808-0234-9. $78.

"This text will complement any home or medical library. It is user-friendly and ideal for the adult reader."
— *American Reference Books Annual, 2000*

Sports Injuries Sourcebook

Basic Consumer Health Information about Common Sports Injuries, Prevention of Injury in Specific Sports, Tips for Training, and Rehabilitation from Injury

Along with Information about Special Concerns for Children, Young Girls in Athletic Training Programs, Senior Athletes, and Women Athletes, and a Directory of Resources for Further Help and Information

Edited by Heather E. Aldred. 624 pages. 1999. 0-7808-0218-7. $78.

Stress-Related Disorders Sourcebook

Basic Consumer Health Information about Stress and Stress-Related Disorders, Including Stress Origins and Signals, Environmental Stress at Work and Home, Mental and Emotional Stress Associated with Depression, Post-Traumatic Stress Disorder, Panic Disorder, Suicide, and the Physical Effects of Stress on the Cardiovascular, Immune, and Nervous Systems

Along with Stress Management Techniques, a Glossary, and a Listing of Additional Resources

Edited by Joyce Brennfleck Shannon. 600 pages. 2002. 0-7808-0560-7. $78.

Substance Abuse Sourcebook

Basic Health-Related Information about the Abuse of Legal and Illegal Substances Such as Alcohol, Tobacco, Prescription Drugs, Marijuana, Cocaine, and Heroin; and Including Facts about Substance Abuse Prevention Strategies, Intervention Methods, Treatment and Recovery Programs, and a Section Addressing the Special Problems Related to Substance Abuse during Pregnancy

Edited by Karen Bellenir. 573 pages. 1996. 0-7808-0038-9. $78.

SEE ALSO *Alcoholism Sourcebook, Drug Abuse Sourcebook*

Transplantation Sourcebook

Basic Consumer Health Information about Organ and Tissue Transplantation, Including Physical and Financial Preparations, Procedures and Issues Relating to Specific Solid Organ and Tissue Transplants, Rehabilitation, Pediatric Transplant Information, the Future of Transplantation, and Organ and Tissue Donation

Along with a Glossary and Listings of Additional Resources

Edited by Joyce Brennfleck Shannon. 628 pages. 2002. 0-7808-0322-1. $78.

Traveler's Health Sourcebook

Basic Consumer Health Information for Travelers, Including Physical and Medical Preparations, Transportation Health and Safety, Essential Information about Food and Water, Sun Exposure, Insect and Snake Bites, Camping and Wilderness Medicine, and Travel with Physical or Medical Disabilities

Along with International Travel Tips, Vaccination Recommendations, Geographical Health Issues, Disease Risks, a Glossary, and a Listing of Additional Resources

Edited by Joyce Brennfleck Shannon. 613 pages. 2000. 0-7808-0384-1. $78.

Women's Health Concerns Sourcebook

Basic Information about Health Issues That Affect Women, Featuring Facts about Menstruation and Other Gynecological Concerns, Including Endometriosis, Fibroids, Menopause, and Vaginitis; Reproductive Concerns, Including Birth Control, Infertility, and Abortion; and Facts about Additional Physical, Emotional, and Mental Health Concerns Prevalent among Women Such as Osteoporosis, Urinary Tract Disorders, Eating Disorders, and Depression

Along with Tips for Maintaining a Healthy Lifestyle

Edited by Heather E. Aldred. 567 pages. 1997. 0-7808-0219-5. $78.

"Handy compilation. There is an impressive range of diseases, devices, disorders, procedures, and other physical and emotional issues covered . . . well organized, illustrated, and indexed." —Choice, Association of College and Research Libraries, Jan '98

SEE ALSO Breast Cancer Sourcebook, Cancer Sourcebook for Women, 1st and 2nd Editions, Healthy Heart Sourcebook for Women, Osteoporosis Sourcebook

■

Workplace Health & Safety Sourcebook

Basic Consumer Health Information about Workplace Health and Safety, Including the Effect of Workplace Hazards on the Lungs, Skin, Heart, Ears, Eyes, Brain, Reproductive Organs, Musculoskeletal System, and Other Organs and Body Parts

Along with Information about Occupational Cancer, Personal Protective Equipment, Toxic and Hazardous Chemicals, Child Labor, Stress, and Workplace Violence

Edited by Chad T. Kimball. 626 pages. 2000. 0-7808-0231-4. $78.

"As a reference for the general public, this would be useful in any library." —E-Streams, Jun '01

"Provides helpful information for primary care physicians and other caregivers interested in occupational medicine. . . . General readers; professionals." — Choice, Association of College & Research Libraries, May '01

"Recommended reference source." — Booklist, American Library Association, Feb '01

"Highly recommended." — The Bookwatch, Jan '01

Worldwide Health Sourcebook

Basic Information about Global Health Issues, Including Malnutrition, Reproductive Health, Disease Dispersion and Prevention, Emerging Diseases, Risky Health Behaviors, and the Leading Causes of Death

Along with Global Health Concerns for Children, Women, and the Elderly, Mental Health Issues, Research and Technology Advancements, and Economic, Environmental, and Political Health Implications, a Glossary, and a Resource Listing for Additional Help and Information

Edited by Joyce Brennfleck Shannon. 614 pages. 2001. 0-7808-0330-2. $78.

"Named an Outstanding Academic Title." —Choice, Association of College & Research Libraries, Jan '02

"Yet another handy but also unique compilation in the extensive Health Reference Series, this is a useful work because many of the international publications reprinted or excerpted are not readily available. Highly recommended." —Choice, Association of College & Research Libraries, Nov '01

"Recommended reference source." —Booklist, American Library Association, Oct '01

Health Reference Series

Adolescent Health Sourcebook

AIDS Sourcebook, 1st Edition

AIDS Sourcebook, 2nd Edition

Alcoholism Sourcebook

Allergies Sourcebook, 1st Edition

Allergies Sourcebook, 2nd Edition

Alternative Medicine Sourcebook,
1st Edition

Alternative Medicine Sourcebook,
2nd Edition

Alzheimer's, Stroke & 29 Other
Neurological Disorders Sourcebook,
1st Edition

Alzheimer's Disease Sourcebook,
2nd Edition

Arthritis Sourcebook

Asthma Sourcebook

Attention Deficit Disorder Sourcebook

Back & Neck Disorders Sourcebook

Blood & Circulatory Disorders
Sourcebook

Brain Disorders Sourcebook

Breast Cancer Sourcebook

Breastfeeding Sourcebook

Burns Sourcebook

Cancer Sourcebook, 1st Edition

Cancer Sourcebook (New), 2nd Edition

Cancer Sourcebook, 3rd Edition

Cancer Sourcebook for Women,
1st Edition

Cancer Sourcebook for Women,
2nd Edition

Cardiovascular Diseases & Disorders
Sourcebook, 1st Edition

Caregiving Sourcebook

Colds, Flu & Other Common Ailments
Sourcebook

Communication Disorders
Sourcebook

Congenital Disorders Sourcebook

Consumer Issues in Health Care
Sourcebook

Contagious & Non-Contagious
Infectious Diseases Sourcebook

Death & Dying Sourcebook

Diabetes Sourcebook, 1st Edition

Diabetes Sourcebook, 2nd Edition

Diet & Nutrition Sourcebook,
1st Edition

Diet & Nutrition Sourcebook,
2nd Edition

Digestive Diseases & Disorder
Sourcebook

Disabilities Sourcebook

Domestic Violence & Child Abuse
Sourcebook

Drug Abuse Sourcebook

Ear, Nose & Throat Disorders
Sourcebook

Eating Disorders Sourcebook

Emergency Medical Services
Sourcebook

Endocrine & Metabolic Disorders
Sourcebook

Environmentally Induced Disorders
Sourcebook

Ethnic Diseases Sourcebook

Family Planning Sourcebook

Fitness & Exercise Sourcebook,
1st Edition

Fitness & Exercise Sourcebook,
2nd Edition

Food & Animal Borne Diseases
Sourcebook

Food Safety Sourcebook

Forensic Medicine Sourcebook

Gastrointestinal Diseases & Disorders
Sourcebook